# Neuroethics

# Neuroethics

## Defining the issues in theory, practice, and policy

Edited by

## Judy Illes

Director, Program in Neuroethics and Senior Research Scholar
Stanford Center for Biomedical Ethics
and
Senior Research Scholar,
Department of Radiology,
Stanford University,
Stanford, CA, USA

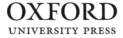

OXFORD
UNIVERSITY PRESS

# OXFORD
## UNIVERSITY PRESS

Great Clarendon Street, Oxford OX2 6DP

Oxford University Press is a department of the University of Oxford.
It furthers the University's objective of excellence in research, scholarship,
and education by publishing worldwide in

Oxford New York

Auckland  Cape Town  Dar es Salaam  Hong Kong  Karachi
Kuala Lumpur  Madrid  Melbourne  Mexico City  Nairobi
New Delhi  Shanghai  Taipei  Toronto

With offices in

Argentina  Austria  Brazil  Chile  Czech Republic  France  Greece
Guatemala  Hungary  Italy  Japan  Poland  Portugal  Singapore
South Korea  Switzerland  Thailand  Turkey  Ukraine  Vietnam

Oxford is a registered trade mark of Oxford University Press
in the UK and in certain other countries

Published in the United States
by Oxford University Press Inc., New York

A catalogue record for this title is available from the British Library

Library of Congress Cataloguing in Publication Data

Neuroethics: defining the issues in theory, practice, and policy / edited by Judy Illes
Includes bibliographical references and index
   1. Brain—Research—Moral and ethical aspects. 2. Neurosciences—Research—Moral
and ethical aspects.
[DNLM: 1. Neurosciences—ethics. 2. Behavior—ethics. 3. Bioethical Issues. 4. Morals.
5. Neurology—ethics. 6. Personal Autonomy. WL 100 N4 934 2005] I. Illes, Judy

RC343.N44 2005      174.2–dc22                                      20005022017

Typeset by SPI Publisher Services, Pondicherry, India
Printed in Great Britain
on acid-free paper by
Biddles Ltd, King's Lynn

ISBN 0 19 8567200 (Hbk)
978–019–856720–2
0 19 8567219 (Pbk)
978–019–856721–9

10 9 8 7 6 5 4 3 2

# Foreword by Colin Blakemore

'Neuro-', like 'Psycho-', 'Cyber-' and 'Retro-', offers itself promiscuously for the creation of neologisms. Put 'Neuro-' into Google and out flood nearly 13 million references. Not just the academic ones, such as 'Neuro-imaging', 'Neuro-linguistics', 'Neuro-semantics', 'Neuro-oncology', 'Neuro-disability' and 'Neuro-philosophy', but also a medley of more dubious 'Neurologisms' – 'Neuro-politics', 'Neuro-technology', and the latest, 'Neuro-marketing'.

'Neuroethics' has evolved so rapidly that its hyphen is now vestigial; yet there is still, rightly, debate about its origin and its validity as a distinct concept or discipline. Judy Illes, editor of this book, traces its pre-history to 1989 (Illes, 2003). The political journalist *William Safire*, Chairman of the Charles A. Dana Foundation, almost certainly coined the word in 2003, and he defined neuroethics as "the field of philosophy that discusses the rights and wrongs of the treatment of, or enhancement of, the human brain." That would make neuroethics a sub-discipline of bioethics, which deals with the ethical implications of biological research and its applications. But, if the brain deserves special attention within the arena of bioethics, why not 'Pulmuno-ethics' (philosophical problems relating to the study or treatment of the lung), 'Phallo-ethics' (moral issues to do with understanding and modification of male sexual function) and so forth?

The answer must surely be that functions associated with the brain, especially intentions, voluntary actions, sentience and feelings of self, guilt, remorse and responsibility, lie at the heart of ethical issues and ethical judgements. Indeed, Michael Gazzaniga, Director of the *Center for Cognitive Neuroscience* at *Dartmouth College* (who has contributed a chapter to this book) has argued in his own recent book *The Ethical Brain* that neuroethics is much broader than Safire's definition implies, and that it deals with "the social issues of disease, normality, mortality, lifestyle, and the philosophy of living, informed by our understanding of underlying brain mechanisms. . . . It is – or should be – an effort to come up with a brain-based philosophy of life" (Gazzaniga, 2005).

If one accepts that the brain, and the brain alone, is responsible for the entirety of consciousness and action, including the sense of right and wrong, and the capacity to contemplate moral values, then it is legitimate to ask whether there is any sort of ethics other than neuroethics. As our understanding of brain function advances, it is surely reasonable to ask how that knowledge illuminates issues that have previously been expressed, formulated, or explained in other terms. Epistemology – the theory of knowledge, legal principles, social and political concepts of rights and responsibilities, religious beliefs and behaviour, the philosophical underpinning of science: all of these are products of our brains, and they deserve reconsideration within the framework of our knowledge of the brain.

This book is a collection of essays from leaders in the burgeoning discipline of neuroethics. It is a comprehensive statement of the state of the field, and it airs all the substantial issues and controversies within the field.

The first section of the book deals with fundamental questions of selfhood and agency, probing the basis of intention, motivation and action, and the extent to which neuroscientific knowledge can, or even could, account for such things. All these chapters, more or less explicitly, address the issue of the contradiction between entirely deterministic accounts of human action and the way that it feels to be a decision-making human being. Tom Buller, in his chapter, describes a challenge, examined by Owen Flanagan (2002) in his book *The Problem of the Soul*, namely to reconcile the humanistic and the scientific views of who we are. "According to the humanistic view we are, for the most part, autonomous intentional rational agents and therefore we are responsible for our actions. Contrariwise, according to the scientific view ... human behavior is not caused by our intentions, beliefs, and desires. Instead, free will is an illusion because the brain is a deterministic physical organ, and it is the brain that is doing the causal work". This is the nub of the issue, and, it is a knotty nub, judging from the fact that Tom Buller, Patricia Churchland and Stephen Morse come to rather different conclusions on the extent to which determinism rules.

The middle section of this book exposes a few of the heavy practical issues to which neuroethics is relevant, and which will certainly increasingly become topics of public concern. These include the possibility of selection of embryos for genes associated with superior intelligence or other mental characteristics, the dilemmas involved in research on people with brain disorders, the moral status of human embryos, the basis of and responsibility for criminal action, and the possibility of enhancement of brain function.

The final section deals with the neuroethical perspective on legal and social issues, and on education and the portrayal of mind in the media.

The coming decades will see not only an explosion of information about the function of the brain, but also increasing sophistication in techniques for probing or altering neural activity related to emotion, motivation and decision-making. We have to look forward to the possibility of a menu of drugs that might be developed for the treatment of disease but which turn out to have enhancing effects on normal function. Brain surgery and other methods of modifying brain activity will continue to develop. The legal profession and the world of education will increasingly look to neuroscience for guidance and clarification about the fundamental underpinnings of what they do.

There can be little doubt that neuroethics is here to stay, whatever the pedantic concerns about its etymology, and that it will impinge directly not only on many areas of academic debate but also on practical issues of immediate importance to ordinary people. This book will stand as a milestone in the development of this endeavour – a statement of the progress of and the challenge for this fascinating subject.

Colin Blakemore

Chief Executive, Medical Research Council, London

and

Waynflete Professor of Physiology, University of Oxford

# References

Illes, J. (2003). Neuroethics in a new era of neuroimaging. *American Journal of Neuroradiology*, **24**, 1739–1741.

Flanagan, O. (2002). *The Problem of the Soul: Two Visions of the Mind and How to Reconcile Them*. Basic Books, New York.

Gazzaniga, M. S. (2005). *The Ethical Brain*. Dana Press, New York.

# Foreword by Arthur L. Caplan

Strange as it may seem neuroethics is not new. It simply got off on the wrong foot. Or rather it had a false start on the wrong hoof.

The misstep occurred when Louis 'Jolly' West and two other researchers at the University of Oklahoma undertook an experiment with the then very poorly understood hallucinogenic drug LSD. They gave a 7000-pound bull elephant named Tusko a huge dose of LSD (297 mg) by shooting the creature with a dart rifle. Five minutes later, the elephant collapsed and went into convulsions.

Twenty minutes after the initial injection of LSD, it was decided that promazine hydrochloride (Thorazine) should be administered in an attempt to counter the above reaction. 2800 mg was injected into the beast's ear over a period of 11 minutes but the drug only partially relieved the seizures. An hour later, in a further attempt to assist the elephant, Dr. West injected Tusko with pentobarbital sodium. The elephant died an hour and 40 minutes after the initial LSD had been administered. The experiment, the death, and what turned out to be a terrible error in computing the dose to use were all reported in the journal *Science.*

What were West and his colleagues up to in conducting this bizarre experiment? Apparently they were involved in an early effort to control the brain by modifying its chemistry.

In the 1950s and '60s West was involved, through the CIA-funded Geschickter Fund for Medical Research, in experiments employing LSD as a means of mind control in animals and humans. The elephant experiment was an attempt to see if LSD could trigger a naturally occurring violent state in elephants known as 'musth'. By understanding the chemistry of the brain, West and our national security agency hoped that pharmacology could be used to control or produce desired behaviors.

Not too long after this strange experiment, in 1965, the Spanish neuroscientist José Delgado conducted another animal study. He implanted electrodes in the brain of a bull, and outfitted the animal with a radiofrequency receiver. Then, while a camera recorded it all, Delgado stood in a bullring in front of the animal and provoked it to charge right at him. Moments before impact, his assistant pushed a button. The animal stopped right in his tracks.

Delgado's demonstration became one of the most famous videotapes in all of science. It was a spectacular example of how knowledge of the brain and its structure could be used to control behavior. Like West, Delgado had ties to the dark world of spies, national security, and dreams about mind-control.

Not much of value came directly out of these two animal studies. But the experiments did trigger the first serious attempt to deal with the ethics of new knowledge of the human brain. A project was undertaken in the early 1970s at the then nearly brand new Hastings Center, the first independent bioethics think-tank in the world, to examine the ethical issues raised by surgical and pharmacological interventions into the brain.

The Hastings project did not quite garner the attention or produce the impact that was intended. Mainly this was due to the fact that the science of the brain from that era was not quite up to the applications and utilizations that would have made for spirited ethical debate. That situation is, as the reader of this book will rapidly learn, no longer true.

Much ethical attention has focused in recent years on the project to map the human genome and the genomes of many other animals, plants, and microorganisms. And this is appropriate since new genetic knowledge raises a host of vitally important questions about genetic testing, engineering, and therapy.

Quietly and with much less fanfare, there has been a parallel explosion in knowledge of the structure and function of animal brains and the human brain. Increasingly sophisticated imaging techniques have made it possible to watch the brain in real time and see how it responds to various stimuli and environmental inputs. Physicians are beginning to find distinctive patterns in the brain indicative of disease and disorder. Great strides are being made in understanding the structure, biochemistry, and organization of the brain.

The science of the brain has advanced quite far since West overdosed his elephant and Delgado shocked the world by stopping a charging bull with a radio signal. There is every reason to believe that in the not so distant future the legal system will have to reckon with claims about normal and abnormal brains as a part of sentencing, parole, and punishment. Employers will want to know their rights to test the honesty and alertness of employees. Drug companies will want to sell potions and pills that can treat a wide range of mental disorders or simply improve mental performance.

Thus, there could not be a more opportune time for bioethics to reengage the brain sciences. The contributors to this book have begun the hard work of both identifying the key ethical questions and formulating regulations, policies, guidelines, and principles that can help answer them. The pace of discovery in neuroscience is guaranteed not to slow down. The emerging field of neuroethics will have to work very hard to keep up.

Arthur L. Caplan

# Preface

Welcome to the first symposium on a two-century-long growing concern: neuroethics—the examination of what is right and wrong and good and bad about the treatment of, perfection of, or unwelcome invasion of and worrisome manipulation of the human brain....It deals with our consciousness—our sense of self—and as such is central to our being. [It involves]...the misuse or abuse of power to change people's lives in the most personal and powerful way, or the failure to make the most of it. (William Safire, 2002)

With this introduction, William Safire, *New York Times* columnist and Chairman of the Charles A. Dana Foundation, charged a group of 150 neuroscience researchers, bioethics scholars, policy-makers, and journalists to map the terrain of neuroethics. He urged the multidisciplinary group to carve out new territory for an old philosophical discipline, a discipline he views as a distinct portion of bioethics, but for which the '...ethics of brain science hits home as research on no other organ does'.

Can widely differing perspectives succeed in informing ethical analysis with powerful themes about promise and benefit in neuroscience, free will and determinism, and individual versus society at the core of the effort? The 2002 "Mapping the Field" meeting was a good start, and the contributors to this volume continue to rise to that challenge. In her chapter in this volume, Adina Roskies writes:

> ...although neuroethics may appear to consist of a collection of diverse and unrelated concerns, the various issues emerging from the confluence of neuroscience and ethics are so densely interconnected that it is defensible, and may even be profitable, to consider them as a unified whole.

As a group of authors here, we strive to inform the neuroethics problem space by capturing the profitability of that potential whole, and harnessing the momentum that has been propelling our efforts forward over the past half-decade.

In defining the ground rules for any new discipline and 'good work' (Gardner *et al.* 2001), contributors to the discipline must first search for a central objective. The objective must recognize societal needs, be supported by the background, traits, values, and commitment of the contributors, and be led, at least in part, by dynamic measures of performance. Can neuroethics (or neuroethicists) yet claim to be grounded by a single objective, a unified identity, and well-defined measures of success? The answer is both yes and no.

Neuroethics can claim a common mission, even if not a singular one; as Safire instructed, that mission is to examine the ethical, legal, and social implications of neuroscience today. This is a lofty multifaceted endeavor and, with an unrelenting stream of innovations in technology and pharmacology for probing and manipulating the brain, there is an enormous amount of ground to cover. While it is as difficult to claim a single identity (or moral framework for that matter) as it is to define a single mission for neuroethics today, strong themes have nonetheless emerged that bring us closer to the task. On the philosophical and bioethical side of the neuroethics continuum, autonomy, determinism, moral agency, and consciousness have been areas of rich discussion so far. On the neuroscience and policy side, frontiers in neurotechno-logy, mind-reading, coercion, enhancement, forensics, and the role of policy and the law have been prevailing topics. These themes recur repeatedly in this volume as the considerable cross-fertilization of ideas and cross-referencing among chapters represent. Therefore the themes can be seen as the first core areas of the new discipline and, whether by coincidence or design, they map neatly onto the original four pillars defined by the 2002 meeting: self, social policy, clinical practice, and communication.

Readers of this volume will appreciate that those who have become active in neuroethics approach it on their own disciplinary paths. Therefore, with widely varying methods and views, measures of success in this young endeavor have appropriately been focused on the numbers of people involved, range of disciplines represented, the frequency with which people gather to meet and expound on topics of interest, the breadth of discussions, and publications. The last of these must be counted not only by number but by the variety of journals publishing them. We have every reason to be optimistic. To date, all these measures for neuroethics have positive slopes.

The Good Work project of Gardner and colleagues also described elements of a profes-sional domain—a discipline—that enable its successful evolution. They showed that a discipline is healthiest when its values are aligned with the knowledge, practice, and skills represented by it, and when expectations of stakeholders and expectations of the domain match. The extent to which internal harmony is achieved in neuroethics over time, how the discipline deals with a potential pull to one professional home in neuroscience or another in bioethics (or somewhere else?), how it withstands natural shifts in the values and priorities of its actors, and how it achieves continued visibility and sustainability will be the measurables of the future.

For the present, we hope that this pioneering anthology of topics in neuroethics—in theory, practice, and policy—succeeds in drawing the reader to the new field with an enthusiasm that reflects our own in participating in its creation. No doubt, we have left some matters untouched and many others that we do cover could easily constitute a volume on their own. Nevertheless, it is a mirror of the first years of dedicated work, thinking, and commitment, and provides an entry way for much that is still to come.

The volume is divided into three major sections: neuroscience, ethics, agency, and the self, neuroethics in practice, and neuroethics at the intersection of justice and social institutions.

In the first section on the neuroscience of ethics, we revisit classic issues in philosophy and bioethics through the neuroethics lens, and examine whether neuroscience helps us to under-stand pre-existing notions about how we function ethically.

Patricia Churchland leads this section with her chapter 'Moral decision-making and the brain'. Here readers are immediately confronted with the question of whether we can have thought without biology. As social animals, 'we [humans] are more like wolves and less like cougars', and our ability to cooperate thoughtfully with one another, divide labor, share, and reciprocate is essential for our well-being. Churchland argues that the question of causality of brain events motivates neuroscientific exploration of brain-based behaviors and ultimately the consequences of 'being in control or not'.

Adina Roskies delves into 'A case study in neuroethics: the nature of moral judgment', with the aim of describing what an in-depth neuroethical analysis of moral control and internalism might look like. She argues that moral belief or judgment is intrinsically motivating and that, in judging morally, one is automatically motivated to act in accordance with one's judgment. As certain patients with prefrontal pathology fail to act reliably in the same way that non-injured people do in ethically charged situations, can moral motivation and moral knowledge be viewed as functionally separable and dependent upon distinct brain systems? Answers to this question bear on both emotional and reward systems that have historically been topics of extensive neuroscience research and, as Roskies convincingly argues, it is incumbent on neuroethics to be concerned with how this research informs empirical investigation of ethical thought and behavior.

When Stephen Morse considers related issues in his chapter 'Moral and legal responsibility and the new neuroscience', he discusses dominant concepts of personhood and responsibility in Western law and morality. He grounds his chapter in the practical example of how to decide whether adolescents who commit capital crimes are sufficiently culpable to deserve the death penalty. What kinds of arguments will help courts make this weighty legal and ethical decision? Morse argues that nothing about the truth of determinism is inconsistent with our view of ourselves as the type of creatures–conscious, intentional, potentially rational–that can be responsible and that determinism is fully compatible with moral and legal responsibility and "other worthy goods such as human dignity." Biological evidence is neither a direct nor an independent measure of diminished responsibility, he asserts; the criteria for responsibility are behavioral and therefore biological evidence can only be indirect confirmation of the behavioral criteria. Therefore Morse urges wariness over routine use of new kinds of neuroscience studies, such as imaging, that may tempt judges and juries into believing they are seeing hard evidence, Neuroscience provides hard, good scientific evidence, but it is not directly relevant to responsibility and decision makers may be wrongly tempted to think it is.

In the next chapter, 'Brains, lies, and psychological explanations', Thomas Buller continues the discussion of ethics, moral agency, and the self with the following question: If we adopt the view that it is the brain that feels, thinks, and decides, then how do we accommodate common-sense explanations of human behavior and the notion that we are intentional rational agents capable of voluntary action? He argues that there are limits to the coexistence of folk psychology (and the notion that we are intentional rational agents) and neuroscience. Buller explores how neuroethics must accommodate both science and ethics and, drawing on contemporary studies of deception, lies, and others, like Morse, he urges an awareness of the limitations of neuroscience in determining thought and defining responsibility for actions.

In her chapter 'On being in the world', Laurie Zoloth illustrates how our ability to unravel the mystery of consciousness can become fundamentally altered as neurobiology increases our understanding of how the brain organizes us. She sees the study of consciousness 'as at once the most elusive and most encumbered of intellectual discourses in philosophy and religion', and that '. . . the nature of ipsity (selfhood), the nature of subjectivity, and the nature of memory are all implicated in its description'. For the ethicist, Zoloth challenges, the problem of being in the world is not only how to describe innately private aspects of our conscious and mental lives in open language, but how to describe and then discern between the rational actions that moral agents take. She examines historical accounts of mind by Descartes, Russell, Parfit, Skinner, Armstrong, Nagel, Dewey, James, Searle, and Koch, and, like Roskies, places memory and motive at the core of the task.

Erik Parens describes different ethical frameworks for engaging us on yet another topic related to agency and the self. In 'Creativity, gratitude, and the enhancement debate: on the fertile tension between two ethical frameworks', Parens discusses interlocking views that can shape our responses to questions about the merits of enhancing cognitive behavior. He uses gratitude and creativity as the two pillars of his framework. Gratitude emphasizes an obligation to remember that life is a gift, one expression of contentment; creativity emphasizes the obligation to transform that gift, possibly to maximize potential. These are not intended to be oppositional; rather, they reflect places on a continuum where one may feel more or less comfortable. For neuroethics, illuminating this continuum toward an understanding of human authenticity and diversity, especially in the face of abundant technological and pharmacological opportunities for self-improvement, is a vital exercise.

In the last chapter of this section, notions of agency and personhood are examined by Agnieszka Jaworska in her chapter 'Ethical dilemmas in neurodegenerative disease: respecting patients at the twilight of agency'. Jaworska contends that the critical interests of a patient with a degenerative brain disorder are the person's values, and that conceptually such values may be understood as independent of the patient's grasp of his or her life. Using Alzheimer's disease as a model, Jaworska draws on two leading theoretical perspectives on agency—Ronald Dworkin's argument that there are compelling reasons to adhere to the earlier wishes and values of demented patients, and Rebecca Dresser's view that decisions affecting a demented person at a given time must take into account the context of that person at that time. Jaworska argues that the capacity to value is central to autonomy, and that significant capacity to value can be preserved far further into the progression of Alzheimer's disease than long-term memory or practical decision-making abilities. She concludes that the retained values of Alzheimer's patients must be respected rather than ignored, and that this respect could involve caregivers promoting the patients' autonomy by assisting them in making decisions that reflect their core values and critical interests. With an eye on caregiving as one's goal, similar analyses would be indispensable for other forms of neurodegenerative disease that are characterized by different trajectories of neurological degeneration and cognitive decline.

The second section of this books deals with neuroethics in practice. It begins with a chapter by Ronald Green, 'From genome to brainome: charting lessons learned', that explores converging and diverging issues between genetic and neuroimaging science research and clinical applications. We see how genetics is intensely communal and familial, while the study of the central nervous system is more focused on the individual. Nonetheless we learn how the 'therapeutic gap', gene hype, and the risk of scientific over-promising from both can lead to advances that may make situations worse before they make them better. We readily grasp that neuroscientists have much to learn from the experiences of others, and that they might as well do so. Geneticists had to 'take their blows through trial and error'. There is no reason for neuroscientists to repeat past mistakes; there is plenty of uncharted terrain for new unknowns.

The chapter by Franklin Miller and Joseph Fins, 'Protecting human subjects in brain research: a pragmatic perspective', elucidates ethical considerations in designing and carrying out clinical research on people with brain disorders based on an approach to research ethics derived from American philosophical pragmatism. With an emphasis on placebo-controlled trials of pharmacological treatments and deep-brain stimulation for psychiatric and neurological disorders, their analysis reflects how moral principles and standards can conflict when applied to contextually complex situations. To guide ethical judgment, they call for a careful balancing of morally relevant considerations and an understanding of moral norms rather than categorical or absolute rules.

The next chapter by Michael Gazzaniga, 'Facts, fictions, and the future of neuroethics', is a force in giving us new ways of conceptualizing social issues of disease, normality, mortality, and a philosophy of life. Committed to an understanding of how the 'brain enables the mind', Gazzaniga describes how cognitive neuroscience has valuable information to contribute to the discussion of many topics that have traditionally been the focus for bioethicists. Issues of enhancement, including selection of genes for intelligence, use of smart drugs to enhance brain performance, when to confer moral status to an embryo, and the search for biological explanations of impaired reasoning in criminals are but a few of these. Gazzaniga describes the intrinsic ability of the brain to adapt and respond to learned rules, social rules and 'built-in rules', and explains that while we may respond in similar ways to similar issues, it is what motivates us to respond in the way we do that differs. As he argues, the differences have roots in our personal narratives and the way we contextualize the world around us—context *is* everything.

Many of the chapters in this book refer to functional neuroimaging as a means of illustrating how far modern capabilities of neurotechnology have advanced for probing human thought. In 'A picture is worth 1000 words, but which 1000?', my co-authors Eric Racine and Matthew Kirschen and I examine the evolution of functional brain imaging over time and the intrinsic power of the image. We explore the underlying meaning of neuroimaging studies in which people make existential choices and solve thought problems, meditate and have religious experiences, and cooperate and compete. As Laurie Zoloth, one of this volume's contributors said at a recent symposium: 'Neuroimaging is heralding a change in the understanding of human life itself' (Stanford University BioX Symposium, 'Watching Life', 25 March 2005). Therefore, given the potential impact of these studies, including the sober reality of possible misuse, we conclude with a scheme for new dimensions of responsibility for responding to the promises on which imaging will surely deliver, and to the real or perceived risks that imaging may bring to our social, legal, and medical institutions.

In the next chapter, 'When genes and brains unite: ethical implications of genomic neuroimaging', Turhan Canli further brings home the real-world potential of neuroimaging by describing his studies of the neurobiology of personality and individual differences, including introversion, extroversion, and neuroticism. He illustrates how data obtained from neuroimaging scans can predict narrowly defined forms of behavior better than self-report and other behavioral measures, and he makes the argument that future integration of genetic and life experience data with neuroimaging data will further enhance this capability. Canli identifies employment screening as the first likely application of this technology. He argues that a statistically informed cost–benefit approach will be needed for the ethical use of this technology across diverse real-life applications in the future.

In 'Engineering the brain', Kenneth Foster examines ethical issues surrounding new technology for invasively stimulating the brain to enhance performance function, including what the boundaries for human brain implants will be. As implants and electrical stimulators for restoring or ameliorating lost functions in conditions traditionally contextualized within the domain of clinical medicine are moved to brain prostheses and pacemakers, mood manipulators, and mood monitors, whose values will prevail? Neuroethics has a key role to play in keeping realities apart from fantasies and in shaping standards that respond to these new developments that lie squarely at the juncture of engineering, neuroscience, and ethics.

Moving to other translational issues, in 'Transcranial magnetic stimulation and the human brain: an ethical evaluation', neuroscientists Alvaro Pascual-Leone and Megan Steven call for scientific engagement in defining an ethical framework for research with and clinical applications of transcranial magnetic stimulation (TMS). In the light of ever-increasing access to this technology for non-invasively stimulating the brain, these authors provide a detailed examination of the technical features of TMS and then explore ethical arguments in favor of and in opposition to neuroenhancement with TMS. Acceptable practices and the evaluation of risk versus benefit for patients must be distinguished unequivocally from non-medical practices in otherwise healthy human populations. The scientific challenge, they argue, is to learn enough about the mechanisms of plasticity to be able to determine the parameters of TMS that will optimally modulate neuronal firing for patients; defining *optimal* is the accompanying and immediate ethical challenge.

Translational principles carry forward in the next chapter, 'Functional neurosurgical intervention: neuroethics in the operating room', by bioethicist Paul Ford and neurosurgeon Jaimie Henderson. Functional neurosurgery presents especially compelling problems given the tensions between optimism and reality in the attempt to restore or normalize brain function. To frame the issues, Ford and Henderson examine the overall challenges of surgical ethics, and then discuss in detail the past, present, and ethical future of functional neurosurgical capabilities.

Robert Klitzman's chapter, 'Clinicians, patients, and the brain', is a natural transition to neuroethics in other clinical scenarios. In this chapter, Klitzman emphasizes the critical dilemmas that physicians face in their role as gatekeepers and shapers of decisions for patients with neurological and psychiatric disease. He tackles key questions for clinicians such as: How should health care providers introduce new neurotechnologies into clinical practice? How will patients incorporate new information into their thinking, the way they comply with treatment, and life expectations, especially as medicine becomes more customized and capabilities for predicting disease (possibly even before it can be prevented) emerge? How will the Internet and direct-to-consumer marketing of medical products and services affect relationships that patients have with their physicians and with science and medicine overall? New national health problems and new health priorities on the world scene will surely bring new challenges to already complex issues in clinical medicine. Clinical neuroethics will have to be alert to historical precedent and respond to these challenges both intuitively and empirically with new educational paradigms.

The final section of this volume is concerned with the interface between neuroethics, justice, and social institutions. It begins with a chapter by Henry (Hank) Greely, 'The social effects of advances in neuroscience: legal problems, legal perspectives', that explores the way in which neuroscience offers possible solutions to many human problems portrayed in (but not limited to) Shakespeare's *Macbeth*. He explores how social changes from advances in neuroscience are likely to have great implications for the law, as they will change both the objects of the law and, in a very direct way, how the legal system functions. Greely explores neuroethical issues surrounding the prediction of behavior, mind reading, enhancement, and legal issues such as regulation, safety, coercion, and distributive justice. With great wit, Greely considers the creation of 'enhancement havens, like the small tax or banking shelter nations scattered around the world', and 'weapons of mass enhancement' in countries hat might embrace technologies banned elsewhere. With a trade in body parts already well underway in certain parts of the world, these possibilities are anything but science fiction.

How could a new kind of educational infrastructure respond to some of our vexing societal challenges? In 'Neuroethics in education', Howard Gardner and his colleagues Kim Sheridan and Elena Zinchenko predict that, in the coming years, educators and the general public will look increasingly to discoveries from the neurosciences for insights into how best to educate young people. To understand the challenges that this may pose, Gardner *et al.* consider how educators navigate change and opportunities of scientific discovery. To respond to the challenges, they propose a new cluster of professionals: neuro-educators. The mission of neuro-educators will be to guide the introduction of neurocognitive advances into education in an ethical manner that pays careful attention to and constructively capitalizes on individual differences. The uniquely honed skills of these neuro-educators will enable them to identify neurocognitive advances that are most promising for specific educational goals and then, even more broadly, to translate basic scientific findings into usable knowledge that can empower new educational policy for a new neurosociety.

In 'Poverty, privilege and the developing brain: empirical findings and ethical implications', Martha Farah, Kimberly Noble, and Hallam Hurt explore how neuroscience can provide a framework for understanding and even solving societal problems, in particular the cognitive impact of poverty across generations. They demonstrate dissociable effects of the socio-economic circumstances of childhood on memory and language systems. Recall the chapters by Churchland, Roskies, Morse, Zoloth, and Buller, and the close links between memory and motivation to agency and selfhood; while cognitive neuroscience focuses on neurocognitive correlates of socio-economic status and provides a platform for testing specific hypotheses about causal mechanisms, neuroethics can respond with ethical analysis. The product of that analysis must be an enabling force in the development of targeted interventions that preserve and promote brain development across society.

Is there an intersection between neuroethics and religion? Paul Root Wolpe explores this question in his chapter 'Religious responses to neuroscientific questions', and demonstrates that, without any doubt, there. Wolpe argues that the questions confronting religious thought are not so much about religion's views on ethical issues, but rather on an understanding of exactly what the religious questions are that neuroscientific findings pose. When the questions of genetics posed by the Human Genome Project and cloning were encountered initially by faith traditions, the resulting dialogue was intense. Now, as he describes, neuroscience has capabilities that some religious traditions oppose or believe should be infused with certain values; these are evident, for example, in stem cell, anti-aging, and anti-cloning debates. However, religion need not be only reactive to the challenges posed by neuroscience; it can also mold science to its needs. Religion can embrace the discoveries of neuroscience and use them in pursuit of religious insight into the human condition. Wolpe has just the right perspective on these issues: while neuroscience may challenge the concept of soul, in doing so, it profoundly reinvigorates our understanding of it.

The last section finishes with 'The mind in the movies: a neuroethical analysis of the portrayal of the mind in popular media' by Maren Grainger-Monsen and Kim Karetsky. In this beautiful chapter, the authors illustrate the critical role that the media play in conveying neuroscience discovery issues in clinical neuropsychiatry and even neuroethics (albeit less directly) to the public. 'Madness', stereotypes and stigma in mental illness, for example, are concepts deeply rooted in historical pictorial media and portrayed in popular films. Grainger-Monsen and Karetsky examine the historical power of these films in reflecting and shaping audiences. Recall the messages of Charly, A Beautiful Mind, Psycho, Silence of the Lambs, and One Flew over the Cuckoo's Nest; consider the heavy burden of the 'pre-cogs' in Minority Report who, after brain changes due to early exposure to drugs of abuse, are able to predict a crime even before a criminal has conceptualized it. The authors further explore changing rules over time about the depiction of mental illness in the movies, and a welcome new trend in independent documentary film-making that has been breaking down negative messages of the past and opening up the image of neurologic and psychiatric illness within the world of storytelling.

Finally, Donald Kennedy anchors this volume with his afterword, 'Neuroethics: mapping a new interdiscipline'. Kennedy's chapter, drawn from the first ever presidential address on the topic of neuroethics at the annual meeting of the Society for Neurosciences (sponsored by the Dana Foundation) takes a look back at the discipline and a look forward. In 2003 Kennedy projected areas of major neuroethical concern—privacy was a particularly big one—and brought attention to their ethical significance and meaning for neuroscience. Here he reflects further on these issues, especially as they are raised in this volume, and brings us closer to realizing how intimately inseparable our science and specifically identity are from our moral world.

Neuroethics has already led to critical and explicit ethical thinking in neuroscience where it existed mostly implicitly before. While we can agree that there is always some risk associated with ethically questioning previously unproblematized issues that involve the brain or central nervous system, it is equally reasonable that we view this proactive movement characteristic of neuroethics as a positive one. Neuroethics has already shed new light on procedures for dealing with unexpected clinical findings in brain imaging research (Olsen 2005). Neuroethics favors professional self-regulation. It may move the meter on policy, but is averse to external regulation that culminates in obstacles that forestall scientific progress. Neuroethics provides fertile ground for discourse, and it opens unprecedented opportunities for academic and public engagement in the issues.

What is next on the horizon? Functional fetal magnetic resonance imaging? Already under-way. The ethics of covert surveillance? Predicting addiction or sociopathy in adolescents? Robotic devices mediated by brain signals—roboethics? Ethics in neuromolecular imaging? Neuroethics in regenerative medicine? Certainly.

How do we move forward from here? Neuroethics must continue to draw on lessons from bioethics of the past and collaborate with modern bioethics to empower neuroscience in the 21st century. We will need neuroethics students, homes for neuroethics training programs that are scientifically-relevant and culturally-sensitive in all corners of the world, reviewers with interdisciplinary grounding in theory and method, and we will require funding to examine the issues that become central to the effort. We will need to take more time to talk with journalists; they are the major conduit of information to the public. To sustain scientific credibility and uphold the highest standards of professional ethics, however, we must resist vetting results in the press prior to peer review, no matter how strong the temptation.

In the same way that there is no singular set of criteria that defines a card-carrying neuroethicist today, there is no predictable single vector for this new field. Like this volume, neuroethics is and should remain a highly intricate web of engaging and passionate interdisciplinary activity.

Judy Illes
Stanford University, Stanford, CA, USA

## References

Olsen S (2005). Brain scans raise privacy concerns, *Science*, **307**, 1548–50.

Gardner H, Csikszentmihalyi M, Damon W (2001). *Good Work: When Excellence and Ethics Meet*. Basic Books, New York.

Safire W. In Marcus SJ (ed.) (2002). *Neuroethics: Mapping the Field*. Dana Foundation, New York.

# Acknowledgments

This book honors Thomas A. Raffin, whose vision as a doctor, scholar, and mentor is surpassed only by his generosity.

To the contributors of this volume—pioneers, risk takers, boundary movers—there are not enough words to describe my gratitude to you.

My deepest thanks to Agnieszka Jaworska, whose effort in helping me shape this volume deserves special acknowledgment.

Many thanks are due to members of the Neuroethics Imaging Group at Stanford University, and in particular to Eric Racine and Marisa Gallo who provided invaluable help with this book. Thanks are also due to the anonymous reviewers who generously contributed their time to help fine tune the content of the volume.

A project like this cannot be achieved without the fundamental support of the organization within which it is realized and the vision of its people: David Magnus, Anne Footer, Mildred Cho, and Maren Grainger-Monsen at the Center for Biomedical Ethics, and Scott Atlas and Gary Glover in the Department of Radiology, Stanford University; and many others at Stanford and elsewhere whose kindness and trust are so appreciated. Thank you.

I am indebted to my husband H. F. Machiel Van der Loos for his unfailing support of yet another major project completed in our extraordinary life together. Thanks are also due to our children Adri and Kiah for their generosity in allowing me the time to put this volume together, and for their own growing insight and curiosity about the challenges emerging in neuroscience and bioethics. To my mother Ibolya, my brother Leslie, and other family, with love, always.

Finally, I extend my deep gratitude to those whose have sponsored my own research in neuroethics to date: the Greenwall Foundation, NIH/NINDS RO1#NS045831, the National Science Foundation, the Children's Health Initiative (Lucile Packard Children's Hospital at Stanford), and the Henry J. Kaiser Family Foundation.

# Contributing Authors

Colin Blakemore, Ph.D., Sc.D., FMedSci, FRS
   (UK)
Waynflete Professor of Physiology
Oxford University, and
Chief Executive
Medical Research Council
London W1B 1AL, UK
colin.blakemore@headoffice.mrc.ac.uk

Tom Buller Ph.D.
Associate Professor and Chair
Philosophy Department
University of Alaska
3211 Providence Drive
Anchorage, AK 99508
aftgb@uaa.alaska.edu

Turhan Canli, Ph.D.
Assistant Professor
Dept. of Psychology
SUNY Stony Brook
Stony Brook, NY 11794-2500
turhan.canli@sunysb.edu

Arthur Caplan, Ph.D.
Emanuel & Robert Hart Professor
   of Bioethics
Chair, Department of Medical Ethics and
   Director Center for Bioethics
University of Pennsylvania
3401 Market St. Suite 320
Phila PA 19104-3308
caplan@mail.med.upenn.edu
http://bioethics.upenn.edu

Patricia Churchland, Ph.D.
University of California President's Professor
   of Philosophy
Department of Philosophy, Chair
Department of Philosophy 0119
University of California, San Diego
La Jolla, CA 92093-011
pschurchland@ucsd.edu

Martha J. Farah, Ph.D.
Director, Center for Cognitive Neuroscience
Professor of Psychology
University of Pennsylvania
3720 Walnut St.
Philadelphia, PA 19104
mfarah@psych.upenn.edu
http://neuroethics.upenn.edu

Joseph J. Fins, M.D., F.A.C.P.
Chief, Division of Medical Ethics
Professor of Medicine
Professor of Public Health
Professor of Medicine in Psychiatry
Weill Medical College of Cornell University
Director of Medical Ethics
New York Presbyterian Hospital-Weill
   Cornell Center
435 East 70th Street, Suite 4-J
NY NY 10021 USA
jjfins@mail.med.cornell.edu

Paul J. Ford, Ph.D.
Associate Staff
Department of Bioethics / JJ60
The Cleveland Clinic Foundation
9500 Euclid Ave.
Cleveland, OH 44195
(216) 444-8720
fordp@ccf.org

Kenneth R. Foster, Ph.D.
Department of Bioengineering
University of Pennsylvania
220 S. 33rd. St.
Philadelphia PA 19104-6392
kfoster@blue.seas.upenn.edu

Howard Gardner, Ph.D.
Hobbs Professor of Education and Cognition
Harvard Graduate School of Education
14 Appian Way
Larsen Hall 201
Cambridge, MA 02138
hgasst@pz.harvard.edu

**Michael S. Gazzaniga, Ph.D.**
David T. McLaughlin Distinguished Professor
Director, Center for Cognitive Neuroscience
6162 Moore Hall
Dartmouth College
Hanover, NH 03755-3569
michael.s.gazzaniga@dartmouth.edu


**Maren Grainger-Monsen, M.D.**
Director, Program in Bioethics and Film
Filmmaker-in-Residence
Stanford University Center for Biomedical
   Ethics
701 Welch Road, Suite A1105
Palo Alto, CA 94304
mmonsen@stanford.edu


**Henry Greely, J.D.**
C. Wendell and Edith M. Carlsmith Professor
Director, Center for Law and Biosciences
Stanford Law School
Crown Quad #333
Stanford, CA, 94305-8610
hgreely@stanford.edu


**Ronald M. Green, Ph.D.**
Eunice and Julian Cohen Professor for
   the Study of Ethics and Human Values
Director, Ethics Institute at Dartmouth
   College
Dartmouth College
Ethics Institute
6031 Parker House
Hanover, NH 03755-3500
Ronald.M.Green@dartmouth.edu


**Jaimie M. Henderson, M.D.**
Director, Stereotactic and Functional
   Neurosurgery
Stanford University Medical Center
300 Pasteur Dr., Edwards Bldg., R-227
Stanford, CA  94305
henderj@stanford.edu


**H. Hurt, M.D.**
Center for Cognitive Neuroscience
University of Pennsylvania
3720 Walnut St.
Philadelphia, PA 19104
http://neuroethics.upenn.edu


**Judy Illes, Ph.D.**
Director, Program in Neuroethics
Senior Research Scholar
Center for Biomedical Ethics and
   Department of Radiology
Stanford University School of Medicine
701 Welch Rd., Suite A1115
Stanford, CA 94304-5748
illes@stanford.edu
http://neuroethics.Stanford.edu


**Agnieszka Jaworska, Ph.D.**
Assistant Professor of Philosophy
Department of Philosophy
Stanford University
Stanford, CA 94305-2155
Building 90nford, CA 94305-2155
jaworska@stanford.edu


**Kim Karetsky, M.B.A.**
Stanford Center for Biomedical Ethics
Program in Neuroethics
701 Welch Rd, Suite A1105
Palo Alto, CA 94304
kimkaretsky@yahoo.com


**Donald Kennedy, Ph.D.**
President, Emeritus
Bing Professor of Environmental
   Science, Emeritus
Stanford University
401 East Encina Hall, 6055
Stanford, California, 94305-6055
kennedyd@stanford.edu


**Matthew P. Kirschen, Ph.D.**
Medical Student
Stanford Center for Biomedical Ethics
Program in Neuroethics
Department of Radiology and Program in
   Neuroscience
Stanford University
701 Welch Rd.
Palo Alto, CA 94304-5748
Kirschen@stanford.edu


**Robert Klitzman, M.D.**
Associate Professor of Clinical Psychiatry
Columbia University
NYSPI-UNIT 15
1051 Riverside Dr.
New York, NY
rlk2@columbia.edu

Franklin G. Miller, Ph.D.
Bioethicist
Department of Clinical Bioethics
National Institutes of Health
Building 10, Room 1C118
Bethesda, MD 20892-1156
fmiller@cc.nih.gov

Stephen J. Morse, J.D., Ph.D.
Ferdinand Wakeman Hubbell Professor of
    Law
Professor of Psychology and Law in
    Psychiatry
University of Pennsylvania Law School
3400 Chestnut Street
Philadelphia, PA 19104
smorse@law.upenn.edu

K. Noble, Ph.D.
Center for Cognitive Neuroscience
University of Pennsylvania
3720 Walnut St.
Philadelphia, PA 19104
http://neuroethics.upenn.edu

Erik Parens, Ph.D.
Senior Research Scholar
The Hastings Center
21 Malcolm Gordon Rd.
Garrison, NY 10524
Parense@thehastingscenter.org

Alvaro Pascual-Leone, M.D., Ph.D.
Associate Professor of Neurology and
Director of the Center for Noninvasive
    Brain Stimulation
Harvard Medical School and Beth Israel
    Deaconess Medical Center
330 Brookline Avenue
Boston, MA 02215
apleone@bidmc.harvard.edu

Eric Racine, Ph.D.
Postdoctoral Fellow
Stanford Center for Biomedical Ethics
Program in Neuroethics
Stanford University
701 Welch Rd.
Palo Alto, CA 94304-5748
eracine@stanford.edu

Paul Root Wolpe, Ph.D.
Director, Program in Psychiatry and Ethics
University of Pennsylvania
3401 Market St., Suite 320
Philadelphia, PA 19104
wolpep@mail.med.upenn.edu

Adina Roskies, Ph.D.
Assistant Professor of Philosophy
207B Thornton Hall
Dartmouth College
Hanover NH 03755
adina.roskies@dartmouth.edu

Megan S. Steven, D.Phil.
Fellow, Center for Cognitive Neuroscience
6162 Dartmouth College
Hanover, NH 03755
megan.steven@alum.dartmouth.org

E. Zinchenko, Ed. M.
Doctoral Candidate
Human Development and Psychology
Harvard Graduate School of Education
11 Appian Way
Cambridge, MA 02138
Elena.zinchenko@gmail.com

Laurie Zoloth, Ph.D.
Director, Center for Bioethics, Science and
    Society Professor of Medical Humanities
    and Bioethics and of Religion Feinberg
    School of Medicine Northwestern
    University,
676 St.Clair St
Chicago, Illinois, 60611
lzoloth@northwestern.edu

# Contents

Part I **Neuroscience, ethics, agency, and the self**

**1** Moral decision-making and the brain  *3*
*Patricia Smith Churchland*

**2** A case study in neuroethics: the nature of moral judgment  *17*
*Adina Roskies*

**3** Moral and legal responsibility and the new neuroscience  *33*
*Stephen J. Morse*

**4** Brains, lies, and psychological explanations  *51*
*Thomas Buller*

**5** Being in the world: neuroscience and the ethical agent  *61*
*Laurie Zoloth*

**6** Creativity, gratitude, and the enhancement debate  *75*
*Erik Parens*

**7** Ethical dilemmas in neurodegenerative disease: respecting
patients at the twilight of agency  *87*
*Agnieszka Jaworska*


Part II **Neuroethics in practice**

**8** From genome to brainome: charting the lessons learned  *105*
*Ronald M. Green*

**9** Protecting human subjects in brain research: a pragmatic perspective  *123*
*Franklin G. Miller and Joseph J. Fins*

**10** Facts, fictions, and the future of neuroethics  *141*
*Michael S. Gazzaniga*

**11** A picture is worth 1000 words, but which 1000?  *149*
*Judy Illes, Eric Racine, and Matthew P. Kirschen*

**12** When genes and brains unite: ethical implications of genomic
neuroimaging  *169*
*Turhan Canli*

**13** Engineering the brain  *185*
*Kenneth R. Foster*

**14** Transcranial magnetic stimulation and the human brain:
an ethical evaluation  *201*
*Megan S. Steven and Alvaro Pascual-Leone*

**15** Functional neurosurgical intervention: neuroethics in
the operating room  *213*
*Paul J. Ford and Jaimie M. Henderson*

**16** Clinicians, patients, and the brain  *229*
*Robert Klitzman*


Part III  **Justice, social institutions, and neuroethics**

**17** The social effects of advances in neuroscience: legal problems,
legal perspectives  *245*
*Henry T. Greely*

**18** Neuroethics in education  *265*
*Kimberly Sheridan, Elena Zinchenko, and Howard Gardner*

**19** Poverty, privilege, and brain development: empirical findings
and ethical implications  *277*
*Martha J. Farah, Kimberly G. Noble, and Hallam Hurt*

**20** Religious responses to neuroscientific questions  *289*
*Paul Root Wolpe*

**21** The mind in the movies: a neuroethical analysis of the portrayal
of the mind in popular media  *297*
*Maren Grainger-Monsen and Kim Karetsky*

Afterword
Neuroethics: mapping a new interdiscipline  *313*
*Donald Kennedy*

Index  *321*

# Part I

# Neuroscience, ethics, agency, and the self

Chapter 1

# Moral decision-making and the brain

Patricia Smith Churchland

## Neuroethics: The coming paradigm

As we understand more about the details of the regulatory systems in the brain and how decisions emerge in neural networks, it is increasingly evident that moral standards, practices, and policies reside in our neurobiology. As we learn more about neural development, the evolution of nervous systems, and how genes are regulated, it has become evident that our neurobiology is profoundly shaped by our evolutionary history. Our moral nature is what it is because our brains are as they are; so too, for our capacities to learn, reason, invent, and do science (Roskies 2002).

Although our moral capacities are prepared during embryological development, they are not wholly configured at birth. One's social and cultural world, with its various regulatory institutions, deeply shapes the exercise of moral capacities in adulthood. These regulatory institutions include the standards prevailing in one's particular family and clan, the prevailing criminal justice system, the organization and style of government, schools, guilds, religions, and professional societies (P.M. Churchland 2000).

Recognition of these various determinants means that the traditional field of ethics must itself undergo recalibration. Philosophers and others are now struggling to understand the significance of seeing morality not as a product of supernatural processes, 'pure reason' or so-called 'natural law', but of **brains**—how they are configured, how they change through experience, how cultural institutions can embody moral wisdom or lack of same, and how emotions, drives, and hormones play a role in decision-making. Some traditional assumptions concerning the roots of moral knowledge have been exposed as untenable. As these assumptions sustain reconfiguration, the beginnings of a new paradigm in ethics can be seen emerging. Owing to the natural and biological roots of morality, this new approach to ethics may be referred to as 'naturalized ethics', or more simply, 'as neuroethics' (P.S. Churchland 1991, 2002; Flanagan 1996; Campbell and Hunter 2000; Illes and Raffin 2002; Roskies 2002; Casebeer and Churchland 2003; Goodenough and Prehn 2004).

The new research on the nature of ethics is located at the interface of philosophy, jurisprudence, and many sciences—neuroscience, evolutionary biology, molecular biology, political science, anthropology, psychology, and ethology. These interdisciplinary inquiries will have profound, and rather unpredictable, social consequences, as people in general rethink their conventional ideas concerning the basis for moral standards and practices. In this context, it will also be important to consider the impact on, and interactions with, organized religion, although I shall not address that matter in this chapter. Here, I shall focus mainly on one central aspect motivating the changing view, namely what we are learning about the neurobiological nature of decisions.

## Decisions and decision-making

Brains incessantly make decisions: some pertain to the immediate future, and others to the distant future; some are trivial, and others are momentous. Some decisions concern only oneself and one's own interest; others concern the interests of offspring, family, clan and distant neighbors; yet others may pertain to the welfare of animals, birds, and the land. From the perspective of the brain, these are all just decisions, involving emotions, memory, prediction, evaluation and temperament. From the perspective of human society, we find it useful to characterize a subset of these, namely the decisions pertaining to the interests of others, as moral decisions. Nevertheless, within the huge domain of practical decision-making, no sharp line demarcates the moral from the non-moral issues. Instead, decisions fall on a continuum, with prototypically non-moral decisions at one end (e.g. Should I have grapefruit or bananas for breakfast?), and prototypically moral decisions at the other end (e.g. How should we punish a juvenile capital offender?). In between, there are many cases where, if inclined, we may argue about whether the matter is best considered genuinely moral or merely pragmatic; whether it concerns justice, or only manners and politeness. All decisions involve some evaluation of the predicted consequences. Such evaluation is anchored by the brain's reward system, by the complex networks supporting emotions, appetites, and moods, and finally by one's background knowledge of the way the world works and one's own varying capacities for acting in it.

In childhood we normally acquire the skills to navigate the physical world of food, danger, and shelter. Acquired in tandem are the skills to navigate the social world; we learn how to please and avoid displeasure, how to find and give comfort, and how to cooperate, share, and benefit from compromise. Children discover the prototypes of exploitation, fairness, cheating, and altruism. They acquire the skills needed to survive and, if they are lucky, to flourish in both the family and the wider social world. Tacitly, they become sensitive to parameters of time to act, and the need to decide on the basis of imperfect and imprecise knowledge, of balancing risk and caution. Contemplation of theoretical knowledge may not require courage, good sense, resolve, or balance, but acting on knowledge surely does. As we all know, a theoretically clever person can, for all that, be a practical fool.

Aristotle (384–322bc) was really the first thoroughly to articulate the idea that the substance of morality is a matter of practical wisdom, rather than a matter of exceptionless rules received from supernatural or other occult sources. On the Aristotelian conception of morality, practical wisdom (praxis) requires development of appropriate habits and character, as well as a thoughtful understanding of what social institutions and judgments best serve human flourishing, all things and all interests considered. Just as theoretical knowledge of the physical world can evolve over generations and through the lifetime of a single person, practical understanding of the social world can evolve likewise (P.M. Churchland 1989, 2000). The evaluation of practices such as child labor, public education, trial by ordeal, trial by jury, income tax, slavery, cannibalism, human sacrifice, separation of church and state, military draft, and so forth occurs as people reflect on the benefits and costs of these institutions.

The role of the brain's reward system in social learning normally fosters respect, or even reverence, for whatever human social institutions happen to exist. Therefore change in those institutions may be neither fast nor linear, and may be vigorously resisted even by those who stand to benefit from the change; for example, women who opposed the vote for women and the poor who oppose taxation of the very rich. Despite the power of social inertia, modifications, and sometimes revolutions, do occur, and some of these changes can reasonably be reckoned as moral progress (P.M. Churchland 1989).

That individuals are to be held responsible for their actions is a common human practice, and typically involves punishment in some manner when actions violate the established standards. By its very nature, punishment inflicts pain (or more generally, dis-utilities) on the punished. Consequently, the nature and justification of punishment, and its scope, mode, and limitations, have traditionally been the locus of much reflection and debate. As science has come to understand the physical basis for insanity and epilepsy, there have been changes in the criminal law to accommodate the scientific facts. Insanity, for example, is rarely considered now to be demonic possession, best treated by isolation to a dung heap. In this century, neuroscientific advances in understanding higher functions inspire renewed reflections on the fundamentals of responsibility and punishment. At the most basic level reside questions about the relation between free choice, punishment, and responsibility.

## Brains, souls, and causes

The brain is a causal machine. Or, perhaps more accurately, given everything that is so far known in neuroscience, it is very probable that the brain is a causal machine. By calling it a causal machine, I mean that it goes from state to state as a function of antecedent conditions. If the antecedent conditions had been different, the result would have been different; if the antecedent conditions remained the same, the same result would obtain. Choices and evaluation of options are processes that occur in the physical brain, and they result in behavioral decisions. These processes, just like other processes in the brain, are very probably the causal result of a large array of antecedent conditions. Some of the antecedent conditions result from the effects of external stimuli; others arise from internally generated changes, such as changes in hormone levels, glucose levels, body temperature, and so forth.

Available evidence indicates that the brain is the thing that thinks, feels, chooses, remembers, and plans. That is, at this stage of science, it is exceedingly improbable that there exists a non-physical soul or mind that does the thinking, feeling, and perceiving, and that in some utterly occult manner connects with the physical brain. Broadly speaking, the evidence from evolutionary biology, molecular biology, physics, chemistry, and the various neurosciences strongly implies that there is *only* the physical brain and its body; there is no non-physical soul, spooky stuff, or ectoplasmic mind-whiffle. For example, there is no reason to believe that the law of conservation of mass/energy is violated in nervous systems, which it would have to be if the non-physical soul could make changes in the physical brain. The most plausible hypothesis on the table is that the brain, and the brain alone, makes choices and decides upon actions. Moreover, it is most likely that these events are the outcome of complex—extremely complex—causal processes (P.S. Churchland 2002).

If an event is caused by antecedent causal factors, does this mean that the event is predictable? Not necessarily. When a system is very complex, and when small changes at one time can be amplified over time to result in large differences in the end result, it is often very difficult to predict exactly the behavior of the system. This characterizes many dynamical systems. For example, it is impossible to predict with great precision exactly whether a tornado will emerge, and exactly when and where it will emerge. Exact predictability is elusive, not because tornadoes are uncaused, but because the weather is a complex dynamical system, there are very many variables to measure, and the values of the variables can change over very short time-scales. Consequently, in practice we cannot make all the measurements and perform all the calculations in real time in order to make precise predictions. The logical point of importance here is that the proposition 'events in system S cannot be precisely predicted in real time' is entirely consistent with the proposition that all the events in system S are caused, i.e. no uncaused events occur in S.

Nevertheless, even when a dynamical system is too complex for exact moment-to-moment prediction, general or rough predictions are certainly possible and technological advances may enhance predictability. Thus satellite photographs and radar maps make it possible to predict roughly where a hurricane will make landfall, at least within several hundred miles, and when, at least within tens of hours. However, greater precision remains impossible with current technology.

Similarly, although it may not be possible to predict exactly what a person may decide on a question regarding which seat to take in a bus, general rough predictions are possible, especially when one knows another person well. In a classroom, students tend to sit in the same seat each time the class meets, and hence I can predict that it is quite likely that Bill will sit in the front row aisle seat, since he has sat there for the last three times the class has met. I can reliably, if imperfectly, predict that another person will be offended if I gratuitously insult him, or that a 6-year-old child will prefer a sweet thing to a bitter thing, that a student will say 'apple' but not 'pomegranate' when asked to name the first fruit he thinks of, or that a person thrown into icy water will want to scramble out quickly. Technology and knowledge allow for improvements in our predictions about people and their behavior. Imaging techniques (functional MRI) showing unusually low levels of activity in orbitofrontal cortex can help us predict that a person is depressed. If a person has a mutation in the gene that normally produces the enzyme monoamine oxidase A (MAOA), and if he has also had an abusive upbringing, we can reliably predict that he will display irrationally violent and self-destructive behavior. An electroencephalogram (EEG) in which electrodes are placed on the scalp can detect brain changes that predict the imminent onset of an epileptic seizure. It has also been shown that criminal recidivism can be roughly predicted by using EEG in a Go–No Go paradigm (Howard and Lumsden 1996).

## To be free, must our choices be uncaused?

A common assumption states that when one's choice is genuinely free, then one created that choice—created it independently of whatever causal events might be occurring in the brain (Van Inwagen 1983; Allison 1990; Kane 2001; Korsgaard 2001; Pereboom 2001). It may be thought that such a choice springs into being as a result of the exercise of pure agency unfettered by any causal antecedents. According to this view, reasons may justify choosing one option rather than another, but reasons do not causally affect the will, for the will acts in a kind of causal vacuum. A free choice will have causal effects, but it has no causal antecedents. This view is known as libertarianism, or the thesis of contra-causal free will.

Looked at in the context of the preceding discussion, the idea of contra-causal free will has very low figures of merit. If choices are brain events, and if brain events have causal antecedents, then choices have causal antecedents. In addition, we can understand quite well why it may seem, introspectively, as though one's choice was uncaused. There are basically two reasons for this. First, our brains are not conscious of all relevant neural events antecedent to choice. From the inside—introspectively, as it were—a person will have no apprehension of non-conscious antecedent causes. Hence one may be inclined to consider the choice as springing from nothing—nothing but his free will. But the fact is, we have no introspective access to many events that happen in our brains. I cannot, for example, introspect the events occurring in the retina, or in the spinal cord. One just feels sexual appetite, without conscious access to the biochemical changes underlying those feelings, and one may imagine that they emerge un-caused. I cannot introspect the processes that typically precede normal unrehearsed speech, and may fancy that speech emerges from the freely acting will, independently of any causal antecedents. But by using imaging techniques such as functional MRI (see also Chapters 11 and 12), the causes can be seen to occur before the conscious awareness of intent.

A second reason helps to explain the introspective sense that choices are innocent of antecedent causes. When a decision is made to move—whether to move the eyes, the whole body, or the attention to a new task—a copy of the command goes back to other regions of the brain. This signal is called efference copy. As Helmholtz observed, one visible demonstration of efference copy consists in observing the difference between moving your eyes to the right and pressing your eyeball to the right. In the latter case, the world seems to move; in the former case, the brain knows, via efference copy, that the movement is my movement, not the world's. Consequently, the conscious visual effect is completely different. The wiring for efference copy means, for example, that it feels different when I lift my arm in deep water and when my arm rises in the water. One might, mistakenly, attribute that difference in feeling to something else: in one case, the buoyancy of the water causes my arm to rise; in the other case, uncaused free will exerts itself so that I raise my arm. However, the actual difference in feeling depends on efference copy or the lack thereof.

Reflecting on libertarianism in the eighteenth century, the Scottish philosopher David Hume realized clearly that the idea of contra-causal free will was muddled (Hume 1739). Hume pointed out, quite correctly, that choices are caused by desires, beliefs, hopes, fears, drives, intentions, and motives. He realized that our preferences are affected by our character, temperament, hormones, and childhood experiences; they are affected by how sleepy or alert we are, by how sick or well we are, by our habits and history. Moreover, and this was the crucial logical point, Hume realized that if a choice could be made independently of all these factors— if, *per impossibile*, it were independent of character, habit, inclination, belief, desire, and so on—the choice would be so bizarre, so 'out of the blue' as to raise the question of whether it was a real choice at all. Those choices we consider free choices, argued Hume, are those that result from our character, needs, habits, and beliefs about duty, among other things. Moreover, these are the choices for which we hold people responsible. If I suddenly choose to throw my phone out of the window, but had no desire, intention, or inclination to do so, if I had no belief that it was my duty to do so, no need to do so, no belief that it was in my self-interest to do so, then, as Hume saw, this would be a rather absurd action. This action would certainly *not* be considered the paradigm of a freely chosen action.

In contrast, consider as a paradigm of free choice President Truman's decision to drop an atomic bomb on Hiroshima in 1945. He believed that the war would continue for a long time if fought in the traditional manner and that American causalities would continue to be extremely high. He believed that Emperor Hirohito would not surrender unless it were starkly clear to him that his civilian losses would be catastrophic. Truman deliberated, reflected, considered the options, weighed the intelligence reports, and finally chose to drop the atomic bomb. His decision appears to have been the outcome of his desires, motives, beliefs, fears, and predic-tions. It is a decision for which he is held responsible. Some historians praise him for the decision and others blame him, but no one doubts that he was responsible. Was he caused to make the decision? Not by coercion or panic or reflex was he caused. Nevertheless, the various states of Truman's brain—states that we call motives, beliefs, and so on—did jointly cause a particular decision. Some of those causes, such as certain beliefs, may also be called reasons.

This does not distinguish them from causes, but is a conventional way of marking certain causes, such as beliefs and goals, as distinct from certain other causes, such as panic and obsession.

Those who find the idea of contra-causal freedom appealing have sometimes looked to quantum physics as providing the theoretical framework for contra-causal free choice. Roughly, the idea is that the indeterminacy at the quantum level—the collapse of the wave function—might provide the physical platform for contra-causal agency. Notice that Hume's argument, although some 200 years old, is sufficiently powerful to sideline this strategy.

If Hume's argument is correct, then free choice is not uncaused; rather, it is caused by certain appropriate conditions that are different from the set of conditions that result in involuntary behavior. Consequently, the appeal to quantum physics is completely irrelevant (P.M. Churchland 2002). As Hume might have said: Why would you consider an act free if it came about through pure randomness, as opposed to coming about as a result of desires, temperament, motives, and goals? Sometimes of course we are flippant about a choice, when there is little to choose between options or when we are indifferent to the consequences of the options, especially if they are trivial. It really does not matter whether I have a blue or a red toothbrush, and so in shopping for a new brush I just take one without deliberation or evaluation of the consequences. However, these sorts of cases are not the paradigm cases of reflective or deliberative or thoughtful choice. They are the minor players, at least in terms of momentous issues of responsibility and punishment.

The further point is that classical physics appears to be entirely adequate to account for the behavior of neurons and their interactions with one another. If uncaused events do actually exist in the neurons, perhaps in tiny structures such as microfilaments, such nanostructural events are unrelated to the level of neural network events that result in mental states, including deliberation and choice. Just as perception and memory storage involve information distributed across many neurons in a network, so a decision to act will be made not by a single neuron, but by many neurons interacting in a network. These interactions at the network level can safely be assumed to overwhelm any non-determined quantum level events that might happen to take place in the inner structures of a single neuron.

Hume's argument against the contra-causal view of rational choice seems to me essentially correct, and, as far as I can determine, no one has ever successfully refuted this argument, or even come close to doing so (see also Dennett 2003). Hume went on to develop a further important point that is especially powerful in the context of the developments in neuroscience that have occurred since about 1980. Assuming the cogency of his argument showing that decisions and choices are caused, Hume went on to propose that the really important question to answer is this: What are the differences between the causes of voluntary behavior and involuntary behavior? What are the differences in causal profile between decisions for which someone is held responsible, and decisions for which someone is excused or granted diminished responsibility? (See also Chapter 3).

From the point of view of civil and criminal law, and of society's interests more generally, these are indeed the important questions. Moreover, at bottom these questions are empirical, for they inquire into the nature of causes of responsible behavior, i.e. for behavior distinguishable on the social criteria that it either does or does not make sense to hold the agent responsible. Hume can be construed as proposing a hypothesis: there are discoverable empirical differences between the causes of accountable behavior and excusable behavior. In the next section, I shall develop Hume's hypothesis using data from the neurosciences. First, however, we need briefly to recall how the law regards choice and responsibility.

# Criteria for accountability and diminished responsibility

In *The Nichomachean Ethics*, Aristotle raises the following question: When should someone be held responsible for his actions? Very insightfully, Aristotle noted that the best strategy is to make responsibility the default condition, i.e. a person is assumed to be responsible for his action unless it can be shown that certain conditions in the person or his environment reduce or excuse responsibility. The main idea was that if punishment in a certain type of case would neither deter nor improve the future behavior of persons, including the defendant—if the punishment in these circumstances fails provide a reason to avoid the action in future—then full responsibility does not apply. To be excused from responsibility, Aristotle reasoned, unusual circumstances must obtain. For example, the person might be insane, and hence completely fail to understand the nature of what he is doing. Or the person might be sleep walking, and injure someone while imagining that he is rowing a boat. If a defendant injured someone while involuntarily intoxicated, for example, then he may be excused, but if he was voluntarily intoxicated, he must be held responsible, since he is expected to have known the dangers of drinking. Aristotle also recognized that responsibility can come in grades and degrees. Depending on conditions, someone may be granted diminished responsibility and therewith, reduced punishment, rather than be excused entirely from responsibility

In many Western countries, standards for determination of responsibility are rooted in the Aristotelian foundation. The standards have been elaborated and revised with the advent of new knowledge concerning defects of decision-making, and the developments in moral standards consequent upon appreciating the significance of the new knowledge. For example, in the USA, Canada, and England, for a person to be convicted of a crime, (a) he have performed the action, (b) the action must be a violation of a criminal statute, and (c) he must have a criminal state of mind. The latter phrase means that the act was willful, knowing, and involved reckless indifference or gross negligence. The state of mind provision is known as *mens rea*. The law assumes as the default condition that adults and mature minors are moral agents, i.e. they are held responsible for the action unless exculpating conditions obtain.

The *mens rea* defense involves trying to prove that the defendant was not, in the conditions under which the action was performed, a moral agent in the full sense. Thus a defendant who can be shown to have acted under duress, who was insane when the act was performed, or who was involuntarily intoxicated will be excused. When the behavior was an automatism, such as sleep-walking or otherwise acting without consciousness, the defendant may be excused. Note also that the excuse from punishment does not entail that the defendant can walk free. Institutions for the criminally insane, for example, will house defendants who are found not guilty by reason of insanity, but who are considered a danger to society nonetheless.

Other factors may show diminished responsibility. These factors do not abolish responsibility. Rather, they play a role in the mitigation of the sentence. Diminished responsibility provisions are complicated, but roughly mean that the person was not in full control of his actions. For example, diminished responsibility may be acknowledged if the person has very low intelligence, or is mentally impaired by disease or injury, or if the action occurred in response to provocation sufficient to make him lose self-control, i.e. where the provocation was such that a reasonable person might well lose self-control. In the UK, this defense can be used only in the charge of murder, and the defense must show that the defendant suffered from an abnormality of mind such as to reduce his ability to have mental responsibility for the murder. If the defense is successful, the charge is reduced to manslaughter. The young are treated differently from adults on the grounds that the capacity for control develops as the child matures, and that we cannot expect the same degree of control in adults and immature minors (Brink 2004).

The insanity defense requires proving first that the defendant is in fact insane or impaired. This requires the testimony of medical experts. In addition, the defendant must prove that the cognitive impairment rendered him unable to appreciate the criminal nature of the act. This requirement is generally known as the McNaghten Rule. In some states, another option is also available, which is to prove that the defendant, although cognitively able to appreciate the criminal nature of the act, was unable to conform his behavior to the requirements of the law. This option concerns volition rather than cognition.

Philosophers such as Van Inwagen (1983) and Allison (1990) argue that no one can justly be held responsible unless contra-causal free will exists. The sustaining assumption is that it would be unjust and immoral to hold someone responsible if his decision were caused by antecedent factors. In contrast, Hume, as we have seen, believed that it would be unjust to hold someone responsible unless the decision were caused—caused by his beliefs, hopes, desires, plans, motives, and so forth. Contemporary philosophers such as Van Inwagen tend to believe that because we do hold people responsible, agents must in fact enjoy contra-causal free will. The trouble with this view is that the facts about the universe, including the facts about the neural basis of choice, cannot be made to conform to our philosophical assumptions about our social institutions and conventions. The neurobiological facts are the neurobiological facts, whatever our social conventions might wish the facts to be.

My hypothesis is that holding people responsible and punishing the guilty is rooted not in some abstract relationship between a Platonic conception of justice and contra-causal willing, but in the fundamental social need for civil behavior. (As someone once whimsically said, there is no *Justice*, there is *just us*.) Humans are biologically disposed to be social animals, and, in general, one's chances of surviving and thriving are better in a social group than if one lives a solitary existence. In this respect, we are more like wolves and less like cougars. In social groups, cooperation, dividing labor, sharing, and reciprocity are essential for well-functioning—the civility of the group. Maintaining civility requires that children come to acquire the social practices of cooperation and so forth, and this acquisition typically involves both inflicting pain and bestowing reward. The young learn to value sharing, for example, and to suffer the consequences of failures to reciprocate.

The criminal justice system is a formal institution that aims to enforce laws regarded as necessary to maintain and protect civil society. To a first approximation, it functions to protect by removing violent offenders from society, to deter people who might otherwise violate the laws, and to provide a formal structure for revenge. The last function is not always emphasized, but its importance derives from recognition that humans who have suffered an injury are apt to retaliate, and that clan feuds can undermine the well-being of the group. Formal mechanisms for revenge are, on the whole, more consistent with civil stability.

## Toward a neurobiology of 'in control' versus 'not in control'

Until the second half of the twentieth century, it was not really possible to explore systematically the neurobiological differences between a voluntary and an involuntary action. However, developments in neuroscience in the last 50 years have made it possible to begin to probe the neurobiological basis for decision-making and impulse control. Emerging understanding of the role of prefrontal structures in planning, evaluation, and choice, and of the relationship between limbic structures and prefrontal cortex, suggests that eventually we will be able understand, at least in general terms, the neurobiological profile of a brain that is in control, and how it differs from a brain that is not in control (Fig. 1.1). More correctly, we may be able to understand the neurobiological profile for all the degrees and shades of dysfunctional control. For the time being, it seems most useful to frame the hypothesis in terms of 'being in control', where this is commonly assumed to involve the capacity to inhibit inappropriate impulses, to maintain goals, to balance long- and short-term values, to consider and evaluate the consequences of a planned action, and to resist being 'carried away by emotion'. Although these descriptions are not very precise, most people roughly agree that they describe what is typical for being in control, and agree on what behaviors are paradigmatic examples of compromised control.

The criminal law recognizes that control is lacking in automatisms, such as sleep-walking or movements made during and shortly following an epileptic seizure. Insanity is also understood to involve disorders of control, for example when the person does not appreciate that his thoughts or actions are in fact his. Other kinds of syndromes implicating compromised control include obsessive–compulsive disorder, where a patient has impaired inability to resist endlessly repeating some self-costly action such as hand-washing, severe Tourette's syndrome,

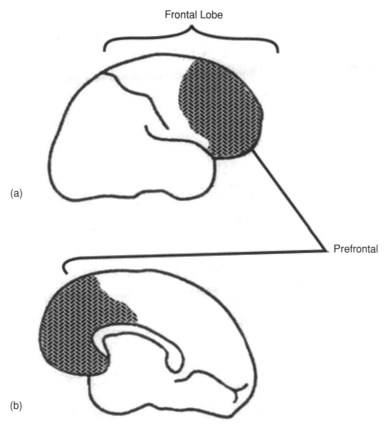

**Fig. 1.1** Schematic drawing showing the regions considered to be the prefrontal cortex: (a) lateral view; (b) medial view. From Damasio 1994.

where the person finds it almost impossible to inhibit particular ticking movements, or leptin disorder, where abnormally low levels of the protein leptin in the hypothalamus cause the person constantly to feel extreme hunger, no matter how much he eats. Obesity is the typical outcome of leptin disorder. Lesions to the prefrontal cortex have long been known to alter the capacity for planning, appropriate emotional response, and impulse control (Stuss and Benson 1984; Damasio 1994). The aim is to advance from a set of cases illustrating prototypical examples of control dysfunction to addressing the neurobiological basis of control and disorders thereof. Consequently, we need to determine whether there is a neurobiological pattern, or a set of common neurobiological themes, underlying the behavioral-level variations in compromised control.

What regions or systems in the brain are particularly important in maintaining control? Cortically, the structures that appear to have a pre-eminent role are anterior and medial: the orbitofrontal, ventromedial frontal, dorsolateral frontal, and cingulate cortices. Subcortically, all those regions that have a role in emotions, drives, motivations, and evaluations are important. These include the hypothalamus, amygdala, and ventral tegmental area (VTA) in the midbrain, and the nucleus accumbens (part of the basal ganglia, and a crucial part of the reward system) (Fig. 1.2). These are part of what is usually referred to as the limbic system, which also includes the cingulate cortex. Circumscribed lesions in these areas have helped reveal the interdependence of cognition, the emotions, and reward, both positive and negative (Stuss and Benson 1984; Damasio 1994; Schore 1994; Panksepp 1998).

Anatomical investigations of the patterns of connectivity among these regions, as well as between these regions and more posterior regions such as the parietal cortex, have begun to fill out the general picture of the dependency relations and the connection to action systems (Schore 1994; Fuster 1995; Panksepp 1998). Imaging studies have produced data that are generally consistent with the lesion data (MacDonald *et al.* 2000; Gray *et al.* 2003). For example, when subjects encounter conflict and must withhold or inhibit the typical response to a stimulus, activity in specific prefrontal and limbic regions increases. For other examples, chronic depression characteristically shows up as reduced activity in orbitofrontal cortex, and

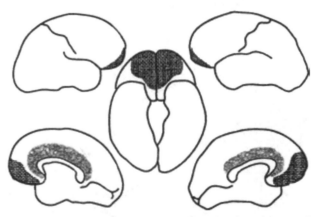

**Fig. 1.2** Schematic drawing showing the location of the orbitofrontal cortex (hatched) and the cingulate cortex (shaded): upper, lateral view of the right and left hemispheres; lower, medial view; center, underside (ventral view). From Damasio 1994.

disruption of connectivity between amygdala and prefrontal cortex results in an absence of normal activity in prefrontal areas in response to fearful or horrifying stimuli.

A common thread linking these anatomical regions is the so-called 'non-specific' neurotransmitter projection systems, each originating in its particular set of brainstem nuclei. There are six such systems, identified via the neurotransmitter secreted at the axon terminals: serotonin, dopamine, norepinephrine, epinephrine, histamine and acetylcholine (Fig. 1.3). These are referred to as the 'non-specific systems' because of their generality of effect and their role in modulating the activity of neurons. Abnormalities in these systems are implicated in mood disorders, schizophrenia, Tourette's syndrome, obsessive–compulsive disorder, social cognition dysfunctions, and disorders of affect. The pattern of axonal projection for each system is unique, and all exhibit extensive axonal branching that yields a very broad distribution of connections. The prefrontal and limbic areas of the brain are universal targets, with proprietary projections to specific subcortical structures such as the substantia nigra (dopamine), the thalamus (acetylcholine, serotonin), and thehypothalamus (norepinephrine, serotonin, acetylcholine).

On the surface, the aforementioned data from lesion studies, anatomy, neuropharmacology and so forth do not seem to coalesce into an orderly hypothesis concerning the neural basis for control. Looking a little more deeply, however, it may be possible to sketch a framework for such a hypothesis. Perhaps we can identify various parameters of the normal profile of being in control, which would include specific connectivity patterns between amygdala, orbitofrontal cortex, and insula, between anterior cingulate gyrus and prefrontal cortex, and so forth. Other parameters would identify, for each of the six non-specific systems, the normal distribution of axon terminals and the normal pattern of neurotransmitter release, uptake, and co-localization with other neurotransmitters such as glutamate. Levels of various hormones would specify another set of parameters. Yet other parameters contrast the immature with the adult pattern of synaptic density and axon myelinization (Sowell et al. 2003). At the current stage of neuroscience, we can identify the normal range for these parameters only roughly, not precisely.

Once a set of $N$ parameters is identified, each can be represented as a dimension in an $n$-dimensional parameter space. Visually, one can depict at most a three-dimensional parameter space, and the extrapolation to $n$ dimensions is conceived via generalization without

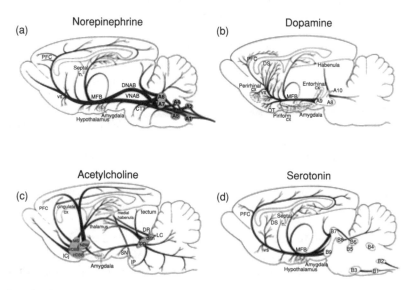

**Fig. 1.3** Projection patterns for four non-specific systems originating in the brainstem.

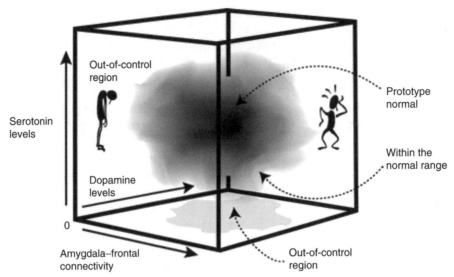

**Fig. 1.4** Cartoon of parameter space showing an inner volume where the values of the parameters mean that the person is in control, and regions outside that volume where the parameter values mean that the person is not in control. Only three parameters are depicted, but in fact the parameter space is multidimensional. Notice that the boundaries are fuzzy rather than sharp. Dynamical properties are omitted.

visualization. Figure 1.4 depicts such a three-dimensional parameter space; for clarity, many dimensions are omitted.

The hypothesis on offer is that within the described *n*-dimensional parameter space, there is a volume such that when a brain's values for those parameters are within that volume, the brain is 'in control', in the sense in which I am using that term, i.e. the person's behavior exhibits those features implying that the person is in control. I suspect that the in-control volume of the control-space is rather large relative to the not-in-control space, suggesting that different brains may be in control by virtue of somewhat different values of the parameters. To put it simply, there may be many ways of being in control. Equally, there are also many very different ways of not being in control, i.e. of being outside the in-control volume. I also assume that the boundaries of the 'in control' volume are fuzzy, not sharp, suggesting that a brain may be 'borderline' in control; it may drift out of the volume, and perhaps drift back in again, as a function of changes in a parameter such as hormone levels.

From the perspective of evolutionary biology, it makes sense that brains normally develop so that they are in the preferred volume (in control). Even simple animals need to be wired so that they flee from a predator, despite being hungry, or that they seek warmth if they are cold, even though they are keen to find a mate. Species with large prefrontal cortex, such as primates, are able to defer gratification, to control impulses, to generate rather abstract goals, and to plan for future satisfactions. Individuals lacking control in these dimensions are at a disadvantage in the struggle for survival (Panksepp 1998; Gisolfi and Mora 2000; Dennett 2003).

Figure 1.4 is a cartoon. It is meant to be a conceptual tool for thinking about 'in control versus not in control' in terms of a parameter space and a preferred volume within that space. So as not to be misled, one must be clear about its limitations. For example, although some of the parameters may interact with one another, this is not reflected in the diagram. Additionally, it is impossible to depict dynamical properties in a static diagram, although dynamical properties, such as changes during early development, adolescence, and senescence, certainly exist. Perhaps there are also diurnal changes or seasonal changes, and there is probably some context-dependency. Despite the many limitations of the diagram, the general concept of a control parameter space lends manageability to the hypothesis that there is a neurobiological basis in terms of which we can understand what is it for a brain to be in control. One can envisage much refinement to the basic conceptual point as neuroscience continues to discover more about prefrontal and limbic functions, and their role in planning, decision-making, self-representation, and evaluation.

## Conclusions

The important core of the idea of free will consists not in the notion of uncaused choice, whatever that might be, but in choices that are made deliberately, knowingly, and intentionally; where the agent is in control. This aspect of our idea of free will is the justifying platform for reward and punishment, both in the informal institutions of childrearing and social commerce, and in the formal institutions of the criminal justice system. Because of developments in neuroscience and cognitive science, it is now possible to formulate a rough hypothesis concerning the neurobiology of 'in-control' brains, and the respects in which it differs from that of 'not-in-control' brains.

My proposal is that we frame this hypothesis in terms of a parameter space, the dimensions of which are specified in terms of neurobiological properties, especially of the prefrontal cortex, the limbic system, and the brainstem. As a consequence, 'in control' can be characterized neurobiologically as a volume within that parameter space. This provides a framework for further research on planning, decision-making, evaluation, and choice in nervous systems.

These developments in the biological sciences give rise to difficult but important issues concerning the possible revision and improvement of particular legal practices, especially in the criminal law (Goodenough and Prehn 2004). A wide range of potential policy changes need careful consideration; options need to be thoroughly articulated, explored, and debated in order for us as a nation to find our way toward wise policy decisions.

No single professional or social group is adequately equipped to solve these problems; no single group or person can claim moral authority to the answers. We will need to count on the thoughtful opinions and solid common sense of people everywhere—in industry, academia, the military, government, the press, religion, and business. Neither dogmatism nor intolerance nor self-righteousness will be an aid progress. Basically, we have to reason together to try to determine how best to proceed.

Aristotle believed in moral progress. In his view, as we search and reason about social life and its perils, as we experience life and reflect on its complexities and surprises, we come to a finer appreciation of what is decent and fair, and of the conditions conducive to human flourishing. We learn from each other, and from those whose lives exemplify the human virtues. We learn from the past—our own, and those in the history of our species. Aristotle's view is not a flashy theory of the Archetypal Good, nor it is the sort of theory to whip up moral zeal. Nevertheless, it is a reasonable and sensible approach to achieving some measure of human good, succumbing neither to invocations of the supernatural, nor to self-destructive skepticism. It is a pragmatic approach anchored by grace, dignity, empathy, and courage (see also A. Roskies, to be published).

# References

Allison H (1990). *Kant's Theory of Freedom*. Cambridge, UK: Cambridge University Press.

Brink DO (2004). Immaturity, normative competence and juvenile transfer: how (not) to punish minors for major crimes. *Texas Law Review* 82, 1555–85.

Campbell R, Hunter B (eds) (2000). *Moral Epistemology Naturalized*. Calgary: University of Calgary Press.

Casebeer, WD (2004). *Natural Ethical Facts*. Cambridge, MA: MIT Press.

Casebeer WD, Churchland PS (2003). The neural mechanisms of moral cognition: a multiple-aspect approach to moral judgment and decision-making. *Biology and Philosophy* 18, 169–94.

Churchland PM (1989). *A Neurocomputational Perspective*. Cambridge, MA: MIT Press.

Churchland PM (2000). Rules, know-how, and the future of moral cognition. In: Campbell R, Hunter B (eds) *Moral Epistemology Naturalized*. Calgary: University of Calgary Press.

Churchland PS (1991). Our brains, our selves: reflections of neuroethical questions. In: Roy DJ, Wynne BE, Old RW (eds) *Bioscience and Society*. New York: Wiley, 77–96.

Churchland PS (2002). *Brain-Wise: Studies in Neurophilosophy*. Cambridge, MA: MIT Press.

Damasio AR (1994). *Descartes' Error*. New York: Grosset/Putnam.

Dennett D (2003). *Freedom Evolves*. New York: Viking.

Flanagan O (1996). *Self-Expressions: Mind, Morals and the Meaning of Life*. Oxford: Oxford University Press.

Fuster JM (1995). *Memory in the Cerebral Cortex*. Cambridge, MA: MIT Press.

Gisolfi CV, Mora F (2000). *The Hot Brain: Survival, Temperature, and the Human Body*. Cambridge, MA: MIT Press.

Goodenough OR, Prehn K (2004). A neuroscientific approach to normative judgment in law and justice. *Philosophical Transactions of the Royal Society of London, Series B* 359, 1709–26.

Gray JR, Chabris CF, Braver TS (2003). *Nature Neuroscience* 6, 316–22.

Howard R, Lumsden J (1996). A neurophysiological predictor of reoffending in special hospital patients. *Criminal Behaviour and Mental Health* 6, 147–56.

Hume D (1739). *A Treatise of Human Nature* (ed. Selby-Bigge LA). Oxford: Clarendon Press, 1967.

Illes J, Raffin T (2002). Neuroethics: a new discipline is emerging in the study of brain and cognition. *Brain and Cognition* 50, 341–4.

Kane R (ed) (2001). *The Oxford Handbook of Free Will*. New York: Oxford University Press.

Korsgaard C (2001). *Self-Constitution: Action, Identity and Integrity*. The John Locke Lectures, Oxford University 2001–2002. Copies of the lecture handouts are available online at http://www.philosophy.ox.ac.uk/misc/johnlocke/index.shtml.

MacDonald AW, Cohen JD, Stenger VA, Carter CS (2000). *Science* 288, 1835–8.

Panksepp J (1998). *Affective Neuroscience: The Foundations of Human and Animal Emotions*. New York: Oxford University Press.

Pereboom D (2001). *Living Without Free Will*. Cambridge, UK: Cambridge University Press.

Roskies A (2002). Neuroethics for the new millennium. *Neuron* 35, 21–3.

Schore AN (1994). *Affect Regulation and the Origin of Self*. Hillsdale, NJ: Lawrence Erlbaum.

Sowell ER, Peterson BS, Thompson PM, Welcome SE, Henkenius AL, Toga AW (2003). Mapping cortical change across the brain. *Nature Neuroscience* 6, 309–15.

Stuss DT, Benson DF (1986). *The Frontal Lobes*. New York: Raven Press.

Van Inwagen P (1983). *An Essay on Free Will*. Oxford; Clarendon Press.

Chapter 2

# A case study of neuroethics: the nature of moral judgment

Adina Roskies

## Introduction

Neuroethics is concerned with how the prodigious advances in our scientific understanding of the workings of the brain will and should affect society, at both a practical and a more abstract conceptual level. It has emerged as a field of inquiry in its own right only in the past few years, and although it is only with hindsight than we can identify with certainty the flowering of a new discipline or the rise of a novel science, the recognition that neuroethics has received of late suggests that we are witnessing the first stirrings of what will be a lasting social and intellectual concern.

The combination of a heightened public moral consciousness, prompted by political and economic current events, and the rapid scientific advances in the biological sciences leads us naturally to ask questions about how to reconcile our burgeoning knowledge of brain functioning, and our increasing technical expertise, with our more general deliberations about how we should live. As evidence of these concerns, papers in neuroethics have appeared in a number of mainstream newspapers and magazines as well as in scientific journals. Despite the subject's recent prominence, neuroethics publications have tended to be rather broad and impressionistic in scope. Therefore my aim in this chapter is to describe one particular neuroethical project in more depth, in order to provide a glimpse of what a neuroethical analysis might look like and the kinds of issues that such an analysis might engender. To this end, I characterize in some detail a body of empirical results from neuroscience, and consider the implications of trying to integrate such knowledge into our social and ethical frameworks. I begin with some preliminaries.

## The structure of neuroethics

It must be stated at the outset that neither the philosophical nor the scientific communities at large yet recognize neuroethics as a legitimate pursuit. Even within the small cadre of professionals that think of themselves as (among other things) neuroethicists, there is no consensus on its scope. Some deny that neuroethics is anything more than a subdomain of bioethics, and thus contend that it is not novel at all; others doubt that the discourse about the brain and body as objects of knowledge and the discourse about the embodied brain as a knowing subject can ever be unified, and consequently they may charge that to unite the two under a single name is merely wishful thinking (Changeux and Ricoeur 2002). I will not respond to either of these arguments directly, nor will I try to prove that neuroethics is a novel and cohesive discipline. I will merely suggest that although neuroethics may appear to consist of a collection of diverse and unrelated concerns, the various issues emerging from the confluence of neuroscience and ethics are so densely interconnected that it is defensible, and may even be profitable, to consider them as a unified whole. Nonetheless, I recognize that it is too early to answer questions about the autonomy or unity of neuroethics with any certainty.

As I see it, neuroethics is an amalgamation of two separately identifiable but interdependent branches of inquiry: the ethics of neuroscience, and the neuroscience of ethics. The ethics of neuroscience is itself composed of two distinct subdomains, which I have termed elsewhere 'the ethics of practice' and 'the ethical implications of neuroscience' (Roskies 2002). The ethics of practice is concerned to elucidate sound ethical principles that should guide our practice of brain research and treatment of neurological disease. The ethical implications of neuroscience, on the other hand, explores the effects that advances in our understanding of brain function have on our social, moral, and philosophical views. This branch of neuroethics has already been the focus of considerable attention. However, the neuroscience of ethics has received rather less. The neuroscience of ethics is, to a first approximation, a scientific approach to understanding ethical behavior. There is a growing recognition that the neuroscientific basis of ethical thought and, more broadly, social interaction is an area amenable to research, and an increasing number of researchers are devoting themselves to exploration of the brain systems involved in these complex behaviors.

While the ethics of neuroscience could arguably be an arena suited more to philosophers and policy-makers than to scientists, the neuroscience of ethics seems, at least initially, straightfor-wardly scientific. Its primary concern is to understand the neurobiology of the representation of value and of moral reasoning and behavior. However, I believe that the ethics of neuroscience will unavoidably extend beyond such purely scientific inquiry into the domain of ethics itself. For example, much philosophical work in meta-ethics is concerned with the nature of value, and in particular with the nature of beliefs or judgments that are ethical. How does our judgment that giving to charity is good differ from our judgment that Sampras is a good tennis player? Is there a difference in kind between judgments of moral rightness and evaluative judgments that lack a moral aspect? A grasp of the brain regions and processing involved in types of cognitive activities such as logical reasoning, decision-making, inductive reasoning, and emotional responses, as well as in moral deliberation, may reveal important similarities and differences between such activities that would form the basis of a classificatory scheme; moral reasoning may in fact turn out to have more similarity to one class of mental processes than to another. With today's modern imaging techniques, such questions can be approached. Here I hope to illuminate the nature of projects in the neuroscience of ethics, as well as how they may impact on issues in the ethics of neuroscience, by illustrating one case in considerable detail.

## A case study: ventromedial frontal damage

Recent investigations into the brain bases of moral reasoning and behavior make it clear that our abilities to think and act morally are not dependent upon a single brain area: there is no 'moral center' in the brain (Casebeer and Churchland 2003). Although we are only in the early stages of research into the neuroscience of ethics, the work of several groups has already given us important insights into the neural basis of ethical thought. For example, recent neuroima-ging studies which posed ethical dilemmas to subjects while scanning them demonstrate that moral reasoning involves widespread brain systems, rather than a single localized area (Greene and Haidt 2002; Greene et al. 2001, 2004; Moll et al. 2002). Widely distributed brain areas are differentially activated during moral reasoning tasks, including cortical regions associated with higher cognitive functions, such as the prefrontal cortex and association areas, as well limbic structures such as the amygdala, hippocampus, cingulate cortex, and thalamus, which are areas canonically thought to be involved in emotional responses. These neuroimaging studies corroborate results from lesion behavior studies, which lead one to expect that emotional systems in the brain play a role in moral reasoning and behavior (Damasio 1995).

Of the many brain areas identified in these studies, I will focus here upon one: the ventromedial frontal (VM) cortex. Paying attention to the contribution that this brain region makes to the functioning of the system can be very instructive, both scientifically and philosophically. An anatomical study of the VM cortex alone might prompt one to think that this region would be an interesting one for moral cognition. The ventromedial frontal part of the brain has extensive connections with areas involved in declarative memory, planning, language, and the limbic system. As such, it is uniquely situated to mediate between the neural systems for arousal and emotion, and those subserving linguistic cognition. Such expectations are vindicated by an extensive series of studies on patients with damage to this region conducted by Damasio and colleagues. Their work suggests that the VM cortex is of central importance in governing moral behavior. Patients with damage to the VM cortex (VM damage) have a fascinating clinical profile, for their deficits in the moral realm contrast starkly with their otherwise normal cognitive functions.

Evidence for the importance of the VM cortex in moral cognition is not new. Phineas Gage, in 1848, was the first person with VM damage described in the medical literature. Gage's VM cortex was destroyed when a spear-like tamping iron rocketed through his skull in a bizarre railway accident (Damasio *et al.* 1994). Amazingly, Gage was able to walk away from his accident and seemed at first to have no permanent deficits. However, it soon became apparent that something was amiss with Gage. Although his memory, reasoning, speech, and motor functions remained intact, his personality seemed altered; the man who was formerly a model citizen now flouted social convention and ignored responsibility. The change was so severe that his friends lamented 'that Gage was no longer Gage' (Damasio *et al.* 1994). Although Gage's story is by far the best known and most dramatic case of VM damage, contemporary cases exhibit similar profiles. The following passage from one of Damasio's case reports nicely illustrates the disorder.

> By age 35, in 1975, EVR was a successful professional, happily married, and the father of two. He led an impeccable social life, and was a role model to younger siblings. In that year, an orbitofrontal meningioma was diagnosed and, in order to achieve its successful surgical resection, a bilateral excision of orbital and lower mesial cortices was necessary. EVR's basic intelligence and standard memory were not compromised by the ablation. His performances on standardized IQ and memory tests are uniformly in the superior range [97–99th percentile]. He passes all formal neuropsychological probes. Standing in sharp contrast to this pattern of neuropsychological test performance, EVR's social conduct was profoundly affected by his brain injury. Over a brief period of time, he entered disastrous business ventures (one of which led to predictable bankruptcy), and was divorced twice (the second marriage, which was to a prostitute, only lasted 6 months). He has been unable to hold any paying job since the time of the surgery, and his plans for future activity are defective. (Damasio *et al.* 1990)

Further studies have enabled Damasio and colleagues to characterize the unique clinical profile associated with VM damage more fully (Saver and Damasio 1991). The main results of this research can be summarized as follows.

1. Moral judgment in VM patients seems to be largely unimpaired.
2. Despite this, VM patients show a marked impairment in their ability to act effectively in 'ethically charged' situations (situations that have a moral component).

3. In addition, VM patients exhibit some defects in their limbic functioning. In contrast with normal subjects, VM patients fail to show a skin-conductance response (SCR) to ethically charged situations, despite the fact that the physiological basis for the SCR is intact.

4. VM patients also report attenuated or absence of affect in situations that reliably elicit emotion in normal subjects.

Point 1 requires further exposition. First, it should be noted that VM patients have deficits in decision-making and prudential behavior in general; their deficit is not purely moral. Nonetheless, the profile of their deficits in the moral realm is striking, and it is on these that I will focus. Until very recently, it was thought that VM patients are normal in their ability to make moral judgments i.e. it was thought that both their reasoning processes and the outcome of those reasoning processes (i.e. their judgments in specific cases) were the same as those of normal people. However, very recent and still unpublished data (R. Adolphs, personal communication) suggest that this is not the case. In certain situations the judgments of VM patients depart from those of normal subjects. As we shall see, the way in which they do turns out to be highly instructive.

The earlier studies which employed Kohlberg's psychological tests of moral reasoning evaluated, in a qualitative way, the level of cognitive sophistication of the VM patient's mode of reasoning about moral situations. They demonstrated that abstract reasoning about moral situations is qualitatively the same in VM patients and normal subjects, and that some VM patients reach the highest level of abstract moral reasoning on the Kohlberg scale. EVR, for instance, was found to have reached the 'late post-conventional stage' of moral reasoning, a level of sophistication that surpasses the highest level reached by many normal people, placing him in the top 11 percent of the population. This does provide reason to think that EVR's abstract moral reasoning is unimpaired, a conclusion that fits nicely with data from other tests showing that his general cognitive reasoning abilities are unimpaired. Nonetheless, even if it is the case that a person's sophistication on moral reasoning tasks is intact, one cannot thereby conclude that his moral judgments are normal.

There are several reasons to question the methodology upon which the earlier claim that VM patients make normal moral judgments was based. First, it is doubtful whether the Kohlberg tests of moral reasoning are sufficiently fine-grained to allow one to conclude that moral reasoning in VM patients is normal as opposed to approximately normal. Secondly, in such tests, subjects are presented with hypothetical scenarios. As a number of researchers have pointed out, moral reasoning about hypothetical scenarios may differ in important ways from moral reasoning *in situ*. Thirdly, the methodology followed in these studies is under-specified. It is unclear exactly how the tests were administered. Were the patients presented with hypothetical scenarios in the first or third person, in indicative or subjunctive mood, etc.? Different ways of administering such tests could plausibly lead to very different results. Finally, it is not clear what role the outcomes of the subjects' judgments played in the experimenters' evaluations of the normalcy of VM moral judgment. To what extent did the experimenters concern themselves only with the process of reasoning, and to what extent did they take into account whether the subjects' judgments of rightness or wrongness corresponded to the judgments that normal people make?

Thus previous tests on VM patients may not have been the ones best suited to determining whether and in what way their moral judgments differ from those of normal subjects. Skepticism about the earlier studies is vindicated by recent evidence that the moral judgments of VM patients do not always parallel those of normal subjects. While current data still suggest that VM patients reason normally about moral situations, and that they usually judge these situations in the same way as normal people (although there are still a number of variables that must be systematically explored in order to make a confident claim of normalcy even in these cases), there is at least one subclass of moral situation in which VM judgments diverge from those of normal subjects. For want of a better way of characterizing them, these situations pose the subject with moral dilemmas that, although hypothetical, normally evoke strong emotion and usually require the subject to imagine himself involved in the situation in an immediate way. This is only a rough pass at a proper characterization of these situations. It is not clear that the actor in such situations has to be the subject, or what counts as 'immediate'. An example may help to delineate these situations from closely related and structurally similar scenarios.

Consider philosophy's famous 'trolley problem', still a matter of much philosophical debate (Fischer and Ravizza 1992). The trolley problem is really a problem about pairs of moral dilemmas, which are in many respects structurally similar but which differ from one another in important ways. The problem lies in determining just how they differ, and how these differences affect moral judgment. Consider the following scenario, which we will call 'switch'.

> **Switch:** A trolley careens down the tracks, out of control. It is heading for a group of five people standing on the tracks, and if something is not done it will kill them all. Coming off the main track, between the out-of-control trolley and the group of five there is a side track upon which one man stands. You could flip a switch to divert the trolley to the side track, killing one and saving five. Should you flip the switch? (It should be understood as built into the scenario that there is no way to alert the five; you have no other options for action, and there is no one else available to do anything.)

Most people say yes, they ought to flip the switch to save the five at the expense of the one. However, when faced with a structurally similar scenario which involves people getting, as Greene says 'up close and personal' (Greene *et al.* 2001), their intuitions change. Therefore consider a second scenario, which we call 'fat man':

> **Fat man:** A trolley careens down the tracks, out of control. It is heading for a group of five people on the tracks, and if something is not done it will kill them all. There is a fat man standing near the track, between the trolley and the group of five. If you push the fat man onto the track, he will stop the trolley. He will be killed, but the five will be saved. Should you push the fat man onto the track?

Here most people's intuitions pull the other way: pushing the fat man onto the track would be impermissible, despite the fact that the lives saved and lost would be the same as in the switch case. The philosophical problem posed by the trolley problem is to explain why our intuitions change. What are the morally relevant facts about the two cases by virtue of which it is permissible (or even required) to kill one to save five in the first case, but in the second case make impermissible the killing of one to save the five? This puzzle and others in this vein have exercised moral philosophers for some time, and have been a source of insight into principles that govern our moral intuitions and moral systems. Moral dilemmas like these have served as good probes for some subtle but important philosophical features of our moral judgment.

What I want to suggest here is that cases of the trolley problem type can also help illuminate our scientific understanding of how moral cognition works. Interestingly, preliminary data suggest that VM patients often depart from normal subjects in their judgments about fat-man-type cases, i.e. VM patients tend to judge that the right thing to do in the fat man case is to push the man onto the track to save the five. Fat man, or 'up close and personal' cases seem to be treated differently by VM patients than by normal subjects, which suggests that a properly functioning VM cortex might be particularly important in the normal deliberation about these 'up close and personal' cases (R. Adolphs and M. Hauser, personal communication).

In what follows I will explore two interrelated trains of thought. The first explores one possible implication that VM data might have for our philosophical understanding of ethics. I will argue that these data have implications for a long-standing but contentious thesis in moral philosophy. That thesis is called 'motive internalism' or, for our purposes, just 'internalism' [for a more detailed discussion of internalism, see Roskies (2003)]. Secondly, I will ask whether these data can significantly enhance our understanding of the neuroscientific basis of moral reasoning. I believe that they fit nicely with a particular model of moral cognition. This model itself has philosophical consequences, for it has a bearing on broader philosophical characterizations of ethical thought.

For clarity, let me provide a brief sketch of the meanings of some central terms in this debate; the actual states or events to which these terms refer is itself a project for neuroethics, and neurophilosophy more generally. Let us call a process of thinking about some issue in order to reach some conclusion a process of deliberation. Usually deliberation centrally involves reasoning, a cognitive process by which thinkers make a transition from one thought content to another, subject to the norms of rationality. Judgments are the outcomes of processes of deliberation, usually evidenced by a verbal report. For the purposes of this discussion, I take it that emotion is an affective component that may be involved in deliberation, distinct from reasoning.

## Internalism

The idea of internalism can be simply stated: moral belief or judgment is intrinsically motivating. That is, in judging morally, one is automatically motivated to act in accordance with one's judgment. The seeds of internalism can be found initially in the writings of David Hume. Hume was responding to the classical picture of our mental landscape, in which the faculty of reason is set against that of emotion or the passions. Moral reasoning was taken to be just one type of exercise of our faculty of reason, just as mathematical or syllogistic reasoning are others. Hume objected to this picture, arguing instead that moral reasoning is fundamentally different from other kinds of reasoning, and cannot be considered part of the faculty of reason at all. This is because moral judgment has the ability to motivate us to act, whereas other types of judgments do not. The fact that judging that something is good or right can suffice to motivate us to act suggests, he claims, that moral judgment is more closely allied with the passions or desires than with reason, for only the passions, and never reason, provide a motive for action. Hume himself was not an internalist, since he denied that what we think of as moral beliefs are really a type of belief. However, a number of subsequent philosophers who accept that moral beliefs are a species of belief have also adopted the Humean intuition that moral beliefs or judgments entail motivation (see also Chapter 1).

Varieties of internalism abound. Elsewhere I consider a number of different internalist theses and argue that many of these are deficient; for instance, they fail to capture the philosophical and intuitive force of Hume's insight, or they are tautological [see Roskies (2003) and Svavarsdottir (1999) for more detailed discussions of varieties of internalism]. Here I consider a version of internalism that is not prey to these problems, and that straightforwardly captures the idea that moral beliefs or judgments are intrinsically motivating. I call this view 'substantive internalism'.

**Substantive internalism:** If an agent believes or judges he ought to X, he will be motivated to X.

This formulation is a strong one, but nonetheless restricts the internalist thesis to a plausible subset of moral scenarios.[1] Substantive internalism is strong because it makes a claim of necessity; it says that, in some sense, moral motivation is constitutive of moral judgment: It cannot be that one can judge morally without being motivated. Substantive internalism is plausible for the following two reasons. First, it only applies to first-person judgments about what one ought to do. Therefore the internalist maintains that if I believe 'I ought to give money to famine relief', I will be, at least to some degree, motivated to give to famine relief. If, on the other hand, I believe 'You ought to give to famine relief', that belief, although moral, does not entail that I will be motivated at all. Secondly, the internalist holds only that a first-person 'ought' belief must *involve* motivation, but not that the motivation implied by the judgment is sufficient to lead to action. We are all intimately familiar with cases of weakness of will, in which our judgments about what it is best to do fail to issue in action because of ennui. We are also aware that in deciding how to act, moral considerations are not the only considerations we take into account. Moral judgment can fail to lead to action because of countervailing reasons. Thus the internalist thesis is *prima facie* plausible; he holds that moral beliefs or judgments about what one ought to do are always and necessarily accompanied by motivation, but he recognizes that this motivation need not issue in action. On the other hand, it is important to recognize that internalism is not merely a contingent claim about what we are like, it is a metaphysical claim about morality. It postulates a sort of special status for moral judgment; unlike other kinds of judgment, moral judgment is intrinsically motivating.

Perhaps a word more should be said about what 'intrinsically motivating' means. Think of it in the following way: it is by virtue of a judgment's being moral that we are motivated. It is the subject matter or content of the judgment that provides its motivational character, and because of internalism's necessity claim, no judgment with the same content or meaning could fail to be motivating. To deny internalism, then, is among other things, to deny that the metaphysical status of moral judgments differs in this way from the status of other judgments.

## An idealization of the data and internalism

How do the neuroscientific results outlined above bear on the truth of internalism? Recall that the moral judgments of VM patients usually accord with those of normal subjects. For ease of analysis, let us assume initially that there is another population of brain-damaged patients (call them VM* patients) who make all the same judgments as normal subjects do, i.e. they do not differ in their 'up close and personal' judgments; indeed, until recently, that is what VM patients were thought to be like. Therefore the clinical picture of VM* patients is as follows. VM* patients retain declarative knowledge related to moral issues and appear to be able to reason morally at a normal level. Significantly, their moral claims accord with those of normal subjects. Nonetheless, they fail to act reliably as normal subjects do in many ethically charged situations. Furthermore, in ethically charged situations, VM* patients seem to lack appropriate motivational and emotional responses, both at the level of their own subjective experience and with regard to normal physiological correlates of emotion and motivation.

Since internalism posits a necessary connection between moral judgment and motivation, a counter-example can demonstrate it to be false. I suggest that VM* patients, if they existed, would be walking counter-examples to the internalist claim (Roskies 2003). VM* patients reason normally and make the same moral judgments that you or I would make, yet they consistently fail to act in accordance with their own first-person moral judgments. We might reasonably conclude that their failure to act stems from a failure to be motivated.

The internalist will respond that merely showing that judgment and action come apart is insufficient to overthrow internalism, which is a claim about judgment and motivation. He might maintain that VM* patients are motivated to act in accord with their moral judgments, but these motivations are overridden by countervailing ones. However, I believe that neuroscientific research can give us a window onto these motivations, and can show the internalist reply to be unconvincing. In normal circumstances we must infer a person's motivation from his actions, since we lack an ability to observe or measure his motivations directly. However, application of scientific techniques enables us to detect many phenomena that might be undetectable in normal circumstances. I believe that motivation is one of these phenomena. Recall that in his experiments with VM patients, Damasio measured the SCR and found that VM patients lack a physiological response that normal subjects demonstrate: the SCR is present in normal subjects but is usually absent in VM patients. In further studies Damasio has reported that occasionally VM patients do exhibit the SCR, and on those occasions they act normally in response to ethically charged situations (Damasio *et al.* 1990). This strong correlation between the presence of the SCR and behavior in both normal subjects and VM patients suggests that the SCR is a sign or a physiological correlate of motivation. If so, then the SCR can help us to distinguish between cases in which action fails to result because of lack of motivation, and those in which it fails because of countervailing motivations. Because the SCR is a unipolar phenomenon (i.e. it occurs regardless of what the motivation is for, or whether it is for or against something), we would expect to see it in cases in which there is motivation to act in accordance with one's moral judgment, as well as in cases in which there is overriding motivation to act in some other way. However, we would not expect to see SCR in cases where motivation is absent. Thus the SCR allows us to distinguish cases in which motivation is lacking from cases in which it is present but overridden; it provides us with a window on motivation that allows us to bypass the usual route of inference from action, enabling us, in a sense, to observe motivation directly. We can conclude from the absence of the SCR in VM patients that they indeed lack motivation to act in accord with their judgments, not merely that they have some motivation but have stronger motivations to act otherwise. Since, by hypothesis, VM* patients are just like VM patients, we can conclude that they too lack motivation, despite their normal moral judgments.

The internalist can respond by arguing that VM* patients do not really make moral judgments all. The argument usually proffered is that although these patients seem to be making moral judgments when they say 'I ought not do X', or 'Doing Y would be morally right', they are not really making moral judgments. They are doing something else—seemingly making judgments or making judgments that are not moral. And since they are not really making moral judgments, the fact that their utterances are phonologically identical to moral judgments in English makes not a whit of difference to our evaluation of the truth of internalism. It remains a statement about the conceptual connection between morality and motivation, immune from the hypothetical picture of VM* patients.

Let us look more closely at the logic behind the internalist's potential defense that VM* patients are not really making moral judgments. Such a defense might rest on a claim about mastery of language. VM* patients do not really make moral judgments because they lack mastery of moral terms; they use the wrong application conditions for words in our language that are related to the moral realm. The opponent of internalism has ample evidence to counter this suggestion. First, as mentioned above, the putative moral beliefs and judgments of VM* patients usually accord with those of normal people. Just as we would not say that a person who categorizes color terms slightly differently from us (e.g. calling a shade of gray a shade of blue) lacks mastery of color language, and so fails to make claims about color, it does not seem correct to say that VM* patients lack mastery of moral terms. Secondly, extensive psychological testing demonstrates that VM patients show no cognitive deficits in either their theoretical reasoning abilities or their declarative knowledge, and that their brain insult does not lead to any type of memory impairment. It would be implausible to argue that they have full mastery of all language but moral language, even though they perform normally on almost all tests of moral reasoning.

Moreover, the typical argument from mastery is inapplicable to the case of VM* patients. The typical argument about mastery is raised in cases in which a person has never demonstrated mastery of a term. For instance, one might reasonably ask of a congenitally blind person whether he ever attains full mastery of the term 'red'. However, in the debate about VM and VM* patients, all parties accept that persons with VM damage had full mastery of moral terms before their accident or surgery. To apply the argument from mastery in this case would be analogous to arguing that a fully sighted person who lost his vision in an accident would no longer know the meaning of the term 'red' immediately following the accident, or perhaps even that we lack mastery of 'red' when we close our eyes! In order for this to be remotely plausible, the internalist would have to offer a compelling story about how mastery of a term's meaning could be affected by damage to the VM cortex, especially since subjects have a demonstrated ability to employ the term correctly. With the mastery argument the burden of proof is shifted to the internalist.

A second possibility is that the internalist can argue that VM* damage results in the loss of moral concepts. This claim is subtly different from the claim about mastery, because here the internalist argues that what is deficient in these patients is not the mapping from language to concepts, but the nature of the underlying conceptual representations themselves. He might argue this on the basis that an emotional or motivational component is essential to a moral concept. Unfortunately, this claim is extremely close to the claim of internalism itself. Just as the internalist cannot justify his claim that VM* patients only seem to be making moral judgments by appeal to the fact that they are not motivated to act in accordance with them (for that would be begging the question), so he cannot simply assert that motivation is essential to a moral concept. He must bring to bear independent arguments for why motivation is essential to a moral concept in order to make the claim of essentialism stick. It is here that the internalist might push, but it is important to see that it is not enough for him to show that the essentialist claim is possible; he must show that it is plausible. For the reasons just defended, it is far more plausible that VM* patients retain the ability to make moral judgments; frontal damage affects neither our mastery of language nor our concepts.

## VM data and internalism

The argument against internalism provided by VM* patients is compelling, and if there were such patients, I believe that substantive judgment internalism would be shown to be false. However, as it turns out, the world has provided us with VM patients, not VM* patients. The difference between these real VM patients and our hypothetical VM* patients is that VM patients occasionally make moral judgments that do not accord with those of normal people. How are we to interpret this difference? Do VM patients threaten internalism as the VM* patients do, or do the differences between VM and VM* patients rescue internalism from the threat of counter-example? In other words, could the internalist make much hay out of the fact that there are circumstances in which normal and VM moral judgments differ?

Given where we have gotten thus far, it is clear that VM patients will pose no threat to internalism only if they do not make moral judgments at all. Does the fact that their judgments about moral situations sometimes differ from those of VM* patients lend support to this interpretation?

One might think, for instance, that the differences between VM and VM* patients prevent one from arguing that VM patients are normal in their moral judgments, and this might lend credence to the claim that they are not really making moral judgments after all. However, the argument about VM* patients does not rest heavily on the fact that VM* moral judgments are always the same as those of normal subjects, but rests more upon the fact that the VM patients' judgments are moral. That VM* judgments are always congruent with those of normal subjects just makes it easier to see that their judgments are moral.

Note, for instance, the important fact that the judgments normal people make are not univocal; when we speak of normalcy, we are making statistical generalizations. A small proportion of ostensibly normal people, noted philosophers among them, also fail to judge trolley problem dilemmas as the majority do; rather, their judgments concur with those of VM patients. We are not tempted to claim that these people lack moral concepts, do not understand moral terms, or fail to make moral judgments. (It would be quite a pickle if it turned out that by virtue of philosophers' dispassionate reasoning about morality, moral philosophy was not really about morality!) On the contrary, it is largely because of variability in normal moral judgments that there are plausible challenges to moral objectivism.

To argue that VM patients do not make moral judgments, one would again have to argue that the content of their judgments is not moral. That is, either they lack mastery of moral terms, or they lack moral concepts. At first glance the argument that they lack mastery of moral terms might seem much more plausible than in the VM* case. After all, one might argue that if someone systematically misapplied a color term, for instance calling gray things blue, but generally agreed with our usage in his application of other color terms, he lacked mastery of the terms 'gray' or 'blue'. However, one would not thereby conclude that he lacked mastery of color terms *tout court*, and therefore failed to make color judgments. Instead, a more plausible interpretation is that his color terms 'gray' and 'blue' had a slightly different extension than our own.

Therefore one plausible evaluation of the fact that VM and normal judgments do not always concur is that although VM patients have a general mastery of moral terms, the content of some terms differs slightly from those of normal subjects. That slight difference in content might account for the differences between normal and VM judgments. Note, however, that this position is of little solace to the internalist, for as long as it is admitted that VM patients make moral judgments yet lack motivation, they stand as counter-examples to internalism. The color case, for instance, does not allow us to claim that our outlier lacks the ability to make color judgments. What we would say is that he makes color judgments, but some are erroneous.

Furthermore, I will suggest that an explanation based on alterations of the content of moral terms is not likely to give an accurate description of what is going on in the case of VM patients. It is difficult, although not impossible, to construct a story whereby normal reasoning processes operating on thoughts whose propositional content is shifted slightly by alterations in moral terms (i.e. terms such as 'wrong', 'ought', 'good') could account for these discrete deviations from normal judgments, while leaving moral judgments in most scenarios unrevised. There is also a genetic difficulty; content shifting seems to be a difficult thing to explain by gross brain damage Finally, such a view would also suggest that we explain the variance in judgment in the normal population as differences in the meaning of moral terms, which also seems unlikely.

Might one argue instead that VM patients lack moral concepts? This is probably the best place for the internalist to push, but again the reasons one can bring to bear in favor of such a position are just reiterations of the internalist claims. VM patients think that they are making moral judgments; they do not think that the content of their terms or extensions of their moral concepts have altered; they are just not motivated to act upon their judgments.

There is further reason to doubt that the proper interpretation of VM damage is that VM patients lack moral concepts. Philosophers and psychologists have made much of the moral–conventional distinction: the idea that 'ought' judgments of a moral nature have a constellation of features which differ from 'ought' judgments of a conventional nature. This is thought to be so because of the nature of the content of those judgments—moral judgments are about moral norms (e.g. 'it is wrong to inflict pain unnecessarily'), and conventional judgments are about conventional norms (e.g. 'it is wrong to talk with your mouth full'). For instance, judgments based on moral norms are often or always held to be motivating, while conventional ones are not; moral norms are authority independent, while conventional ones are authority dependent; and transgressions of moral norms are taken to be more serious than transgressions of conventional norms (Nichols 2002). Nichols, in some interesting studies, has shown that conventional judgments that have an emotional component, such as judgments of disgust, share the characteristic features of moral judgments (Nichols 2002). Even more surprising, judgments that are clearly not moral can take on the features that are thought to characterize moral judgments if they are accompanied by high arousal (S. Schnall et al. 2004, unpublished observations; T. Wheatley and J. Haidt 2004, unpublished observations). This suggests that features thought to mark moral judgments are not dependent on the judgment's content, but on the level of emotional arousal that accompanies the judgment. It seems clear that content of a judgment about a convention remains unchanged by whether or not that judgment is made in an aroused state; a judgment about proper table manners does not become a moral judgment just because it takes on characteristics usually attributed to moral judgments. By parity of reasoning, the content of a moral judgment does not change if made in conditions of low arousal, regardless of whether it loses some of the features usually attributed to moral judgments, such as its motivational status. I think that VM patients are just instances of such cases. So although these arguments about the malleability of characteristics of judgments by arousal levels do not rule out the possibility that a judgment cannot be a moral judgment unless it is motivating, they support the idea that the content of an 'ought' judgment can be dissociated from its motivational character.

In short, appeal to the fact that there are circumstances in which VM and normal judgments differ does not seem to provide the internalist with the resources necessary to argue convincingly that VM patients do not make moral judgments, and thus defuse the challenge to internalism. Although admittedly VM patients do not definitively refute internalism, they do place the burden of proof firmly upon the internalist. The types of responses open to the person who holds this substantive internalist thesis might involve a denial that the SCR data reflect motivation, and thus a denial that motivation is absent in cases in which VM patients fail to act. In this case the deficits illustrated by VM patients must be interpreted to fall more on the side of action than of motivation. Alternatively, the internalist may deny that VM patients perceive moral situations as moral in relevant respects, either because of a general deficit in perception, or because they do not view moral situations as binding upon them (I am indebted to A. Jaworska for this suggestion). However, it is doubtful that perceiving something as moral is really a type of perception, rather than a type of cognition; insofar as perceptual and cognitive deficits both seem to be absent in these patients, this does not look like a promising avenue for the internalist to pursue.

There are no knock-down arguments in philosophy; however, there are more and less plausible ones. As J.J.C. Smart recently noted in Canberra, plausibility in the light of total science is an important tool in metaphysics. The most plausible interpretation of the VM data, given what we know about the brain, is that VM patients do make moral judgments and that, consequently, internalism is false. I believe that there is a coherent explanation of what is going on with VM patients which accounts for all the data. This account supports the interpretation that VM patients make moral judgments, and the picture it paints is incompatible with internalism. So, let us move on to the positive account.

## A positive picture of moral judgment

Based on the above considerations it is reasonable to hold, provisionally, that VM patients really do make moral judgments. Can we construct a good explanation of what goes on in moral judgment, harnessing what is known about the brain and VM damage, according to which people with damage to the VM cortex make judgments about moral situations which usually accord with those of normal subjects, but deviate from them in just those situations in which the VM patients' judgments deviate, (namely judgments about 'up close and personal' situations?) I think we can, and what is striking is the coherence and simplicity of the resulting account. A number of aspects of the VM data make perfect sense once one has in place a particular understanding of how moral judgments are made. What is more, if an account of the data yields a picture of normal moral judgment in which moral judgments are not intrinsically motivating, we have additional reason to think that internalism provides an erroneous picture of the nature of moral judgment.

My proposal is this. The general cognitivist picture of morality is correct: moral judgments are a subspecies of judgment; moral reasoning is a type of reasoning; moral concepts are an ordinary type of concept, and there is nothing intrinsically motivating about either moral concepts or moral judgments. However, in normal people, emotion plays an important role in modulating reasoning about morality, and this modulating influence is apparent in the different judgments that people make in high-affect and low-affect situations, such as in the fat man and switch versions of the trolley problem. It is this affective ingredient that so often accompanies our moral deliberation that leads to the impression that it is the moral judgment itself that is motivating. The affective component is most strongly harnessed in situations in which we imagine ourselves personally and physically involved in what can be thought of as an emotionally charged situation, and in these cases the affective component can bias processes of moral evaluation that are rather more dispassionate. What VM patients illustrate is an important feature of the functional organization of the neural systems that subserve judgment in moral situations. They show that this emotional–motivational component can be dissociated from the process of reasoning and judgment. VM patients have demonstrably impaired levels of emotional arousal, as is known both from self-report, brain imaging studies, and measurements of skin conductance. The failure of these depressed or absent emotional responses to affect the reasoning process results in the deviation of the VM patients' moral judgments in cases of the fat man type from the intuitions of normal subjects; in such cases VM reasoning about moral situations continues to be dispassionate, and thus they reach a different conclusion than do normal subjects. As some have described it, VM patients' judgments in the trolley problem cases seem to reflect utilitarian calculations across the board, while the majority of normal people seem to employ different standards in the two types of scenarios. However, importantly, the emotional component that often accompanies moral judgment in normal subjects is a contingent feature of moral judgment—it does not affect the content or meaning of the judgment, and just as the motivating features of judgments of disgust do not thereby turn judgments of disgust into judgments of morality, so judgments of morality do not become something else when lacking this motivating force.

This view fits with a number of features of VM patients, and with what is known about normal moral cognition. First, the differences in judgment between normal subjects and VM patients are attributable to the VM patients' demonstrated emotional deficits. Such deficits also account for their lack of SCR in emotionally charged situations. It is also consistent with the surprising finding that in cases in which VM patients can recover a normal SCR (albeit by a different route than normal), they also demonstrate a motivation to act in accord with their judgments. Thus artificial manipulation of the arousal system reinstates the commonly seen connection between moral judgment and motivation. Furthermore, this picture is consistent with recent findings from neuroimaging, documenting the involvement of systems known to be important in emotional responses during moral reasoning tasks.

Thus the differences in moral judgment between normal subjects and VM patients is seen to provide further evidence about *how* reason and emotion commonly interact in the issuance of moral judgment, and not as evidence for the claim that VM patients do not 'really' make moral judgments.

## Further implications

As I have argued, neuroscientific research has enabled us to evaluate from a different perspective a long-standing thesis in moral philosophy—that moral judgments are intrinsically motivating. It has provided strong evidence that substantive internalism is false. The research also suggests that moral motivation and moral knowledge are functionally separable and depend upon distinct brain systems. In addition, lesion and neuroimaging studies indicate that moral motivation is dependent upon limbic structures typically involved in emotion and reward learning. Both emotional and reward systems are topics of intensive neuroscientific research, and it behooves us to examine these fields to see to what extent the results there are applicable to questions about neuroethics. These insights provide us with a starting point for further empirical investigation in the neuroscience of ethics.

A thorough neuroethical treatment moves beyond the merely scientific to explore the ethical ramifications of scientific discovery. If indeed it is the case that substantive internalism is false, and that moral motivation and moral judgment can come apart, what are the neuroethical consequences? I will suggest here one area for which this study may have radical implications: moral education. Education in our society has a twofold purpose. Part of the reason we educate ourselves is to promote our future success. But we also view education as a way of improving ourselves as people, and as a way to make us better citizens (see also Chapter 18). Moral education is an important component in this process. Historically, moral education has usually proceeded in a relatively unstructured way. However, recently more emphasis has been placed on formal moral education. For instance, Harvard University now requires all undergraduates to complete a course in moral reasoning. Does our insight into the neural systems involved in moral behavior contribute anything to our pursuit of moral education? Possibly so. As I have argued, moral behavior requires both the declarative knowledge structures of morality and the proper linking of our motivational system to those cognitive structures. Recognition of moral obligation alone does not a moral person make. Thus, if we want a moral citizenry, it is probably insufficient merely to teach what is right and wrong. We need a two-pronged view of moral education: one that will satisfy the cognitive requirements of moral life by instilling moral knowledge, and one that will reinforce an internal drive to act in accord with the moral. This seems to be an aspect of moral education that has been absent in the formal curriculum; it is unknown to what extent it plays a role in informal moral education. Of course, the importance of such an approach will depend upon the type and degree of contingency between moral judgment and motivation, and this is still an open question.

Neuroscientific research into reward learning has shown that brain circuits involved in reward learning overlap extensively with those seen in moral cognition. Current research is aimed at discovering how external rewards become internally represented, and how internalization of reward is associated with learning and behavior. Perhaps with a deeper understanding of how internal systems of reward work, and how they are developed, we can come up with practical recommendations for how to structure more effective programs of moral education, whether formal or informal. If we can, we must also address difficult ethical issues that arise in this context: What sorts of learning paradigms are ethical? What sorts of brain manipulations can be countenanced with the goal of developing a more morally responsive citizenry? Such manipulation can clearly be used for good or ill. What is the difference between learning and indoctrination? What sorts of teaching and learning are compatible with the value we place in personal autonomy? Is deliberate shaping of our moral sensibility permissible? Is it obligatory?

It should be apparent that what we have learned about the neural basis of ethical reasoning also has implications for legal questions. Laws often codify consensus intuitions of moral rightness and wrongness. For example, in some states for a defendant to be convicted of a crime it must be shown that he knows the difference between right and wrong. However, if science reveals that moral behavior requires the proper operation of two neural systems, is the knowledge requirement, which only mentions one, sufficient? Is it even just? For example, should our laws be altered to take into account cases in which the motivational system malfunctions as well? These questions merely scratch the surface of the ethical implications of neuroscientific discovery.

## Summary

I have tried to illustrate in detail one line of research in the neuroscience of ethics, and to show how research in the neurosciences and ethics are interdependent. This project began in moral philosophy and the neuroscience of ethics, but it has implications for wider issues. By focusing upon what is currently known about moral judgment and behavior, I have tried to illustrate how brain research can affect our philosophical views, as well as to suggest how the results of such inquiries can raise challenging ethical questions. An empirical investigation in the neuroscience of ethics into the neural basis of moral action has led us to a position on a matter generally thought to belong to the purview of meta-ethics. It has suggested potential directions for further research, as well as raised the possibility that we could deliberately manipulate the neural pathways underlying moral behavior. These developments themselves raise further important questions regarding the ethical implications of neuroscience, about what sorts of interventions in people's cognitive lives can be justified and how.

Early in this chapter I noted that many have expressed skepticism about the claim that neuroethics is a coherent discipline. I hope that, by considering a particular case, the importance of the interaction between the neuroscience of ethics and the ethics of neuroscience has become more apparent, and that the possibility of dissociating them completely appears more remote. These interactions provide reason to think of neuroethics as a coherent, if not a unified, discipline, and one distinguishable from bioethics in general. The problem for the status of neuroethics, if there is one, is not a lack of coherence or unity; it is a lack of clear-cut boundaries. It is because of its wide-ranging implications that it is critical that all sorts of people, not just neuroscientists and philosophers, but also lawyers, medical professionals, policy-makers, educators, journalists, and the public, engage in the neuroethical debates that are sure to be a part of our future.

## Acknowledgments

This work was supported in part by an ARC fellowship from the RSSS, Australian National University, and in part by the McDonnell Project in Neurophilosophy.

## Notes

1. The view discussed here is relatively simple but is the basis for many more sophisticated versions of internalism in the literature. A version of internalism similar to the one considered here is the focus of discussions by Roskies (2003) and Svavarsdottir (1999), and appears in the writings of, for example, Frankena, Smith, Nagel, Miller, and Mele. Many of these philosophers ultimately argue for (or against) modifications of this strong internalist thesis. Roskies (2003) discusses the viability of some of these modifications, and suggests that many of these weaker versions of internalism suffer from philosophical deficiencies. The discussion also notes that some varieties of internalism, such as internalism about reasons, are not subject to the criticisms levied here.

## References

Casebeer WD, Churchland PS (2003). The neural mechanisms of moral cognition: a multiple-aspect approach to moral judgment and decision-making. *Biology and Philosophy* 18, 169–94.

Changeux JP, Ricoeur P (2002). *What Makes Us Think? A Neuroscientist and a Philosopher Argue about Ethics, Human Nature, and the Brain.* Princeton, NJ: Princeton University Press.

Damasio AR (1995). *Descartes' Error: Emotion, Reason and the Human Brain.* New York: Avon Books.

Damasio AR, Tranel D, Damasio H (1990). Individuals with sociopathic behavior caused by frontal damage fail to respond autonomically to social stimuli. *Behavioral Brain Research* 41, 81–94.

Damasio H, Grabowski T, Frank R, Galaburda AM, Damasio AR (1994). The return of Phineas Gage: clues about the brain from the skull of a famous patient. *Science* 264, 1102–5.

Fischer JM, Ravizza M (eds) (1992). *Ethics: Problems and Principles.* Fort Worth, TX: Harcourt Brace Jovanovich.

Greene J, Haidt J (2002). How (and where) does moral judgment work? *Trends in Cognitive Sciences* 6, 517–23.

Greene JD, Sommerville RB, Nystrom LE, Darley JM, Cohen, JD (2001). An fMRI investigation of emotional engagement in moral judgment. *Science* 293, 2105–8.

Greene JD, Nystrom LE, Engell AD, Darley JM, Cohen JD (2004). The neural bases of cognitive conflict and control in moral judgment. *Neuron* 44, 389–400.

Moll J, de Oliveriera-Souza R, Eslinger PJ, *et al.* (2002). The neural correlates of moral sensitivity: a functional magnetic resonance imaging investigation of basic and moral emotions. *Journal of Neuroscience* 22, 2730–6.

Nichols S (2002). Norms with feeling: towards a psychological account of moral judgment. *Cognition* 84, 221–36.

Roskies A (2002). Neuroethics for the new millenium. *Neuron* 35, 21–3.

Roskies A (2003). Are ethical judgments intrinsically motivational? Lessons from 'acquired sociopathy'. *Philosophical Psychology* 16, 51–66.

Saver JL, Damasio AR (1991). Preserved access and processing of social knowledge in a patient with acquired sociopathy due to ventromedial frontal damage. *Neuropsychologia* 29, 1241–9.

Svavarsdottir S (1999). Moral cognitivism and motivation. *Philosophical Review* 108, 161–219.

Chapter 3

# Moral and legal responsibility and the new neuroscience

Stephen J. Morse

## Introduction

Let us begin with an exemplary case. How should we decide if adolescents who commit capital murder when they are 16 or 17 years old are sufficiently culpable to deserve the death penalty? The Supreme Court of the United States approved the death penalty in such cases in 1989 in *Stanford* v. *Kentucky*, but during the October 2004 term the Court will reconsider and decide this question in *Roper* v. *Simmons*. What kinds of arguments will be good arguments to help the Court make this weighty decision?

In *Thompson* v. *Oklahoma* (1988), the Supreme Court barred capital punishment of murderers who killed when they were 15 years old or younger, and in *Atkins* v. *Virginia* (2002), the High Court categorically prohibited capital punishment of convicted killers with mental retardation. Although the Court provided many reasons for its *Thompson* and *Atkins* holdings, crucial to both was the conclusion that younger adolescents and persons with retardation are categorically less culpable and less responsible, and therefore do not deserve capital punishment. The operative language in *Atkins* concerning culpability and responsibility is instructive. The Court wrote:

> Mentally retarded persons frequently know the difference between right and wrong ... Because of their impairments, however, by definition they have diminished capacities to understand and process information, to communicate, to engage in logical reasoning, to control impulses, and to understand the reactions of others ... Their deficiencies do not warrant an exemption from criminal sanctions, but they do diminish their personal culpability ... With respect to retribution—the interest in seeing that the offender gets his 'just deserts'– the severity of the appropriate punishment necessarily depends on the culpability of the offender. (*Atkins* v. *Virginia* 2002)

All the criteria that the Court mentions are behavioral (broadly understood to refer to cognitive and control functioning). Advocates of abolition in *Roper* have seized on this language to make similar arguments concerning 16- and 17-year-old killers. Although apparently normal adolescents do not suffer from abnormal impairments, lack of full developmental maturation allegedly distinguishes them from adults on behavioral dimensions, such as the capacity for judgment, that are relevant to responsibility.

What is striking and novel about the argument in *Roper*, however, is that advocates of abolition are using newly discovered neuroscientific evidence concerning the adolescent brain to bolster their argument that 16- and 17-year-old killers do not deserve to die. The *New York Times* editorial page encouraged the High Court to consider the neuroscientific evidence to help it reach its decision (*New York Times* 2004). Although neuroscience evidence had been adduced in earlier high-profile cases, such as the 1982 prosecution of John Hinckley Jr for the attempted assassination of President Reagan and others, *Roper* is the most important case in which the new neuroscience has been used to affect responsibility questions. Indeed, the American Medical Association, the American Bar Association, the American Psychiatric Association, and the American Psychological Association, among others, have all filed *amicus* ('friend of the court') briefs in *Roper* urging abolition based in part on the neuroscience findings. Although some deny the validity of this evidence, let us assume that it is valid. The potentially legitimating use of neuroscience in *Roper* is likely to be the beginning of a movement to use such evidence generally when considering responsibility. The question is whether the new neuroscience is relevant to responsibility ascriptions and just punishment, even if it is valid.

This chapter contends that neuroscience is largely irrelevant if the concept of responsibility is properly understood and evaluated. It begins with a positive description of the dominant conception of personhood and responsibility in Western law and morality. Then it considers and rejects the challenge to this conception that any materialist scientific understanding of behavior, including neuroscientific explanation, creates. It next argues that unless brain science evolves to such a stage that it radically undermines current conceptions of personhood, the brain will largely be irrelevant to ascriptions of moral and legal responsibility. The chapter concludes by returning to *Roper* and suggesting the proper way that the case should be argued.

## Personhood and responsibility in morals and law

This section provides a description and analysis of the dominant model of personhood and responsibility in Anglo-American positive morality and law, i.e. the morality and law that seem to exist in practice today. This section tries to give the best account of morality and law as we find it. Of course, no universal theory of morality or jurisprudence is consensually accepted, but virtually all current conceptions share certain features that this section will try to describe. The next section addresses fundamental challenges to the coherence and desirability of existing morality and law.

### The nature of morality and law

Morality and law are socially constructed or invented, intensely practical, and evaluative systems of rules and institutions that guide and govern human action, that help us live together. Although both create and identify value, their primary purpose is guidance. Although questions such as the source of morality or whether there are necessary and sufficient conditions for something to be a law and what gives law its authority are intensely controversial, virtually all commentators would agree with the foregoing emphasis on guidance. For example, law gives people good reason to behave one way or another by making the consequences of non-compliance clear or through people's understanding of the reasons that support a particular rule. In what follows, for ease of exposition I shall focus on legal conceptions of personhood and responsibility, but most of the analysis will apply equally to morality. As an action-guiding system of rules, law shares many characteristics with other sources of guidance, such as morality and custom, but law is distinguishable because its rules and institutions are created and enforced by the state.

### The concept of the person and action

The law's concept of the person flows from the nature of law itself and may be usefully contrasted with a more mechanistic view of the person. To introduce the issues, allow me to describe a demonstration with which I often begin a presentation to neuroscientists and psychologists. I ask the audience to assist me with a demonstration that is loosely based on Wittgenstein's famous question: 'What is left over if I subtract the fact that my arm goes up from the fact that I raise my arm?'(Wittgenstein 1958). I vary the instructions somewhat, but the usual request is to ask people who have brown hair and who wear eyeglasses to raise their non-dominant arm. Although I have never rigorously observed and calculated the rate of cooperation, watching my audiences closely suggests that I receive total cooperation. No one who believes that he has brown hair (the instructions clarify that the current color is brown) and wears eyeglasses (the instructions clarify that anyone who wears eyeglasses at any time is included) and is able to identify his non-dominant arm (I assume that everyone in a professional audience can perform this task) fails to raise that arm. I then tell the participants that they may lower their arms and I politely thank them for their cooperation. Next I ask participants to explain what caused their arms to rise. I usually then paraphrase this question as: 'Why did you raise your arms?' How should one answer such a question?

Bodily movements that appear to be the results of intentions, i.e. actions, unlike other phenomena, can be explained by physical causes and by reasons for action. This is also true of intentionally produced mental states or feelings, although we do not tend to term the production of such states actions. Although physical causes explain the structure and mechanisms of the brain and nervous system and all the other moving parts of the physical universe, only human action and other intentionally produced states can also be explained by reasons. Therefore when one asks about human action, 'Why did he do that?', two distinct types of answers may be given. The reason-giving explanation accounts for human behavior as a product of intentions that arise from the desires and beliefs of the agent. The second type of explanation treats human behavior as simply one more part of the phenomena of the universe, subject to the same natural physical laws that explain all phenomena.

Only human action, the intentional bodily movements of persons, is explained by reasons resulting from desires and beliefs, rather than simply by mechanistic causes. I recognize that there is no uncontroversial definition of action in any of the relevant literatures (Audi 1993). Nonetheless, the account I am giving is most consistent with the law's view of the person, action, and responsibility, as is explained below. Only human beings are fully intentional creatures. To comprehend fully why an agent has particular desires, beliefs and reasons requires biophysical, psychological, and sociological explanations, but to ask why a person acted in a certain way is to ask for reasons for action, not for reductionist and mechanistic biophysical, psychological, or sociological explanations. I assume, controversially, that mental states are not identical to brain states even though the former depend on the latter (Searle 2004). In the argot of philosophy of mind, I am assuming that material reductionism is not the best explanation of the relation between mental states and brain states. In any case, my assumption is consistent with the law's view of the person. Only persons can deliberate about what action to perform and can determine their conduct by practical reason.

Suppose, for example, that we wish to explain why the participants in the demonstration described above raised their non-dominant arms. The reason-giving explanation might be that they desired the presentation to go well and believed that if they cooperated, they would increase the probability that this would happen. Therefore they formed the intention to raise their non-dominant arms and executed that intention. This type of causal explanation, which philosophers and some psychologists refer to as 'folk psychology', is clearly the dominant type of explanation we all use every day to understand ourselves, other people, and our interactions with others in the world.

The mechanistic type of explanation would approach these questions quite differently. For example, those who believe that mind can ultimately be reduced to the biophysical workings of the brain and nervous system or that mental states have no ontological status whatsoever would believe that the participants' arm-raisings are *solely* the law-governed product of biophysical causes. Therefore desires, beliefs, intentions, and choices, if they exist at all, are simply correlational or epiphenomenal, rather than genuine causes of behavior. According to this mode of explanation, human behavior is indistinguishable from any other phenomenon in the universe, including the movements of molecules and bacteria. In short, there is nothing really special about people; we are just a piece of particularly complicated biophysical flotsam and jetsam. It is always rather amusing and disconcerting to observe neuroscientists struggle to explain arm-raising in the language of mechanisms, as they sometimes do, especially if I push them, because they so clearly do not have a real clue about how it happens. I am not implying the unduly skeptical claim that we have no neurological and musculoskeletal understanding of the necessary conditions for bodily movements. It is simply true, however, that, despite the extraordinary progress in neuroscience, how human action occurs—the so-called mind–body problem—remains fundamentally mysterious.

The social and behavioral sciences, including psychology and psychiatry, are uncomfortably wedged between the reason-giving and mechanistic accounts of human behavior. Sometimes they treat behavior 'objectively' as primarily mechanistic or physical; at other times, social science treats behavior 'subjectively' as a text to be interpreted. At yet other times, social science engages in an uneasy amalgam of the two. What is always clear, however, is that the domain of the social sciences is human action and not simply the movements of bodies in space or the mechanisms of the brain and nervous system. One can attempt to assimilate folk psychology's reason-giving to mechanistic explanation by claiming that desires, beliefs, and intentions are genuine causes and not simply rationalizations of behavior. Indeed, folk psychology proceeds on the assumption that reasons for action are genuinely causal. But the assimilationist position is philosophically controversial, a controversy that will not be solved until the mind–body problem is solved.

At present, however, we have no idea how the brain enables the mind, but when we solve this problem, if we ever do, the solution will revolutionize our understanding of biological processes (McHugh and Slavney 1998). On the other hand, some philosophers deny that human beings have the resources ever to solve the mind–body problem and to explain consciousness, which is perhaps the greatest mystery (McGinn 1999). Assuming that these problems can be unraveled, our view of ourselves and all our moral and political arrangements are likely to be as profoundly altered as our understanding of biological processes. For now, however, despite the impressive gains in neuroscience and related disciplines, we still do not know mechanistically how action happens even if we are convinced, as I am, that a physicalist account of some sort must be correct.

Law, unlike mechanistic explanation or the conflicted stance of the social sciences, views human action as governed by reason and treats people as potentially rational intentional agents, not simply as biophysical mechanisms in a thoroughly causal universe. It could not be otherwise because law is concerned with human action. It makes no sense to ask a bull that gores a matador, 'Why did you do that?', but this question makes sense and is vitally important when it is addressed to a person who sticks a knife into the chest of another human being. It makes a great difference to us if the knife-wielder is a surgeon who is cutting with the patient's consent or a person who is enraged with the victim and intends to kill him.

Law is a system of rules that at the least is meant to guide or influence behavior and thus to operate as a potential cause of behavior. According to Searle (2002, p. 35):

> Once we have the possibility of explaining particular forms of human behavior as following rules, we have a very rich explanatory apparatus that differs dramatically from the explanatory apparatus of the natural sciences. When we say we are following rules, we are accepting the notion of mental causation and the attendant notions of rationality and existence of norms ... The content of the rule does not just describe what is happening, but plays a part in *making it happen.*

But legal and moral rules are not simply mechanistic causes that produce 'reflex' compliance. They operate within the domain of practical reason. People are meant to and can only use these rules as potential reasons for action as they deliberate about what they should do. Thus moral and legal rules are action guiding primarily because they provide an agent with good moral or prudential reasons for forbearance or action. Unless people were capable of understanding and then using legal rules as premises in deliberation, law would be powerless to affect human behavior (Shapiro 2000). People use legal rules as premises in the practical syllogisms that guide much human action. No 'instinct' governs how fast a person drives on the open highway, but among the various explanatory variables, the posted speed limit and the belief in the probability of paying the consequences for exceeding it surely play a large role in the driver's choice of speed. I am not suggesting that human behavior cannot be modified by means other than influencing deliberation or that human beings always deliberate before they act. Of course it can and of course they do not. But law operates through practical reason, even when we most habitually follow the legal rules. Law can directly and indirectly affect the world we inhabit only by its influence on practical reason.

For the law, then, a person is a practical reasoner. The legal view of the person is not that all people always reason and behave consistently rationally according to some pre-ordained normative notion of rationality. It is simply that people are creatures who are capable of acting for and consistently with their reasons for action and who are generally capable of minimal rationality according to mostly conventional, socially constructed standards of rationality.

There is a perfectly plausible evolutionary story about why human beings need rules such as those that law provides. We have evolved to be self-conscious creatures who act for reasons. Practical reason is inescapable for creatures like ourselves who inevitably care about the ends we pursue and about what reason we have to act in one way rather than another (Bok 1998). Because we are social creatures whose interactions are not governed primarily by innate repertoires, it is inevitable that rules will be necessary to help order our interactions in any minimally complex social group (Alexander and Sherwin 2001). Human beings have developed extraordinarily diverse ways of living together, but a ubiquitous feature of all societies is that they are governed by rules addressed to beings capable of following those rules. The most basic view of human nature is that we are rational creatures. As I shall discuss below, the new neuroscience does not yet pose a threat to this fundamental conception and all that follows from it, including the concept of responsibility, to which this chapter now turns.

## The concept of responsibility

The law's concept of responsibility follows logically from its conception of the person and the nature of law itself. Law can only guide action if human beings are rational creatures who can understand and conform to legal requirements through intentional action. Therefore legally responsible or legally competent agents are people who have the general capacity to grasp and be guided by good reason in particular legal contexts, who are generally capable of properly using the rules as premises in practical reasoning (Wallace 1994). As I shall discuss below, responsibility, properly understood, has nothing to do with what most people understand by 'free will'. The capacity for rationality is the touchstone of responsibility. What rationality demands will of course differ across contexts. The requirements for competence to contract and for criminal responsibility are not identical. The usual legal presumptions are that adults are capable of minimal rationality and responsibility and that the same rules may be applied to all.

The law's requirement for responsibility—a general capacity for rationality—is not self-defining. It must be understood according to some contingent normative notion both of rationality and of how much capability is required. For example, legal responsibility might require the capability of understanding the reason for an applicable rule, as well as the rule's narrow behavior command. These are matters of moral, political, and ultimately legal judgment, about which reasonable people can and do differ. There is no uncontroversial definition of rationality or of what kind and how much is required for responsibility in various legal contexts. These are normative issues, and, whatever the outcome might be within a polity and its legal system, the debate is about human action—intentional behavior that is potentially rationalized and guidable by reasons.

## The criteria for responsibility

Virtually all legal responsibility and competence criteria depend on assessment of the agent's rational capacities in the context in question. For example, a person is competent to contract if he is capable of understanding the nature of the bargain; a person is criminally responsible if the agent was capable of knowing the nature of his conduct or the applicable law. To continue the example, some people who commit crimes under the influence of mental disorder are excused from responsibility because their rationality was compromised, not because mental disorder played a causal role in explaining the conduct. The rationality criterion for responsibility is perfectly consistent with the facts—most adults are capable of minimal rationality virtually all the time—and with moral theories concerning fairness and justice that we have good reason to accept.

Coercion or compulsion criteria for non-responsibility also exist in civil and criminal law, although they much less frequently provide an excusing condition. Properly understood, coercion obtains when the agent is placed through no fault of his own in a threatening 'hard choice' situation from which he cannot readily escape and in which he yields to the threat. The classic example in criminal law is the excuse of duress, which requires that the criminal must be threatened with death or serious bodily harm unless he commits the crime and that a person of 'reasonable firmness' would have yielded to the threat. The agent has surely acted intentionally and rationally. His completely understandable desire to avoid death or grievous bodily harm fully explains why he formed and executed the intention to commit the crime. The reason we excuse the coerced agent is not that determinism or causation is at work, for it always is. The genuine moral and legal justification is that requiring human beings not to yield to some threats is simply too much to ask of creatures like ourselves. Now, how hard the choice has to be is a moral normative question that can vary across contexts. A compulsion excuse for crime might require a greater threat than a compulsion excuse for a contract. As the section on neuroscience, personhood and responsibility explains, however, in no case does compulsion have anything to do with the presence or absence of causation *per se*, contra-causal freedom, or free will.

A persistent vexed question is how to assess the responsibility of people who seem to be acting in response to some inner compulsion, or, in more ordinary language, seem to have trouble controlling themselves. Examples from psychopathology include impulse control disorders, addictions, and paraphilias (disorders of sexual desire). If people really have immense difficulty in refraining from acting in certain ways through no fault of their own, this surely provides an appealing justification for mitigation or excuse. But what does it mean to say that an agent who is acting cannot control himself? I have explored this question at length elsewhere (Morse 1994, 2002), and so I shall be brief and conclusory here. People who act in response to such inner states as craving are intentional agents. A drug addict who seeks and uses drugs to satisfy his craving does so intentionally. Simply because an abnormal biological cause played a causal role, and neuroscientific evidence frequently confirms this (Goldstein and Volkow 2002; Potenza *et al.* 2003), does not *per se* mean the person could not control himself or had great difficulty in doing so. Nor does the presence of an abnormal causal variable mean that the person was acting under compulsion.

One can draw an analogy between one-party cases and cases of duress, treating the agent's intense arousal and desire as if it were a gun to the head. This is a misleading metaphor, however, and I believe that cases in which we want to say that a person cannot control himself and should be excused for that reason can be better explained on the basis of a rationality defect. In short, at certain times or under certain circumstances, states of desire or the like make it supremely difficult for the agent to access reason. In either case, however, lack of control can only be finally demonstrated behaviorally, by evaluating action. Neither causation nor free will is the issue or provides the criteria for mitigation or excuse. Although neuroscientific evidence may surely provide assistance in performing this evaluation, neuroscience could never tell us how much control ability is required for responsibility. That question is normative, moral, and ultimately legal.

To explore the ramifications of the foregoing analysis for the new neuroscience, let us consider the example of brain abnormalities and violent or aggressive conduct. Accumulating evidence from increasingly sophisticated diagnostic techniques, such as functional and structural imaging, demonstrates that various abnormalities predispose people to engage in violent conduct (Cummings and Mega 2003). Such information may have both predictive and therapeutic implications, although mandatory screening and any form of involuntary intervention, no matter how benignly motivated, would raise serious civil liberties issues. It might also have the effects of deflecting attention from other, equally powerful and perhaps remediable, social causes and of treating the problem as solely within the individual rather than as the product of an interaction between the individual and his environment. In the remainder of the discussion, however, I shall focus solely on the relevance of such information to individual responsibility.

The easiest case arises when the abnormality causes a state of severely altered consciousness. Criminal responsibility requires action and rationality, and in such instances the law holds either that the person did not act because the definition of action requires reasonably intact consciousness or that the action was not rational because rationality requires the potential for self-reflection that altered consciousness undermines. Note that the presence of altered consciousness must be evaluated behaviorally, although biology will surely play a causally explanatory role (Vaitl *et al.* 2005). Indeed, the law concerning the relevance of consciousness to responsibility was developed and the law was able to evaluate such claims before any of the modern neuroscientific investigative techniques were invented. If the agent was clearly fully conscious, no legal problem arises, whatever the neuroscience may purport to show. If the agent was acting in a state of impaired consciousness, some claim for mitigation or excuse is possible despite the absence of neuroscientific findings. However, neuroscientific evidence might well be relevant in such cases to assess the validity of the defendant's claim about his mental state. Thus neuroscience teaches us nothing new morally or legally about these cases, but it may help us adjudicate them more accurately.

The more problematic cases are those in which the defendant's consciousness was intact and he clearly acted, but an abnormality was present that may have played a causal role in the criminal conduct. As sophisticated people understand, abnormalities do not cause violent conduct directly and they are not excusing conditions *per se* simply because they played a causal role. Instead, they produce behavioral states or traits, such as rage, impulsiveness, or disinhibition generally, that predispose the agent to commit violent acts and that may be relevant to the agent's responsibility. After all, such states and traits can compromise rationality, making it more difficult for the agent to play by the rules. For example, younger children and people with developmental disability are not held fully responsible because it is recognized that their capacity for rationality is not fully developed. Again, it is a rationality consideration, and not lack of free will, that is doing the work in these cases. Note, too, that if the capacity for rationality is compromised by non-biological causes, such as child-rearing practices, the same analysis holds. There is nothing special about biological causation (Richards 2000). Once again, the law was cognizant of the relevance of diminished rationality to responsibility and developed its doctrines of mitigation and excuse long before modern neuroscience emerged. Neuroscience will surely discover much more about the types of conditions that can compromise rationality, and thus may potentially lead to a broadening of current legal excusing and mitigating doctrines or to a widening of the class of people who can raise a colorable claim under current law. Further, neuroscience may help to adjudicate excusing and mitigating claims more accurately.

We must remember, however, that it is unlikely that there will ever be a precise correlation between any neuroscientific finding and a legal criterion (except in extreme cases in which neuroscience will not be necessary to aid legal decision-making). For example, much as there is no gene for violation of any section of the penal code, there will be no single brain finding or set of findings that demonstrate that a defendant did not form the intent to perform a prohibited action or lacked sufficient capacity for rationality to be found legally insane. As honest brain scientists know and admit, the relation between the brain and complex but discrete intentional conduct is mostly mysterious. Neuroscience will not be very precisely helpful even in those cases in which it is relevant. We will need to be very cautious (Cacioppo *et al.* 2003).

In principle, no amount of increased causal understanding of behavior, from any form of science, threatens the law's notion of responsibility unless it shows definitively that we humans (or some subset of us) are not intentional, minimally rational creatures, and no information about biological or social causes shows this directly. It will have to be demonstrated behaviorally. Even if a person has undoubted brain abnormalities or has suffered various forms of severe environmental deprivation, if he behaves minimally rationally, he will be responsible. Indeed, some abnormalities may make people 'hyper-responsible'. Consider, for example, a businessperson with hypomania who is especially energetic and sharp in some stages of his illness. Such a person is undoubtedly competent to contract in this state, even though the abnormality is playing a causal role in his behavior. It is of course true that many people continue mistakenly to believe that causation, especially abnormal causation, is *per se* an excusing condition, but this is quite simply an analytic error that I have called 'the fundamental psycholegal error' and will discuss below. It leads people to try to create a new excuse every time an allegedly valid new 'syndrome' is discovered that is thought to play a role in behavior. But syndromes and other causes do not have excusing force unless they sufficiently diminish rationality in the context in question. In that case, it is diminished rationality that is the excusing condition, not the presence of any particular type of cause.

Now that we have addressed the concepts of personhood, action, and responsibility and its criteria in law and morality, let us turn to more general external challenges to personhood and responsibility that neuroscience and other materialistic explanatory variables present.

## The neuroscience challenge to personhood and responsibility

Neuroscience and other materialistic disciplines (see also Chapter 5) that adhere to the notion that the phenomena of the universe can be explained in terms of matter and laws that affect matter pose two potential challenges. First, they might demonstrate that, contra our inflated view of ourselves, people are not conscious, intentional, and potentially rational agents. That is, the alleged criteria for personhood cannot be satisfied by people as they are; in turn, because personhood is necessary for responsibility, responsibility is impossible. Secondly, even if we descriptively are in fact conscious, intentional, and potentially rational agents, the concept of responsibility is nonetheless unsupportable, even for creatures such as ourselves or any others. This is the challenge from determinism or universal causation. In this section, I address these two challenges in order.

### The challenge to personhood

The seriousness of neuroscience's potential challenge to the traditional legal concepts of personhood and responsibility is best summed up in the title of an eminent psychologist's recent book, *The Illusion of Conscious Will* (Wegner 2002). In brief, the thesis is that we delude ourselves when we think that our intentions are genuinely causal. In fact, we are just mechanisms, although the illusion of conscious will may play a positive role in our lives (see also Chapter 1). Wegner's evidence and arguments are not all based on neuroscientific findings, but the claim that we are purely mechanisms is often thought to follow from all physicalist, naturalist, and scientific views of the person. If this is right, our conception of human nature must change and the foundations of law and morality appear insupportable. This ominous prospect is not imminent, however. Advances in neuroscience and related fields have revealed hitherto unimagined biological causes that predispose people to behave as they do (Caspi *et al.* 2002; Goldstein and Volkow 2002; Potenza *et al.* 2003; Stein *et al.* 2002), but the science typically supporting claims that conscious will is an illusion—that we do not act and therefore cannot be responsible—is either insufficient empirically to support such a claim or does not have the implications supposed.

The philosophy of mind and action has long contained arguments for various forms of material reductionism and for eliminative materialism (Churchland 1988). Reductive accounts hold, simply, that mental states are as they seem to us, but that they are identical to brain states. Eliminative accounts hold that our beliefs about our mental states are radically false and, consequently, that no match-up between brain states and mental states is possible. Both types of views are conceptual and existed long before the exciting recent discoveries in neuroscience and psychology that have so deepened our understanding of how the brain and nervous system are constructed and work. Needless to say, both are extremely controversial. Most philosophers of mind believe that complete reduction of mind to biophysical explanation is impossible (G. Strawson 1989; Searle 1992, 2004). Again, until the conceptual revolution that allows us to solve the mind–body problem occurs, science cannot resolve the debate, although it can furnish support for conceptual arguments. At present and for the foreseeable future, we have no convincing conceptual reason from the philosophy of mind, even when it is completely informed about the most recent neuroscience, to abandon our view of ourselves as creatures with causally efficacious mental states.

Even if we cannot solve the mind–body problem, and thus determine if reductive accounts are true, it is possible, however, that we might make empirical discoveries indicating that some parts of our ordinary understanding about action and agency are incorrect. Much recent argument based on current neuroscience and psychology takes this position, arguing that mental causation does not exist as we think it does. For ease of exposition, let us call this the 'no action thesis' (NAT). However, the logic of these arguments is often shaky. Discovering a brain correlate or cause of an action does not mean that it is not an action. If actions exist, they have causes, including those arising in the brain.

The real question is whether scientific empirical studies have shown that action is rare or non-existent, that conscious will is an illusion after all. Two kinds of evidence are often adduced. First, demonstrations that a very large part of our activity is undeniably caused by variables that we are not in the slightest aware of, and, second, studies indicating that more activity than we think takes place when our consciousness is divided or diminished. Neither kind of evidence offers logical support to NAT, however. Just because a person may not be aware of all the causes of why he formed an intention does not entail that he did not form an intention and was not a fully conscious agent when he did so. Even if human beings were never aware of the causes of their intentions to act and actions, it still would not mean that they were not acting consciously, intentionally and for reasons that make eminent sense to anyone under the circumstances.

Human consciousness can undeniably be divided or diminished by a wide variety of normal and abnormal causes (Cummings and Mega 2003; Vaitl *et al.* 2005). We have known this long before contemporary scientific discoveries of what causes such states and how they correlate with brain structure and processes. Law and morality agree that if an agent's capacity for consciousness is non-culpably diminished, responsibility is likewise diminished. Some believe that it is diminished because bodily movements in the absence of fully integrated consciousness are not actions (American Law Institute [sec. 2.01] 1962; Moore 1993,1994). Others believe that apparently goal-directed behavior that is responsive to the environment, such as sleep-walking, is action, but that it should be excused because diminished consciousness reduces the capacity for rationality (Morse 1994; Williams 1994). Let us assume that the former view is correct, however, because it offers more direct moral and legal support to NAT. Let us also assume that studies have demonstrated that divided or diminished consciousness is more common than we think. To demonstrate that divided or partial consciousness is more common than it appears certainly extends the range of cases in which people are not responsible or have diminished responsibility, but such studies do not demonstrate that most human bodily movements that appear intentional and rational, that appear to be rational actions, occur when the person has altered consciousness. One cannot generalize from deviant cases or cases in which a known abnormality is present.

What is needed to support NAT is thus a general demonstration that causal intentionality is an illusion *tout court*, but I believe that no such general demonstration has yet been produced by scientific study. The most interesting evidence has arisen from studies done by Benjamin Libet (1999), which have generated an immense amount of comment (Wegner 2002). In extreme brief, Libet's exceptionally creative and careful studies demonstrate that measurable electrical brain activity associated with intentional actions occurs about 550 msec before the subject actually acts and for about 350–400 msec before the subject is consciously aware of the intention to act (see also Gazzaniga, this volume). Let us assume, with cautious reservations (Walter 2001; Zhu 2003), the validity of the studies. Even if they are valid, it does not follow that conscious intentionality does no causal work. They simply demonstrate that non-conscious brain events precede conscious experience, but this seems precisely what one would expect of the mind-brain. It does not mean that intentionality played no causal role and Libet concedes that people can 'veto' the act, which is another form of mental act that plays a causal role. Libet's work is fascinating, but it does not prove that persons are not conscious, intentional agents (see also Crane 2005).

NAT provides no guidance about what we should do next and is potentially incoherent. Let us suppose that you were convinced by the mechanistic view of persons that you were not an intentional, rational agent after all. (Of course, the notion of being convinced would be an illusion, too. Being convinced means that you were persuaded by evidence or argument, but a mechanism is not persuaded by anything. It is simply neurophysically transformed or some such). What should you do now? You know that it's an illusion to think that your deliberation and intention has any causal efficacy in the world. (Again, what does it mean according to the purely mechanistic view to know something? Persons know things; brains don't know any-thing. But enough.) You also know, however, that you experience sensations such as pleasure and pain and that you care about what happens to you and to the world. You cannot just sit quietly and wait for your neurotransmitters to fire. You will of course deliberate and act. Even if pure mechanism is true–about which, once again, we will never be certain until we solve the mind–body problem–human beings will find it almost impossible not to treat themselves as rational, intentional agents unless there are major changes in the way our brain works. Moreover, if you use the truth of pure mechanism as a premise in deciding what to do, this premise will entail no particular moral, legal or political conclusions. It will provide no guide to how one should live, including how one should respond to the truth of NAT.

Finally, the argument from common sense in favor of the justified belief that we are conscious, intentional creatures is overwhelming. Consider again, for example, the nature of law itself. As we have seen, law is a system of rules that at the least is meant to guide or influence behavior and thus to operate as a potential cause of behavior. In brief, it would be impossible at present for us to abandon the well-justified belief that action may be influenced by reason and that our intentions are causally efficacious. As Fodor (1987, p. xii) writes,

> ... if commonsense intentional psychology were really to collapse, that would be, beyond compari-son, the greatest intellectual catastrophe in the history of our species; if we're that wrong about the mind, then that's the wrongest we've ever been about anything. The collapse of the supernatural, for example, doesn't compare ... Nothing except, perhaps, our commonsense physics ... comes as near our cognitive core as intentional explanation does. We'll be in deep, deep trouble if we have to give it up ... But be of good cheer; everything is going to be all right.

Is it really an illusion for Professor Wegner to believe that he deserves the credit (and royalties) for *The Illusion of Conscious Will* because, really, it was his brain that wrote the book and brains don't deserve credit and royalties?

The new neuroscience does not yet pose a threat to our fundamental conception of personhood and all that follows from it, including the concept of responsibility and related concepts, such as *mens rea* [the mental states, such as intention or knowledge, that are part of the definitional criteria for most crimes]. At the very least, we remain entitled to presume that conscious intentions are potentially rational and causal and to place the burden of persuasion at a very high level on proponents of NAT. At present, the case is not close to meeting the burden. We are fully entitled to continue to believe that we are the sorts of creatures we believe ourselves to be.

In conclusion, it is reasonable to assume that the task of neuroscience is not to reduce mind entirely to matter or to explain away conscious intentionality. Rather, the task of a robust neuroscience will be to explain how human consciousness, intentionality and rationality are enabled by the brain.

## The challenge of determinism

For reasons similar to those just adduced, the new neuroscience casts little doubt on responsibility generally. People often think that the discovery of causes of behavior over which people have no control suggests that determinism or universal causation is true, at least for caused behavior, and undermines free will, which in turn is thought to be a precondition for responsibility and other worthy goods such as human dignity. This thought is what terrifies people about scientific understanding of human behavior, which relentlessly exposes the numerous causal variables that seem to toss us about like small boats in a raging sea storm. They are afraid that science will demonstrate that we are nothing but mechanisms. To see why this view is mistaken, however, and why the new neuroscience does not threaten responsibility generally requires a brief general discussion about the concept of free will.

Before discussing the threat to responsibility generally, it is first important to understand that neuroscientific or other biological causes pose no more challenge to responsibility than non-biological or social causes. As a conceptual matter, we do not necessarily have more control over social causal variables than over biological causal variables. In a world of universal causation or determinism, causal mechanisms are indistinguishable and biological causation creates no necessarily greater threat to our life hopes than social causation (Richards 2000). For purposes of the free will debate, a cause is just a cause, whether it is biological, psychological, sociological, or astrological.

There is no uncontroversial definition of determinism and we will never be able to confirm that it is true or not. As a working definition, however, let us assume, roughly, that all events have causes that operate according to the physical laws of the universe and that were themselves caused by those same laws operating on prior states of the universe in a continuous thread of causation going back to the first state. Even if this is too strong, the universe seems sufficiently regular and lawful that it seems we must adopt the hypothesis that universal causation is approximately correct (G. Strawson 1989) which Strawson terms the 'realism constraint'. If this is true, the people we are and the actions we perform have been caused by a chain of causation over which we had no control and for which we could not possibly be responsible. How would responsibility be possible for action or anything else in such a universe?

No analysis of this problem could conceivably persuade everyone. There are no decisive analytically incontrovertible arguments to resolve the metaphysical question of the relation between determinism and responsibility. And the question is metaphysical, not scientific. Indeed, the debate is so fraught that even theorists who adopt the same general approach to the metaphysical challenge substantially disagree. Nevertheless, the view one adopts has profound consequences for moral and legal theory and practice. After describing the debate in extremely brief and conclusory terms, I shall turn to why ordinary responsibility is eminently plausible even in a thoroughly material causal universe.

## The metaphysics of free will versus determinism

The first standard answer to the claim that the universe is deterministic, incompatibilism, comes in two forms, hard determinism and metaphysical libertarianism, both of which hold that determinism is inconsistent with responsibility. The former admits that mechanism is true—that human beings, like the rest of the universe, are entirely subject to and produced by the physical states and laws of the universe—and therefore claims that no one is responsible for anything. The latter denies that mechanism is a true explanation of human action, and therefore responsibility is possible. The second standard answer, compatibilism, also embraces mechanism, but claims that responsibility is nonetheless possible. Some philosophers, such as Dennett (2003), believe that the debate should be abandoned and that responsibility can be justified without taking a position. I believe, however, that although the debate is unresolvable, considering responsibility requires taking a position and that writers such as Dennett have not avoided the debate. I argue that only compatibilism can explain and justify our moral and legal responsibility doctrines and practices, including the uniqueness of human action, and that it insulates responsibility from the challenges that scientific understanding seems to pose.

Hard determinists and libertarians agree that real or ultimate responsibility is possible only if human beings have contra-causal freedom, i.e. the freedom to originate action uncaused by prior events and influences. This is what is typically meant by free will. Otherwise, both agree, human beings have no real freedom, even if reasons are undeniably part of the causal chain that leads to action. Contra-causal freedom also appears to be the type of freedom that most ordinary people intuit or perceive that they in fact possess and that makes them responsible. Of course, incompatibilists disagree about whether we have contra-causal freedom. Hard determinists believe that determinism or mechanism is true, that we lack contra-causal power, that acting for reasons is ultimately as mechanistic as other causes, and therefore that we are not responsible. Metaphysical libertarians believe that human beings are unique because we do have contra-causal power—at least normal adults do—and that acting for reasons originates uncaused new causal chains. This god-like power of agent origination is the libertarian foundation of responsibility for action.

Hard determinism generates an external, rather than an internal, critique of responsibility. That is, hard determinism does not try either to explain or to justify our responsibility concepts and practices. It simply assumes that genuine responsibility is metaphysically unjustified. Even if an internally coherent account of responsibility and related practices can be given, it will be based on an illusion (Smilansky 2000). To see why hard determinism or mechanism cannot explain our responsibility attributions, remember that such causal accounts 'go all the way down'; determinism or mechanism applies to all people, to all events. Causation is not partial and lack of knowledge about how something is caused does not mean that it is uncaused. Determinism is not a degree or continuum concept. To say, as many do (Committee on Addictions of the Group for Advancement of Psychiatry 2002) that there is a continuum between determinism and free will is simply a conceptual error. Thus, if determinism is true and is genuinely inconsistent with responsibility, then no one can ever be really responsible for anything and responsibility attributions cannot properly justify further attitudes or action. Western theories of morality and the law do hold some people responsible and excuse others, however, and when we do excuse, it is not because there has been a little local determinism at work. Hard determinism can produce an internally coherent, forward-looking consequential system that treats human action specially and might possibly encourage good behavior and discourage bad behavior. Nevertheless, hard determinism cannot tell us which goals we should pursue and it cannot explain or justify our present practices, which routinely pursue non-efficiency goals such as giving people what they deserve, even if doing so is not the most efficient outcome.

The libertarian concedes that determinism or mechanism may account for most of the moving parts of the universe, but argues that human action is not fully subject to causal influence. Thus the libertarian is able to distinguish action from all other phenomena and to ground responsibility in contra-causal freedom. If the libertarian is correct, the 'buck' really does stop with human intentions, at least if intentional action is both rational and not influenced by coercive threats. The difficulty is that libertarianism produces a worthless view of responsibility or it depends on a 'panicky' metaphysics, to use Strawson's phrase (P.F. Strawson 1982).

One form of libertarianism holds that human actions are the product of indeterministic events in the brain, but why should such events ground responsibility? In what way are actions produced by indeterminate or random brain events 'ours' or an exercise of a freedom worth wanting? If our brain states and the world in general are truly random or indeterministic, then it is difficult to imagine how responsibility could be possible. Such randomness is deeply implausible, however. We could not explain the regularity of physical events and of human interactions, nor could we explain the dependable relation between intentions and actions, unless there was a cosmic coincidence of astounding proportion that accounted for the regularity. More important, brains would be akin to random number generators and our behavior would be equivalent to the random numbers generated. This is scarcely a secure foundation for responsibility or for any form of moral evaluation because rational intentions would be random rather than the product of genuine practical reason. In a sense, nothing would be up to us. In sum, if rational action is simply a product of biophysical indeterminacy, no one should be responsible for any action.

An apparently more plausible version of libertarianism concedes that prior events and experiences affect our mental states, but alleges that our actions are ultimately uncaused by anything other than ourselves. To begin, such a theory cannot specify the nature of the causal relation between an agent and an act that he causes (Moore 2000). Furthermore, there is no observational evidence that would confirm that agent-causation is true. Our experience of psychological freedom when we act intentionally is often cited, but such arguments from experience for contra-causal freedom have been properly criticized on many grounds (Mill 1979). Perhaps most important, our experience might simply be a psychological fact about us rather than good evidence to justify the truth of agent-origination. Moreover, why would we choose to adopt such an implausible theory when there are no good non-observational grounds, such as coherence or parsimony, for doing so (Bok 1998)? Finally, our desire to believe that agent-causation is true or the importance of this truth to our self-conception is not an independently good reason to accept that truth if the metaphysical foundation is false. Metaphysical libertarianism is simply too extravagantly implausible to be a secure foundation for responsibility.

Compatibilism, which accepts that universal causation is true, offers the most plausible causal metaphysics and the only coherent positive explanation of our current legal (and moral) practices. I also believe that a satisfactory normative defense of compatibilism is possible, based on conceptions of personhood, dignity, and the like. Compatibilist responsibility treats human beings as moral agents and provides for moral communities that enrich our lives (Oldenquist 1988). For the purpose of this chapter, however, which is concerned with the implications of one class of causal explanation within a thoroughly material world view—neuroscientific explanation—a positive account is sufficient. The next subsection addresses whether neuro-science or other materialistic explanations might compel abandoning this positive account.

The form of compatibilism most consistent with the legal view of responsibility is not concerned with whether we have ultimate responsibility. Instead, it treats responsibility practices as human constructions concerning human action and asks if they are consistent with facts about human beings that we justifiably believe and moral theories that we justifiably endorse. As the previous subsection argues, until currently unimaginable scientific advances convince us otherwise, we are fully entitled to believe that we are ordinarily conscious, intentional, and potentially rational creatures, who sometimes suffer from rationality defects when we act or who sometimes act under compulsion. These are simply true facts about the human condition, even if determinism is true. Moreover, concepts of responsibility and of desert that are based on the capacity for rationality and the absence of compulsion are fully justifiable by moral theories of fairness and justice that we confidently accept. Determinism does not compel us to abandon current responsibility criteria and practices.

Although legal cases and commentary are replete with talk about free will being the basis for responsibility, especially if a biological abnormality seemed to affect the legally relevant behavior in question, the presence or absence of contra-causal freedom or something like it is not part of the criteria for any legal doctrine that holds some people non-responsible. If the realism constraint is true, all behavior is caused, but not all behavior is excused because causation *per se* has nothing to do with responsibility. If causation negated responsibility, no one would be morally responsible and holding people legally responsible would be extremely problematic. An assertion that free will was or was not present is simply a conclusory statement about responsibility that had to have been reached based on other criteria. Finally, causation is not the equivalent of a compelling condition that ought to excuse conduct. All behavior is caused, but only some behavior is compelled. When intentional action is excused because we consider it compelled—think of a gun to one's head—the action is excused because it meets hard choice compulsion criteria, not because it is caused.

In sum, neuroscientific explanations of behavior are fully consistent with ordinary notions of responsibility.

## Brave new world

I am often asked how our conception of responsibility would be affected in the brave new world in which neuroscience and allied disciplines fully reveal how the brain enables the mind, allowing hitherto ungraspable ability to understand, predict, and control all human behavior. The short answer is that I have no idea. As McHugh and Slavney (1998) argue, such discoveries would profoundly alter our understanding of biological processes and our view of ourselves as creatures. The new understanding would certainly drastically alter concepts of personhood and action that are the foundations of responsibility, but precisely how they would do so is entirely speculative. For the nonce, however, such discoveries do not seem possible and perhaps, as many philosophers suggest, they are unachievable in principle. Until the brave new world becomes a reality, ordinary notions of responsibility are secure, although neuroscience may provide evidence to support the claim that some excusing conditions are more prevalent than we think.

## *Roper* revisited: neuroscience in legal decision-making

Here is the opening of the summary of the *amicus* brief filed by, *inter alia*, the American Medical Association, the American Psychiatric Association, the American Academy of Child and Adolescent Psychiatry, and the American Academy of Psychiatry and Law (American Medical Association 2004).

> The adolescent's mind works differently from ours. Parents know it. This Court [the United States Supreme Court] has said it. Legislatures have presumed it for decades or more.

Precisely. The brief points to evidence concerning impulsivity, poor short-term risk and long-term benefit estimations, emotional volatility, and susceptibility to stress among adolescents compared with adults. These are common-sense fireside conclusions that parents and others have reached in one form or another since time immemorial. In recent years, common sense has been bolstered by methodologically rigorous behavioral investigations that have confirmed ordinary wisdom. Most important, all these behavioral characteristics are clearly relevant to responsibility because they all bear on the adolescent's capacity for rationality. Without any further scientific evidence, advocates of abolition would have an entirely ample factual basis to support the types of moral and constitutional claims that they are making.

As the introductory section indicates, however, *Roper* briefs are filled with discussion of new neuroscientific evidence that confirms that adolescent brains are different from adult brains in ways consistent with the observed behavioral differences that bear on culpability and responsibility. Again assuming the validity of the neuroscientific evidence, what does it add? The rigorous behavioral studies already confirm the behavioral differences, or at least arguably do so. No one believes that these data are invalid because adolescent subjects are faking or for some other reason. The moral and constitutional implications of the data may be controversial, but the data are not. At most, the neuroscientific evidence provides a partial causal explanation of why the observed behavioral differences exist and thus some further evidence of the validity of the behavioral differences. It is only of limited and indirect relevance to responsibility assessment, which is based on behavioral criteria. Rationality is a property that persons manifest, not brains. Brains do not kill and deserve punishment; persons, i.e. beings capable of conscious intentionality, kill and potentially deserve punishment.

The neuroscience evidence in no way independently confirms that adolescents are less responsible. If the behavioral differences between adolescents and adults are slight, it would not matter if their brains were quite different. Similarly, if the behavioral differences are sufficient for moral and constitutional differential treatment, then it would not matter if the brains were essentially indistinguishable.

Assuming the validity of the findings of behavioral and biological difference, the size of that difference entails no necessary moral or constitutional conclusions. Even if one concedes that adolescents as a group are less rational than adults, the question is whether at least some of them may be sufficiently responsible to deserve execution. Whether the mean differences are large enough and whether the overlap between the two populations is small enough to warrant treating adolescents differently categorically as a class is a normative moral, political, social, and ultimately legal constitutional question about which behavioral science and neuroscience must finally fall silent.

As the *New York Times* admonishes, the Court may nonetheless give weight to the emerging neuroscience evidence. Doing so will indicate only that the Court is unjustifiably swayed by seemingly hard science rather than by a full understanding of its limited indirect relevance. The Court should properly focus primarily on the behavioral evidence and should use the neuroscience only as indirect confirmation of what the crucial behavioral studies disclose.

If, contrary to this chapter's advice, the Supreme Court gives great weight to the neuroscientific evidence in *Roper*, suggesting that these findings are a direct or independent measure of diminished responsibility, the Court will legitimate a confused understanding of responsibility and encourage the general admission of mostly irrelevant neuroscience evidence in criminal and civil cases concerning responsibility. Needless and expensive imaging studies will become routine, and judges and juries will be swayed by hard science which may be valid, but which will seldom be relevant for the purpose of evaluating responsibility. This will create a fearful new legal world that we should strive to avoid.

## Postscript: *Roper* v. *Simmons*

On 1 March 2005 the Supreme Court decided *Roper* v. *Simmons*, holding that the Eighth and Fourteen Amendments forbid imposition of the death penalty on offenders who were under the age of 18 when they committed murder. The Court cited many reasons for its decision, including the abundant common-sense and behavioral science evidence that adolescents differ from adults. This evidence demonstrates, said the Court, 'that juvenile offenders cannot with reliability be classified among the worst offenders', for whom capital punishment is reserved. The Court cited three differences: adolescents have 'a lack of maturity and an underdeveloped sense of responsibility'; adolescents are more 'vulnerable or susceptible to negative influences and outside pressures, including peer pressure', a difference in part explained by the adolescent's weaker control or experience of control over his own environment; adolescents do not have fully formed characters. As a result of these factors, juvenile culpability is diminished and the penological justifications for capital punishment apply to adolescents with 'lesser force.'

Characteristically, the Court did not cite much evidence for the empirical propositions that supported its diminished culpability argument. What is notable, however, is that the Court did not cite any of the neuroscience evidence concerning myelination and pruning that the *amici* and others had urged them to rely on. Perhaps the neuroscience evidence actually played a role in the decision, but there is no evidence in the opinion to support this speculation. As the body of this chapter argued, the behavioral science was crucial to proper resolution of the case and the neuroscience was largely irrelevant. The reasoning of the case is consistent with this argument. In my view, *Roper* properly disregarded the neuroscience evidence and thus did not provide unwarranted legitimation for the use of such evidence to decide culpability questions generally.

## References

Alexander L, Sherwin S (2001). *The Rule of Rules: Morality, Rules and the Dilemmas of Law*. Durham, NC: Duke University Press, 11–25.

American Law Institute (1962). *Model Penal Code*, sec. 2.01. Philadelphia, PA: American Law Institute.

American Medical Association (2004). Brief *Amicus Curiae* in Support of Respondent in *Roper* v. *Simmons*.

*Atkins* v. *Virginia*, 536 U.S. 304 (2002).

Audi R (1993). *Action, Intention and Reason*. Ithaca, NY: Cornell University Press, 1–4.

Bok H (1998). *Freedom and responsibility*, Princeton, NJ: Princeton University Press, 75–91, 129–31, 146–51.

Cacioppo JT, Berntson GG, Lorig T, *et al*. (2003). Just because you're imaging the brain doesn't mean you can stop using your head: a primer and set of first principles. *Journal of Personality and Social Psychology*, 85, 650–61.

Caspi A, McClay J, Moffitt TE, *et al*. (2002). Role of genotype in the cycle of violence in maltreated children. *Science*, 297, 851–4.

Churchland PM (1988). *Matter and Consciousness* (revised edn). Cambridge, MA: MIT Press, 26–34, 43–49.

Committee on Addictions of the Group for the Advancement of Psychiatry (2002). Responsibility and choice in addiction. *Psychiatric Services*, 53, 707–713.

Crane T (2005). Ready or not. *Times Literary Supplement*, 14 January, p. 26.

Cummings JL, Mega MS (2003). *Neuropsychiatry and Behavioral Neuroscience*. Oxford: Oxford University Press, 333–43, 360–70.

Dennett DC (2003). *Freedom Evolves*. New York: Viking, 1–22.

Fodor J (1987). *Psychosemantics: The Problem of Meaning in the Philosophy of Mind*. Cambridge, MA: MIT Press, xii.

Goldstein RZ, Volkow ND (2002). Drug addiction and its underlying neurobiological basis: neuroimaging evidence for the involvement of the frontal cortex. *American Journal of Psychiatry*, 159, 1642–52.

Libet B (1999). Do we have free will. In: Libet B, Freeman A, Sutherland, K (eds) *The Volitional Brain: Towards a Neuroscience of Free Will*. Thorverton, Devon, UK: Imprint Academic, 47–58.

McGinn C (1999). The Mysterious Flame: Conscious Minds in a Material World. New York: Basic Books, 1–76.

McHugh PR, Slavney PR (1998). *The Perspectives of Psychiatry* (2nd edn). Baltimore, MD: Johns Hopkins University Press, 11–12.

Mill JS (1979). An examination of Sir William Hamilton's philosophy. In: Robson, J.M (ed) *Collected Works of John Stuart Mill*, Vol. 9. Toronto: University of Toronto Press, 449–57.

Moore MS (1993). *Act and Crime*. Oxford: Clarendon Press, 49–52, 135–155, 257–58.

Moore MS (1994). More on act and crime. *University of Pennsylvania Law Review*, 142, 1749–1840.

Moore MS (2000). The metaphysics of causal intervention. *California Law Review*, 88, 827–78.

Morse SJ (1994). Culpability and control. *University of Pennsylvania Law Review*, 142, 1587–1660.

Morse SJ (2002). Uncontrollable urges and irrational people. *Virginia Law Review*, 88, 1025–78.

*New York Times* (2004). Juveniles and the death penalty. 13 October, p. A:26.

Oldenquist A (1988). An explanation of retribution. *Journal of Philosophy*, 85, 464–78.

Potenza M, Steinberg MA, Skudlarski P, *et al.* (2003). Gambling urges in pathological gambling: a functional magnetic resonance imaging study. *Archives of General Psychiatry*, 60, 828–36.

Richards JR (2000). *Human Nature After Darwin: A Philosophical Introduction*. London: Routledge.

*Roper* v. *Simmons*, 124 S. Ct. 2198 (*2004*).

*Roper* v. *Simmons*, 125 S.Ct. 1183 (2005).

Searle JR (1992). *The Rediscovery of the Mind*. Cambridge, MA: MIT Press.

Searle JR (2002). End of the revolution. *New York Review of Books*, 28 February, 35.

Searle JR (2004). *Mind: A Brief Introduction*. New York: Oxford University Press, 88–92, 111–32.

Shapiro SJ (2000). Law, morality and the guidance of conduct. *Legal Theory*, 6, 127–70.

Smilansky S (2000). *Free Will and Illusion*. Oxford: Oxford University Press, 40–73, 145–219.

*Stanford* v. *Kentucky*, 492 U.S. 361 (1989).

Stein MB, Jang KL, Taylor S, *et al.* (2002). Genetic and environmental influences on trauma exposure and posttraumatic stress disorder symptoms: a twin study. *American Journal of Psychiatry*, 159, 1675–81.

Strawson G (1989). Consciousness, free will, and the unimportance of determinism. *Inquiry*, 32, 3–27.

Strawson PF (1982). Freedom and resentment. In: Watson G (ed). *Free Will*. Oxford: Oxford University Press, 59–80.

*Thompson* v. *Oklahoma*, 487 U.S. 815 (1988).

Vaitl D, Birbaumer N, Gruzelier J, *et al.* (2005). Psychobiology of altered states of consciousness. *Psychological Bulletin*, 131, 98–127.

Wallace RJ (1994). *Responsibility and the Moral Sentiments*. Cambridge, MA: Harvard University Press.

Walter H (2001). *Neurophilosophy of Free Will: From Libertarian Illusions to a Concept of Neural Anatomy*. Cambridge, MA: MIT Press, 250–2.

Wegner DM (2002). *The Illusion of Conscious Will*. Cambridge, MA: MIT Press.

Williams B (1994). The *actus reus* of Dr Caligari. *University of Pennsylvania Law Review*, 142, 1661–73.

Wittgenstein L (1958). *Philosophical Investigations* (3rd edn). Part I, Section 621. New York: Macmillan.

Zhu J (2003). Reclaiming volition: an alternative interpretation of Libet's experiment. *Journal of Consciousness Studies*, 10, 61–7.

## Chapter 4

# Brains, lies, and psychological explanations

Tom Buller

## Introduction

As the contributions to this book attest, neuroscience is a hot topic. Advances in neuroscience, particularly in neuroimaging and psychopharmacology, now enable us to correlate psychological states with specific brain functions, and to alter psychological states by modifying neurochemistry. As Farah and Wolpe (2004) put the matter succinctly, we are now able to 'monitor and manipulate' our brain function and thereby to affect our thoughts and actions by intervening at the neurobiological level.

In broad terms, these advances have two sorts of implications for ethics. As Roskies (2002) describes, we can distinguish the 'ethics of neuroscience' from the 'neuroscience of ethics'. In the first category we can place a host of ethical questions, some of which are familiar to us from earlier parallel advances and discussions in genethics, for example those pertaining to the ethics of enhancement (Parens 1998; see also Chapter 6), or to the predisposition and prediction of behavior (Raine *et al*. 1998), or to concerns about privacy (Kulynych 2002). In the second category we can place discussions about how these advances in neuroscience are providing us with a scientific naturalized account of how we make moral judgments and, more controversially, the extent to which the neuroscientific evidence suggests a revision of the belief that we are intentional rational agents who are capable of voluntary action.

The challenge neuroscience presents for neuroethics is that there is a tension between the two categories. The types of issues raised by the 'ethics of neuroscience', for example whether cognitive enhancement diminishes respect for persons (Kass 2003), rest on the belief that our folk psychological understanding of ourselves as intentional rational agents is correct. Cognitive enhancement raises ethical questions because it is consistent with agency and psychological explanations; we want new drugs to enhance our memories, desires, and actions. However, the types of issues raised by the 'neuroscience of ethics', for example the discovery of the neural correlates for our personality, preferences, or attitudes appears to challenge the notion that our behaviors are the result of intentional rational decisions. The neuroscience of ethics, like the neuroscience of anything, is a normative enterprise that purports to achieve an explanation of this phenomenon through a naturalistic view of psychobehavioral states in terms of their underlying neurobiology. Prior to the identification of the neural correlate for a particular psychobehavioral state we would attempt to explain the behavior in terms of the person's psychological states, for example lying in terms of intentional deception; subsequent to the identification of the neural correlate, lying is explained in terms of the neurobiology of this behavior. Unless we are prepared to accept neuroscientific explanations merely in terms of token-neurobiological states, and thereby lose any explanatory gain, our naturalistic account must explain psychobehavioral states in terms of type-neurobiological states, rather than in the context of this person's particular beliefs and intentions. The tension between these two categories could be released if we could formulate a naturalized neuroscientific account of human behavior that could accommodate the belief that we are intentional rational agents. My goal in this chapter is to argue that such an accommodation will be hard to find.

## Two visions of the mind

Until comparatively recently, neuroscience did not generate much public discussion or controversy. Within the philosophical community, neuroscience has been a familiar topic to philosophers of mind; however, it has been largely ignored by those working in ethics. The explanation for this is twofold: first, discussion about finding the neural correlate for belief, emotion, consciousness, or depression was based on expectation rather than on evidence; secondly, doctrinaire philosophy maintained that descriptive neuroscience had little to do with normative ethics.

A wealth of new data suggests that we have moved from expectation to evidence, and even if we are skeptical that we will reach a comprehensive mature neuroscience as claimed by some, there is little doubt that neuroscience will continue to find important correlations between neurological and psychological states. Since it is not an empirical claim like the first, the second of the two explanations above appears less susceptible to revision by advances in neuroscience. Is neuroethics merely the latest attempt at a naturalized ethics? Following Hume (1739) and Moore (1902) it has been customary to insist on the distinction between fact and value and to avoid committing the naturalistic fallacy, the error of drawing normative conclusions from descriptive empirical facts (Held 1996); although a number of recent discussions that have re-examined this issue (Johnson 1993; May *et al.* 1996; Casebeer 2003). If neuroethics amounts to no more than the 'science of ethics' and the grounding of moral judgments on empirical facts, then perhaps we should be dismissive of the entire enterprise. However, as noted above, this is only half the picture. If we consider some of the issues that have provoked discussion in the neuroethical literature (e.g. cognitive enhancement, psychopharmacology, and forensic neuroimaging), it is not the case that we have simply identified the neurological basis for intelligence or depression or truth-telling and, on the basis of this, set our ethical parameters; rather, it is that these new technologies and abilities raise ethical questions.

As Flanagan (2002) argues, the challenge we face is to reconcile two 'grand images of who we are, the humanistic and the scientific'. According to the humanistic view we are, for the most part, autonomous intentional rational agents and therefore we are responsible for our actions. Contrariwise, according to the scientific view, we are animals, exhaustively described in physical terms and constrained by the ordinary laws of cause and effect. Thus on the scientific view human behavior is not caused by our intentions, beliefs, and desires. Instead, free will is an illusion because the brain is a deterministic physical organ, and it is the brain that is doing the causal work.

The reconciliation of these two visions is essential for neuroethics. Neuroethics has emerged because advances in the neurosciences present us with ethical questions; however, there would be no questions at all if we believed that ethics and neuroscience were incompatible. Consider, for example, the question as to whether neuroimaging for lie detection should be admissible in court. This is an ethical question only if there is nothing incompatible about holding (a) that we are intentional agents who sometimes attempt to deceive, and (b) that we can determine whether a person is being deceptive by directly observing brain activity. If one held that these two claims were incompatible, then there can be no ethical question; that is, if the identification of the neural correlate of lying were taken as evidence that psychological states are just neurological states, and hence that our folk psychological concepts are, in fact, false, then it is incoherent to suppose that neuroimaging could reveal whether a person is lying. Similarly, Patricia Churchland's claim that neuroscience will be able to distinguish 'in-control' from 'out-of-control' behavior makes sense only if there is no contradiction between neuroscience and intentional voluntary human action. (Moreno 2003; P.S. Churchland 2002; see also Chapter 1). Thus neuroethics is possible, in a transcendental sense, if and only if the scientific and humanistic visions can be reconciled. In other words, neuroethics makes sense only if eliminativism and determinism are rejected (Moreno 2003; see also Chapter 3).

## Consciousness and rationality

What is to say that we are intentional rational agents capable of voluntary action? Broadly, this means that we act on the basis of our conscious (and, perhaps, unconscious) beliefs and desires, that we are capable of weighing alternatives, and choosing and executing a course of action, and that the resulting actions follow directly from our thoughts and reasons for action. It is evident that consciousness and rationality are necessary conditions of agency; in order for a person to be an agent the person must be able to make conscious decisions, i.e. be *aware* of his own motivations, intentions, and beliefs, and the consequences of these actions to a meaningful extent. In this regard, agency requires self-consciousness. There are, of course, degrees of consciousness and rationality in this context, but if a person were substantially unaware of his own motivations, intentions, and beliefs, or was incapable of weighing alternatives and choosing a course of action, then it would be difficult to maintain that this person qualified as an agent. Therefore it would be difficult to hold this person responsible for action.

As Davidson (1980) has argued, an important component of rationality is the interconnectedness of psychological states and the role that individual psychological states play within a person's overall psychology. If we know that John is feeling cold and desires to get warm, and that he believes that closing the window will help, then (other things being equal) John will close the window. In a similar vein, if Sally hates cats and she has to visit her friend who has 20 of them, we can predict her opinion of the experience. This normative component of rationality plays an important role when we consider responsibility. If John knows that throwing a rock will harm the children playing and he goes ahead and throws the rock, then, other things being equal, we may conclude that he must have wanted to harm the children.

Can these conceptions of consciousness and rationality that underlie agency be accommodated by neuroscience? The last 30 years have witnessed a vast number of articles and books on the topic of consciousness, and there is a spectrum of positions on this topic. These range from eliminativists and reductionists on the one side (P.S. Churchland 1989, 2002; P.M. Churchland 1992) to non-reductionists (Chalmers 1996; Davidson 1980), dual-aspect theorists (Nagel 1974, 1986), and 'mysterians' (McGinn 1993). According to neuroscientific reductionism, empirical discoveries will identify elements in the reducing theory (neuroscience) that correspond to elements in the reduced theory (folk psychology) in conjunction with 'bridge laws' connecting the elements of both theories (P.S. Churchland 1989, 2002; Bickle 2003). It is customary to think of reductionism as making both ontological claims about the identity of properties between the reduced and the reducing theories, and explanatory claims about the appropriate way to describe the world. Ideally, neuroscience will provide us with a more accurate and successful way of explaining human behavior than folk psychology, for we will be able to explain in greater and more accurate detail why a person is feeling depressed or paranoid or has a constant craving for food. It is for these reasons, one supposes, that Ramachandran (2003) claims that psychiatry will be reduced to neurology. As Ramachandran discusses in the case of hysteria and other 'psychological disturbances', this disturbance can be usefully explained in terms of what is happening in the person's brain.

The goal of a reductive neuroscience is to provide us with greater explanatory success. In principle, this is achieved by identifying correlations between psychological states and neur biological states, and the added predictive and explanatory value of neuroscience; for instance, the identification of the function and role of neurotransimitters such as dopamine and serotonin provide us with us with a better way of explaining and understanding depression. As part of this reduction, it is predicted that neuroscience will reveal that some parts of our folk psychology are mistaken. This might occur, for example, if we were to find that our folk psychological notions of consciousness and free will do not correlate with the emerging neuroscientific evidence (P.S. Churchland 1989; Ramachandran 2003; Greene and Cohen 2004). As one example we can consider the research by Libet (1985) that appears to undermine the notion of free will through the identification of neurological activity that precedes a conscious decision to act. For the sake of argument, let us accept that Libet's studies do show that my conscious decision to raise my arm was preceded by brain activity—the 'readiness potential'. What impact should these results have on the conceptions of rationality and consciousness that underlie agency and responsibility? Should we revise these in order to match the neuroscientific facts? While revision may be the appropriate course of action to take, why should we choose this course of action rather than draw conclusions about the limitations of neuroscience? What we are faced with is not simply a choice between the scientific and humanistic visions but a philosophical dispute about the meaning of terms such as 'free will', 'rationality', and 'consciousness.' According to the reductionist neuroscientific approach, empirical evidence will either show that these terms refer to particular neurobi logical states or that they are dispensable terms belonging to an outdated mysticism. According to the non-reductionist humanistic approach these terms refer to psychobehavioral states, and therefore the fact that they have no neurobiological correlate is, frankly, unimportant. To put the matter differently, if we think that free will can be confirmed or denied by empirical evidence, then we should be concerned about Libet's findings; however, if we do not believe that free will is an empirical notion, then these findings are irrelevant. To repeat, this is not to deny these neurobiological findings; it is only to say that their importance depends upon a prior commitment to the ontological and explanatory success of neuroscientific reductionism.

As Morse (2004) argues, emerging neuroscientific information is relevant if it provides an explanation of why a person is capable of acting rationally; however, without further argument, there is little justification as to why this new information should be used as a determination that the person is incapable of acting rationally, independent of any social or pragmatic reasons (see also Chapter 3). Suppose that neuroscience will further reveal how a person's decision-making capacities are adversely affected by stress or depression. What relevance does this information have for our notion of rationality? Perhaps new neurobi logical information will ead us to consider revising our moral and legal notions of rationality. However, if we do decide to do so, it would be for social or pragmatic reasons. Independent of such reasons, it is difficult to see how this new information could be used without committing the naturalistic fallacy. Certainly, there are good parsimonious reasons why one might wish to argue for the ontological reduction of psychological states to neurobiological states but, particularly in the context of neuroethics, one needs further arguments to show that such a reduction will have an appropriate degree of explanatory success.

## Minds, brains, and agents

In the first chapter of his book *Descartes' Error*, Damasio (1994) recounts the now well-known story of Phineas Gage. Gage was a hardworking, even-tempered, and respected construction foreman who worked laying track for the Rutland and Burlington Railroad. On 13 August 1848, Gage was helping to set detonations used to clear rock from the future course of the rail track. Momentarily distracted, Gage forgot to put sand into the hole in the rock in which the explosive powder had already been placed. He then inserted the tamping iron, a 3ft 7in iron bar weighing 13 pounds (Macmillan 2004) into the hole to pack down the sand but the iron caused a spark which ignited the explosive powder. The explosion sent the tamping iron up through the base of Gage's skull, through the front of his brain and out through the top of his head, eventually landing more than 100 ft away (Damasio 1994). Remarkably, Gage was not killed by the accident; however, after he recovered it became clear that 'Gage was no longer Gage.' His personality and behavior had changed, and he became profane, impatient, irreverent, and unreliable.

The tragic accident that befell Phineas Gage has helped us to understand better how injury to a particular part of the brain can lead to specific types of behavioral effect. As Damasio states, '[T]here is no question that Gage's personality change was caused by a circumscribed brain lesion in a specific site' (Damasio 1994; see also Chapter 2). Recent advances in neuroimaging have greatly increased our ability to locate brain abnormalities and have helped to identify these abnormalities as explanations of psychological and behavioral changes (P.S. Churchland 2002; Ramachandran 2003). Furthermore, through the identification and study of abnormal cases, we are able to gain a clearer understanding of the relationship between brain function and behavior. In this regard, one can see an obvious parallel between the growth of knowledge in genetics and in neuroscience; abnormal states of affairs (diseases, disorders) have been linked to damage to a particular gene or part of the brain which, in turn, has enabled us to identify the function of the gene or part of the brain in the normal case.

As Patricia Churchland (2002) has argued, the distinction between being in control and being out of control is not a sharp one but a matter of varying degrees. A person may have greater ability for freedom of choice with regard to some types of decisions than others, and this ability may be affected by a variety of factors, including damage to particular parts of the brain, and the levels of neuromodulators and hormones. It is plausible to contend, as Churchland does, that we will be able to identify the major neurobiological factors that underlie a person's ability to be in control and, conversely, those that undermine it. On the basis of the above neuroscientific evidence we may be able to identify the factors that impede a person's ability to be in control, and hence, in the absence of such factors, we will by default have an account of the neurobiological factors that are consistent with being in control; nevertheless, I want to argue that this does not warrant the claim underlying Churchland's hypothesis.

To begin, the neuroscientific evidence cannot on its own be the basis for the distinction between being in control or out of control. The evidence is not sufficient for this task because being in control or having freedom of choice are normative notions distinct from the neuroscientific facts. Independent of social standards and expectations, it is difficult to understand what it would mean to say that one type of neurological functioning is any more or less in control than any other, or that a behavior is any more or less rational. We are able to gain some idea of the normal level of the neuromodulators because, *ex hypothesi*, we have discovered in an important set of cases that individuals who were not in control had abnormal levels. In the absence of these behaviors and society's judgment of them, one neuromodulator level is no more normal than any other.

Furthermore, what counts as being in control or being out of control will vary according to time and place; what is viewed in Richmond as refined self-possession may in Reyjkjavik be regarded as wanton excess. Less figuratively, different cultures may have different ideas as to what constitutes depression or hyperactivity. If this is correct, then it is either the case that the notion of being in control cannot be grounded in neuroscientific terms, or we have to be generous in these terms and admit a range of possible neurological states as underlying this notion. The first of these options suggests that we should abandon or revise our hopes for a successful ontological reduction of psychobehavioral states to neurobiological states; and the second questions the possibility of successful explanatory reduction. If the neuroscientific evidence does not match up with our social or ethical notions of what constitutes decision-making capacity, then it is difficult to see how neuroscience can successfully explain this capacity in neuroscientific terms.

Moreover, it is not at all clear what we gain in explanatory terms by being able to distinguish in-control from out-of-control behavior in neuroscientific terms. For the sake of argument, let us grant that for each and every psychological state or activity there is a correlative neurophysical state. Accordingly, we should not be surprised that the distinction between being in control and being out of control correlates with neurophysical states. But correlation is not the same as explanation. It does not follow from the fact that psycho-behavioral differences correlate with neurophysical differences that differences at the neuro-physical level explain the differences at the psychobehavioral level. We might discover that there are neurophysical differences that correspond to the distinction between introverts and extroverts. Does this mean that the neurophysical differences explain the difference between introverts and extroverts? Not necessarily, because the neurological differences may have no relation to the psychological aspects that are relevant to a person's being an introvert or an extrovert.

Neuroscience can inform our notion of intentional rational action by revealing how abnor-mal brain function can explain a person's behavior. In this way a judge might decide that Smith is not responsible for his actions if Smith's actions or volitions are beyond his control. In such a case we think it appropriate to explain Smith's behavior in these terms not only because we believe that the cause of his actions and/or volitions was not intentional, but also because we believe that this enables us to better predict what he will do. However, in the normal course of events we do not attempt to explain behavior in neurophysical terms because we simply take it for granted that neurophysical explanations are irrelevant. If Jones throws a brick through a shop window it is no excuse to say that his brain did it. Since all our psychobehavioral states correlate in some fashion with neurophysical states, we should either jettison completely the belief that we are intentional rational agents or deny neuroscience any broad explanatory role in the normal case. Neuroscientific explanations become relevant only in those cases where we have independent reasons for claiming that the person's behavior is not intentional or the person is not capable of acting rationally. In such cases, neuroscience can provide an explan-ation of why this is so.

# Neuroimaging and 'brain-reading'

Neuroscientific reductionism can be appropriately categorized as an internalist theory since the theory claims that the content of a person's psychological state can be individuated according to the state of that person's brain (see also Chapter 2). For example, to say that Sally believes that it is snowing is to make a remark about the current state of he brain; if the content of her psychological states were to change, then, according to our best neuroscientific theory, we could infer that the state of her brain had changed.

This internalist perspective underlies an issue that has already provoked considerable discussion in the neuroethics literature, namely the use of neuroimaging to 'read' a person's mind. Discussion of this issue has divided into two topics: firstly, the use of neuroimaging to detect whether a person is telling the truth (Farah 2002; Langleben et al. 2002; Farah and Wolpe 2004) or to identify a person's attitudes or preferences (Hart et al. 2000; Phelps et al. 2000); secondly, the threat that neuroimaging poses to our privacy (Kulynych 2002; Farah and Wolpe 2004; Wolpe et al. 2005; Illes and Racine 2005).

Two potential examples of lie detection by neuroimaging have been discussed in the literature. First, Langleben and his colleagues performed a study that involved subjects bluffing versus telling the truth about symbols on playing cards (Langleben et al. 2002). As a result of the experiments, they identified the anterior cingulate cortex and superior frontal gyrus as 'components of the basic neural circuitry of deception', and they drew the conclusion that 'cognitive differences between deception and truth have neural correlates detectable by fMRI' (Langleben et al. 2002). Secondly, Farwell has described a brain fingerprinting device that, according to him, can detect whether a person recognizes a word or phrase shown on a computer screen according to changes in the P300 event-related potential (Farewell 1991; Knight 2004). Farwell claims that, using this device, one can determine whether a suspect was familiar with the details of a crime scene, and hence the device could be used to determine whether the person was telling the truth. With regard to attitudes and preferences, two studies have reported finding neurological evidence that our brains respond differently to faces from our own or a different racial group (Hart et al. 2000; Phelps et al. 2000).

As Illes and Kulynych have argued (Illes and Raffin 2002; Kulynych 2002; Illes 2003; Illes et al. 2003), neuroimaging raises important concerns about a person's right to privacy and confidentiality. These concerns apply not simply to the accidental revelation of medical information (e.g. a fMRI scan inadvertently revealing an abnormality) but also to a person's preferences or knowledge. If neuroimaging can reveal a person's psychological states (thoughts, attitudes, or preferences), then it is clear that privacy concerns are raised. (One need only consider the potential use of such machines by security services, law enforcement, or marketing firms).

As described, the ethical questions raised by neuroimaging depend upon an internalist conception of the mind, for these questions are predicated on the understanding that, in principle or in fact, we can determine what a person is thinking by examining that person's brain. Clearly, there are privacy concerns associated with neuroimaging, but is the notion of 'brain-reading' coherent and a legitimate cause for concern? I think that there are a number of reasons why one might challenge the internalist conception of the mind that underlies some of the ethical concerns associated with neuroimaging. In a recent paper discussing the 'promises and perils' for emerging lie-detection technologies, Wolpe et al. describe various neuroimaging technologies and research, including that of Langleben. As the authors thoroughly discuss, there are good reasons to be cautious about the conclusions that one can draw about lie detection and neuroimaging outside the parameters of the study design. Nevertheless they are prepared to conclude that 'there are fundamental neurological differences between deception and truth at the neurological level...' (P. Wolpe *et al.* 2005).

I want to raise a number of reasons why one might resist this internalist picture and the conclusion drawn above. First, one might object to this conclusion on the grounds that the tests reveal not truth-telling or lying but our beliefs about how society views lying. For example, Langleben *et al.* (2002) report that subjects did not report being anxious during the test. However, the state of anxiety is distinct from the belief (albeit perhaps false) that one ought not to lie. Perhaps the neurological feature that the tests reveal is not lying, but the belief or sentiment that one ought not to do something that is generally condemned. In a society of liars, would the neurological features associated with deception be associated instead with truth-telling?

More importantly, perhaps, there are many different types of lies: prevarication, tact, 'white lies', self-deception, and lies told as part of a game or a play (Illes 2004). If there were a neurological feature that correlated with the distinction between truth-telling and deception, then we would expect all these types of lying to be correlated with this neurological feature. It is, of course, an empirical question whether we will find such a correlation, but given earlier remarks about how our normative notions are culturally variable, I believe that the class of psychobehavioral states classified as lying will have no useful explanatory correlation at the neurophysical level. And if we do not find the appropriate correlations between neuroscience and the psychobehavioral states, then what implications does this have for our folk psychological notion of lying? Furthermore, problems are raised by mistaken cases of lying. Imagine that Jones believes that John Kerry won the last US Presidential election but lies to his wife and tells her that George W. Bush won. Technically, we might suppose that neuroimaging would reveal that Jones was lying, but even if he is shown to be doing so by this technology, the question of whether, in fact, he is lying is still open. A related objection is that we might find that one type of lie may be realized by different neurophysical states—the problem of multiple realizability. In this case it would still be true that each type of lying corresponds to a neural correlate but we gain little or no explanatory advantage by identifying lying in this way.

Finally, there is also a perhaps more fundamental concern about neuroimaging and 'brain-reading' that pertains directly to the internalist perspective. In their book *Philosophical Foundations of Neuroscience*, Bennett and Hacker (2003) criticize neuroscientific reductionism on the grounds that it commits a 'mereological fallacy', i.e. the fallacy of ascribing properties to parts that should be ascribed to the whole. According to their Wittgensteinian perspective, terms such as 'believes', 'reasons', 'understands', or, for that matter, 'lies' should be properly thought of as descriptions not simply of mind but of behavior. To say that Smith understands Spanish or believes that it is going to rain is to say something about how Smith will behave, what other beliefs Smith will have, and what statements Smith will agree to. All of this is to say that we should understand particular psychological states in terms of the role that they play within a person's overall psychology.

Bennett and Hacker's conclusion bears directly on neuroimaging studies that claim to detect a neurological basis for certain preferences or attitudes (Hart *et al.* 2000; Phelps *et al.* 2000). In their study, Hart and colleagues report neurophysical differences between how individuals respond to images of members of their own racial group and how they respond to images of members of a different group. As a result of this neuroscientific evidence, would we be justified in claiming that a person's racial preferences have a neurobiological basis?

Imagine that a neuroscientific study revealed that there was a neurological difference between how people respond to accents that are similar to or different from their own. The results of this study do not warrant any general conclusions about people's preferences about accents because it is not clear that there is any obvious connection between how a person's brain might respond to a certain auditory event and that person's moral or general preferences. There is nothing incoherent about the possibility that someone might respond differently (more favorably?) in neuroscientific terms to English accents than to Welsh accents, yet believe that Welsh accents are much more pleasant.

The objection here pertains to the interconnectedness of our psychological states, preferences, and attitudes. If we know that Davis prefers Welsh accents, then we can plausibly infer that, other things being equal, he would prefer to live in Wales or to be surrounded by his Welsh friends—this is all part and parcel of what it means to have a preference. But this interconnectedness of psychological states has no echo at the neurological level. Detecting neurologically that Davis responds differently (more favorably?) to Welsh accents than to English ones has no implications for any other neurophysical states, including those that correlate with the other psychological states that are the substance of his preference.

## A modest accommodation

In this chapter I have attempted to argue that there are challenges to a successful accommodation between a naturalized neuroscientific account of human behavior and the belief that we are intentional rational agents. In particular, I have tried to show, first, that the internalist perspective that underlies reductionist neuroscience and some of the current neuroethical issues is at odds with our folk psychological notions. Secondly, I have argued that the relevance of neuroscience to our notion of agency is derivative upon prior normative considerations, and hence that the impact of neuroscientific advances on matters of agency and responsibility is limited.

As advances in neuroscience improve our ability to monitor and manipulate brain function, so the discussion of the ethics of such actions will continue. These advances are also ensuring that the discussion continues on fundamental philosophical questions regarding the status of folk psychology and the reach of science. It is these two sets of discussions that make neuroethics such an exciting field and, as long as we can continue to distinguish normative from metaphysical questions, neuroethics will continue to grow.

## References

Bennett MR, Hacker PMS (2003). *Philosophical Foundations of Neuroscience*. Oxford: Blackwell.

Bickle J (2003). *Philosophy and Neuroscience: A Ruthlessly Reductive Account*. New York: Springer.

Casebeer WD (2003). *Natural Ethical Facts: Evolution, Connectionism, and Moral Cognition*. Cambridge, MA: MIT Press.

Chalmers DJ (1996). *The Conscious Mind: In Search of A Fundamental Theory*. New York: Oxford University Press.

Churchland PM (1992). *A Neurocomputational Perspective: The Nature of Mind and the Structure of Science*. Cambridge, MA: MIT Press.

Churchland PS (1989). *Neurophilosophy: Toward a Unified Science of the Mind–Brain*. Cambridge, MA: MIT Press.

Churchland PS (2002). *Brain-Wise: Studies in Neurophilosophy*. MIT Press, Cambridge.

Churchland PS (2004)

Damasio AR (1994). *Descartes' Error: Emotion, Reason and the Human Brain*. London: Picador.

Davidson D (1980). *Mental Events: Essays on Actions and Events*. Oxford: Clarendon Press.

Farah MJ (2002). Emerging ethical issues in neuroscience. *Nature Neuroscience* 5, 1123–9.

Farah MJ, Wolpe PR (2004). Monitoring and manipulating brain function: new neuroscience technologies and their ethical implications. *Hastings Center Report* **34**, 34–45.

Farwell and Donchin (1991). The truth will out: Interrogative Polygraphy ('lie-detection') with event-related potentials, *Psychophysiology* **28**, 531–547.

Flanagan O (2002). *The Problem of the Soul: Two Visions of the Mind and How to Reconcile Them*. New York: Basic Books.

Greene J, Cohen J (2004). For the law, neuroscience changes nothing and everything. *Philosophical Transactions of the Royal Society of London, Series B* **359**, 1775–1885.

Hart AJ, Whalen PJ, Shin LM, McInerney SC, Fischer H, Rauch SL (2000). Differential response in the human amygdala to racial outgroup vs ingroup face stimuli. *Neuroreport* **11**, 2351–5.

Held V (1996). Whose Agenda? Ethics versus Cognitive Science. In L. May, M. Friedman and A. Clark eds. Mind and Morals: Essays on Ethics and Cognitive Science, MIT Press, Cambridge, 6–87.

Hume D (1739). *A Treatise of Human Nature* (ed. Selby-Bigge LA). Oxford: Clarendon Press, 1967.

Illes J (2003). Neuroethics in a new era of neuroimaging. *American Journal of Neuroradiology* **24**, 1739–41.

Illes J (2004). A fish story? Brain maps, lie detection and personhood. *Cerebrum* **6**, 73–80.

Illes J, Racine E (2005). Imaging or imagining? A neuroethics challenge informed by genetics. *American Journal of Bioethics* **5**, 1–14.

Illes J, Raffin TA (2002). Neuroethics: an emerging new discipline in the study of brain and cognition. *Brain and Cognition* **50**, 341–4.

Illes J, Kirschen M, Gabrieli JD (2003). From neuroimaging to neuroethics. *Nature Neuroscience* **6**, 205.

Johnson M (1993). *Moral Imagination: Implications of Cognitive Science for Ethics*. Chicago, IL: University of Chicago Press.

Kass L (2003). *Beyond Therapy: Biotechnology and the Pursuit of Happiness*. New York: Harper Collins.

Knight J (2004). The truth about lying. *Nature* **428**, 692–694.

Kulynych J (2002). Legal and ethical issues in neuroimaging research: human subjects protection, medical privacy, and the public communication of research results. *Brain and Cognition* **50**, 345–57.

Langleben DD, Schroeder L, Maldjian JA, *et al.* (2002). Brain activity during simulated deception: an event-related functional magnetic resonance study. *NeuroImage*, **15**, 727–732.

Libet B (1985). Unconscious cerebral initiative and the role of conscious will in voluntary action. *Behavioral and Brain Sciences* **8**, 529–66.

McGinn C (1993). *The Problem of Consciousness*. Oxford: Blackwell.

Macmillan M (2004). The Phineas Gage homepage. http://www.deakin.edu.au/hbs/GAGEPAGE/ (accessed 22 April 2005).

May L, Friedman M, Clark A (eds) (1996). *Mind and Morals: Essays on Ethics and Cognitive Science*. Cambridge, MA: MIT Press.

Moore GE (1902). *Principia Ethica*. London: Prometheus Books, 1988.

Moreno JD (2003). Neuroethics: An agenda for neuroscience and society. *Nature Reviews Neuroscience* **4**, 149–53.

Morse SJ (2004). *Neuroscience and the Law: Brain, Mind, and the Scales of Justice*. New York: Dana Press.

Nagel T (1974). What's is it like to be a bat? *Philosophical Review* **83**, 435–50.

Nagel T (1986). *The View From Nowhere*. New York: Oxford University Press.

Parens E (1998). *Enhancing Human Traits: Ethical and Social Implications*. Washington, DC: Georgetown University Press.

Phelps EA, O'Connor KJ, Cunningham WA, *et al.* (2000). Performance on indirect measures of race evaluation predicts amygdala activation. *Journal of Cognitive Neuroscience* **12**, 729–38.

Raine A, Meloy JR, Bihrle S, *et al.* (1998). Reduced prefrontal and increased subcortical brain functioning assessed using positron emission tomography in predatory and affectivemurderers. *Behavioral Science and Law* **16**, 319–32.

Ramachandran VS (2003). *The Emerging Mind*. London: Profile Books.

Roskies A (2002). Neuroethics for the new millenium. *Neuron* **35**, 21–3.

Wolpe RP, Langleben DD, Foster, K (2005). Emerging neurotechnologies for lie detection: promises and perils. *American Journal of Bioethics* **5**, 15–26.

Chapter 5

# Being in the world: neuroscience and the ethical agent

Laurie Zoloth

## Introduction

As the science of neurobiology increases our understanding of how the brain sees, organizes,.and communicates, our ability to unravel the puzzle of consciousness is fundamentally altered. Consciousness is at once the most elusive and most encumbered of intellectual concepts in philosophy and religion, for the nature of ipsity, the nature of subjectivity, and the nature of memory are all implicated in its description. For the ethicist, however, the problem of being a being in the world is not only how to describe the innately private qualia in language that is public, but also how to describe and then discern between the rational actions that moral agents take. Consciousness is interesting for the philosopher, for whom the existence of persons, the nature of reality, and the nature of matter are imperative notions. It is critical for the ethicist as well, for understanding the self is improbable without understanding the self as a moral agent, capable of the interesting free will and the capacity for good and evil.

This chapter will summarize several classic arguments about consciousness and the nature of the mind, it will argue that a coherent view of consciousness will include a way to understand memory and rational action, and it will suggest areas for future research on ethics in a world in which traditional ideas about duty, covenant, ipsity, and relationality are rapidly being re-understood in biological terms. It is my contention that ethics depends on narrative structures that give meaning to norms. Hence the way that minds (and brains, to be precise) structure story and rule is critical to how we know and discern. At the core of this is memory and motive, yet for the ethicist, it will be the publicity of the moral gesture, the play out in history and social space, that is the final criterion of what beings mean to one another. In a world that is fundamentally hospitable, our question is how the autonomous self that is so determinative in ethics is newly understood and hence newly shaped by emerging science. The ten classic arguments I will summarize are Descartes, Russell, Parfit, Skinner, Armstrong, Nagel, Dewey, James, Searle and Koch. The core ethical problem I will explore is the problem of the moral meaning of reduction: if the self is a place in the brain, which can be mapped genomically and imaged by MRI and CT scans, then it can be altered by design or deliberacy, and what are the consequences of this for our moral imagination? There are four related ways to explore these core ethical issues: memory, agency, morality, and justificatory sentences.

## Selected Classic Arguments

### Descartes

All accounts of what it means to be conscious begin with noting the seminal contributions of René Descartes. Prior to Descartes (1596–1650), the texts of the self, perception of phenomena, the sense of being aware were primarily expressed religiously, largely attributing such a sense to the nature of the embodied person, whose soul, or *nefesh* (literally 'breath') was an attribute of his non-animal connection to God. For members of faith traditions, what was at stake was the nature of our limited mortal self. Increasingly, in the medieval period, the problem called the mind–body problem arises. How is it that the soul, or species-being, or self inhabits the actual animal body of the human person? The tension between the nature of logos and the nature of the corporeal troubled the medieval mind, especially when the aspirational goals of faith seemed so far from the world of scarcity, death, plague, and desire. Descartes, thinking both rationally (seeking to base the argument for one's own existence in a primary knowable fact) and politically (seeking to allow a science of the material body and fact-based world to proceed) posited a finality: a cognito. This cognito was a thinking being, aware of his own perceptions and rational arguments. How to know that one's senses are not deceiving one? How to know if one is awake or dreaming?

> Thought is an attribute that belongs to me; it alone is inseparable from my nature. I am, I exist—that is certain; but for how long do I exist? For as long as I think; for it might perhaps happen, if I totally ceased thinking, that I would at the same time completely cease to be...I am therefore to speak precisely, only a thinking being, that is to say, a mind, an understanding, or a reasoning being....a thing that thinks. (Descartes 1641)

The mind or cognito was not like the body, but in relationship to the body, this mind–body split (dualism) allowed for Church doctrine of an afterlife to proceed along with developments in medicine, and allowed for a flourishing spiritualism, a deep belief in supernaturalism, and a profound account of reward and punishment well into the nineteenth century.

### James and Dewey

For American pragmatists of the mid-nineteenth century, the expanding realm of science challenged fundamental ideas of theism and society. James was among the first to understand how the new study of cognition would impact on philosophy, i.e. how the study of the physical brain would impact on the study of wisdom, knowledge, and the experience of experience. For James, the theory of 'reflex action' will 'trace new consequences'.

> ...The acts we perform are always the result of outward discharges from the nervous centers, and that these outward discharges are themselves the result of impressions from the external world, carried on along one or another of our sensory nerves...every action, whatever, even the most deliberately weighed and calculated does, so far as its organic conditions go, follow the reflex type....The only use of the thought...is to determine the direction to whichever of these organs shall, on the whole, under the circumstances actually present, act in the way most propitious to our welfare. The willing department of our nature, in short, dominates both the conceiving department and the feeling department; or in plainer English, perception and thinking are only there for behavior's sake. (James 1881)

American pragmatists were intrigued with the biological basis both for perception and for the language that set meaning into signs for perceived objects. For Dewey, this fact of language allowed for acts of aesthetic and interpretive meaning, drawn from experiential cognition. For Dewey, the quintessential moment that defined consciousness was the 'having' of the experience.

> Experience occurs continuously, because the interaction of live creatures and environing conditions is involved in the very process of living. Under conditions of resistance and conflict, aspects and elements of the self and the world that are implicated in this interaction qualify as experience with emotions and ideas so that conscious intent emerges. (Dewey 1881)

But such consciousness is only real to us, complete to us, when it is 'fulfilled'. In this, Dewey means something like 'becomes a narrative with meaning'. It is then 'An Experience'. Consciousness for these thinkers is 'not just doing and undergoing in alternation but in relationship'. This idea—that the reflex action must be organized, patterned, and in a sense renegotiated to be called into awareness opens the door for later research on memory. James and Dewey set the stage for the malleability of consciousness. For Dewey, this would take the form of education via empirical method. For both James and Dewey, consciousness is 'a continuous stream of consciousness that involves attention, intentionality and self-awareness. Self-awareness includes both perception, *per se*, and the awareness of experiencing perceptions, often referred to as "qualia" ' (Schwartz 2000).

## Russell

For Bertrand Russell, the core question of mind was to ask if the self was an entity—for if it was, this self could survive death. His seminal essay, written in 1936, is heavily inflected by the problem of Nazism and its competing truth claims about the proper ends of history (Russell 1957). Let us turn to his text. After noting that all cells of the body, all atoms, are constantly in a state of flux and change, merely appearing to be continuous, he notes that the same biological principle applies to the mind.

> We think and feel and act but there is not, in addition to thoughts and feeling and action, a bare entity, the mind or the soul, which does or suffers these occurrences. The mental continuity of a person is a continuity of habit and memory: there was yesterday one person whose feelings I can remember, and that person I regard as myself of yesterday; but in fact, myself of yesterday was only certain mental occurrences which are now remembered and regarded as part of the person who now recollects them. All that constitutes a person is a series of experiences connected by memory and by certain similarities of the sort we call habit. (Russell 1957)

Persons need thinking and acting brains to re-call them; without an event in the future-which-is-now-present, the thinking of the past does not occur. Memory and habit need the physical structure of a brain, much as, notes Russell, 'the river needs a riverbed' (Russell 1957). The body and its integration allow the formation of habits—which for Russell can be shaped, and obliterated. Useful emotions (for Russell, the fear of death) can be cultivated or overcome, and hence what one thinks of as consciousness is the sense memory (habits) or the conscious speaking of memory. For Russell, Darwinism shapes morality as well.

> Our feelings and beliefs on the subject of good and evil are like everything else about us, natural facts developed in the struggle for existence and not having any divine or supernatural origin. (Russell 1957)

Hence his account of the nature of consciousness and the nature of morality are the same: such a being is the being that is needed for existence.

## Parfit

Parfit's reflections on the problem of consciousness begin, he notes, in the study of neuroscience ['It was the split-brain cases which drew me into philosophy' (Parfit 1987)]. He reflects on work by Donald MacKay on how people whose hemispheres are severed surgically can have two perceptions and visual sensations and hence recount two narratives about the nature of reality before them. In reflecting on what this means, Parfit argues that it is evident that there are not two persons, nor one person, but no 'person' at all. For Parfit, as for Russell, consciousness is not an ego, that would exist without a brain or body; consciousness is a 'bundle' of a long series of mental states, thoughts, sensations, and 'the like' held together by memories, which we then call a life. While we cling to the idea of a self, for Parfit even the self of a self as located in a brain is a fiction that we must 'let go of'. A replica, cell by cell, would work as well—it would be 'you' to the extent that it would match the bundled series of events, yet not 'you' in the sense that we want to mean this.

Consciousness is of interest to Parfit in its unity despite the reality (for him) that ordinary people are 'aware any time, of having several different experiences. Our consciousness is always and already "split" '. Hence, for Parfit, what would matter is merely the perception of continuity of consciousness—for his theory the actual physical structures of the brain are of little importance.

## Skinner

B.F. Skinner extends the work of pragmatism in both his theory of consciousness and his use of education to shape it. Skinner has to incorporate, as do all post-Freudians, the idea of an 'unconscious' along with the early sense of the qualia or consciousness of 'being', and, for Skinner, this is done by positing mental states, some of which are public (shown in action and know to the agent) and some of which are unknown. The idea that there is a self in a real world is also a possible illusion.

> The heart of the behaviorist position on conscious experience may be summed up in this way: seeing does not imply something seen. We acquire the behavior of seeing under stimulation from actual objects, but it may occur in the absence of these objects under the control of other variables. [So far as the world within the skin is concerned it always occurs in the absence of such objects.] (Skinner 1964)

Skinner argues that consciousness is contingent on essentially private sensations, and could only be noted as a set of behaviors. We do not need the world as much as we need the behavior of perceiving the world so as to act upon it.

## Armstrong

As neuroscience continued to expand its methods from the data derived from electrophysiological, genetic, and chemical etiologies, philosophers of consciousness followed closely. Armstrong and others began to argue for a 'materialist theory of mind–brain'.

> For me, then, and for many philosophers who think like me, the moral is clear. We must try to work out an account of the nature of the mind which is compatible with the view that man is nothing but a physico-chemical mechanism'.

In contrast to the behaviorists, this view of consciousness sees behavior as an 'outward manifestation' of this 'inner principle' which brings behavior into being. 'The mind is an inner principle apt for bringing about a kind of behavior'. (Armstrong 1981) Consciousness is:

'nothing but the perception or awareness of the state of our own mind . . . This consciousness of our own inner state may be assimilated to our own mental state and like other perceptions, it may then be conceived of as an inner state or event giving a capacity for selective behavior, in this case selective behavior towards our own mental state . . . consciousness of our own mental state becomes simply scanning of one part of our nervous system by another . . . a self-scanning mechanism in the central nervous system'. (Armstrong 1981)

## Nagel

Yet for Thomas Nagel, and for Colin McGinn, such a 'self-scan' is logically impossible, for consciousness is irreducibly subjective, first person-specific and in this privacy, unlike any other sort of event one could observe in nature using the scientific method.

'This bears directly on the mind–body problem. For if the facts of experience—facts about what it is like for the experiencing organism—are accessible only from one point of view, then it is a mystery how the true character of experience could be revealed in the physical operation of that organism'.

Here there seems to be a troubling problem—the more one relies on evidence, objectivity, and method, the less possible the determination of 'consciousness' seems. For McGinn, such a quest is not only methodologically impossible, it is linguistically, possibly, and causally impossible as well (we will return to this later). Perhaps, argue these theorists, the idea of persons understanding the mind is like 'monkeys understanding particle physics'—surely a difficult rendering for the field (Schwartz 2000). For others, like Dennett, the mind is largely an abstraction—our capacity for mind is in our brains, but not particular to brains—it is a feature of complex information processing systems that likewise cannot understand their own circuitry (Dennett 1992).

## Searle

A related development in our story about consciousness as understood by philosophy is that of the development of artificial intelligence and increasingly sophisticated computers. Dennett and others found the idea of mind as a computer increasingly compelling. Perhaps consciousness, they argued, was like a computer program—very complicated but largely computational, whose output, or sensations, or qualia, were the result of programming by self-updating systems of representations.

For Searle, this account is absurd, and he struggles to construct an account of consciousness that is grounded (as Armstrong) in the physicality of the brain—'neurons, chemistry and genes, for it is all we have to understand consciousness' (J. Searle, 'Consciousness', a debate with A. Wallace at Northwestern University, Evanston, IL, 13 January 2005). For Searle, the way to research consciousness is complex, for it will have to account for much beyond the discovery of rules—it will have to account for values, sense, and meaning, some of which is found in the structure of language, which is, if not inherent, suggested by the sort of structures that brains have. In this, he has increasingly turned to the work of Crick and Koch, in which 'consciousness is an integration of neural activity similar in mechanism to the binding of different aspects of sensation that occurs to produce a unified perception' (Schwartz 2000).

The famous mind–body problem, the source of so much controversy over the past two millennia, has a simple solution. This solution has been available to any educated person since serious work began on the brain nearly a century ago, and in a sense, we all know it to be true. Here it is: mental phenomena are caused by neurophysiologic processes in the brain and are themselves features of the brain...Mental events and processes are as much a part of our biological natural history as are digestion, mitosis, meiosis or enzyme secretion. (Searle 2002)

## Koch, Kandel, Crick, and Edelman

Searle directs us toward neuroscience in the final analysis, telling his readers that philosophers ought now to turn to issues of social theory, as neuroscientists work out the specifics of how the neural correlates of consciousness could be found. Indeed, contemporary work on this topic is proceeding rapidly. Kandel, for example,has identified simple pathways in simple organisms for memory and learning. Others have noted the capacity for the early basic sense of being the subject of a life—the behaviors for defining self from non-self. Finally, Edelman has described the complexities of consciousness as a property of the neural circuitry, the ability for 're-entry' and feedback of stimulation so that it can be integrated and interpreted (Edelman and Tononi 2000).

Crick and Koch argue that the specific site for such activity, called the neural correlate of consciousness (NCC), could be located and studied and have proposed a mechanism and method. By studying the visual cortex, one's finite sense could be used to work out the mechanisms of 'core consciousness'—the perceptions of the here and now (Koch 2004). For Koch, what needs to be explained is:

What is the relation between the conscious mind and the electro-chemical interactions in the body that give rise to it? The puzzle is, how can a physical structure have qualia? (Koch 2004)

## Unanswered questions

In his book on mind and brain, Pinker (1997) sets out six core questions for future research:

- the problem of subjectivity and empathy, or the problem of other minds—how is sentience explained?
- the problem of the self, with worth and identity—how is a self continuous?
- the problem of free will
- the problem of linguistic meaning for finite beings
- the problem of epistemology
- the problem of morality.

Pinker notes, following McGinn, that there are four 'solutions' to these problems, but that none is satisfactory. The first is a belief in faith (which Pinker dismisses without fully explaining the complexities of that claim, to be sure); the second is simply to declare the problem irreducible—a force in the universe akin to say, 'gravity' or 'matter'; the third is to deny that such problems are only constructs of the limits of language; the fourth is to reduce it to mere electrons—describing only the structure and function of the parts of the brain wherein the events of recognition take place (Pinker 1997). Pinker concludes that such problems are 'cognitively closed' to us, as many aspects are closed to other perfectly nice conscious animals (like algebra to golden retrievers, as far as we can tell.) Pinker ends his book, as do Koch (2004) and Kandel et al. (2000), with the sort of description that I have provided by my brief and partial summary of the history of the problem—it is the logical way to conclude, yet I will argue that it may still leave us room for a fruitful exploration of some other concerns in bioethics.

## What else needs to be explained? What ought we to question?

If neuroscience can bring us to this point in our story, 'fleshing out', as it were, the narrative begun by the identification of the cognito and proceeding to the NCC, what is now left to do for ethicists who watch science? Let me suggest some fruitful directions for further research.

First, the obvious: bioethics comes of age along with the insights of modern neuroscience and this means that the field is pulled along with several theories of knowledge. Such theories bear directly on our ability to have a field—for what is epistemology, if we cannot understand discernment? What is narrative ethics if we cannot trust memory (S. Rubin S and L. Zoloth, 'Recovered memory and the problem of truthful telling', presented at Society for Health and Human Values Annual Conference, San Diego, CA, 1997)? What are we to make of the formation of rules and norms, much less law and regulation, if we cannot agree on the nature of free will?

Secondly, also plainly expressed in the first literature of 'neuroethics' is the problem of regulation. Long a feature of all research ethics, the problem is that if one can understand how behavior or cognition works, then one can manipulate it toward specific ends. If the controlling entity is malevolent then classic problems, such as those identified by Foucault and others, emerge: How can a Kafkaesque state, or indeed the sort of state that did emerge historically in totalitarian regimes, keep from using new powers of understanding cognition to enslave or coerce? The classic response to this problem was first articulated in post-Nuremberg codes, and has been carefully delineated in the literature on informed refusal and consent. Linked to the problem of a coercive state that might use neurobiology to confound or control a newly found NCC is the problem that a cunning marketplace might seduce one's NCC for manipulative ends. This issue too is not new, for every novel insight about neurobiology and cognition has indeed been used for manipulation, seduction, and persuasion. It is a premise as old as art, when illusion, masks, and theater made use of the brain's ability for narrative over gaps— a feature of all fiction.

Thirdly, several authors have raised as an ethical issue that problem of the reduction—that if we understand consciousness to be neurally correlated, we destroy our humanness, our wonder, our quirky human mystery. For such authors as Alan Wallace, the taboo of science is the taboo of subjectivity, and hence science is not fully equipped to lead such a discovery. Such a mystery is best understood by, for example, monks in the meditative tradition whose praxis of inward reflection may reveal the ontology of the mind. Reducing this task to neuronal firing, goes this argument, thins the task into meaninglessness. Searle has a forceful response to this, noting that this was precisely what an earlier generation held to be the case about the mechanism of biological life, and Watson has made such a point about the way that generations inherit traits, or viruses mutate and transform, all equally mysterious and seemingly sacred or magic activity best left to those concerned with spirituality. Here, the use of functional MRI (fMRI) is questioned and needs to be further researched.

Finally, concern has been raised about the dangers of enhancement to our consciousness— and here, perhaps, the strongest concern about the search for consciousness is at stake. At play in this debate are the concerns about enhancement via gene therapy—in neuroethics literature, the concern centers on selective serotonin-reuptake inhibitors (SSRIs), implantable devices, and memory 'chips' or proteomics, as well as on genetic manipulation (see also Chapters 6 and 13). Yet the philosophic arguments made in the earlier enhancement debate are the same. Are natural limits natural? Should individuals be able to choose what characteristics or physicalities they want? Should the marketplace or a separate system of justice prevail in such cases?

Most ethicists can agree on two central things. First, unlike Kant, whose final ethical question about a social practice could be said to be 'For what can I hope?', in our era, one fraught with anxiety, the question must also be 'For what must I fear?' It is not absurd in the twenty-first century to have doubts about science, and such doubts and skepticism are not marks of superstition or ignorance. Secondly, ethicists call for oversight and transparency in research— I might call this 'open source/open telos' for the data ought to emerge from all corners of the bright and curious world, and the ends ought to be openly debated as well.

These concerns are not new, nor are their solutions—they have been so well articulated in earlier literature about basic research questions that they will stand us in good stead as we turn to what many now claim is the new core question. How will the combined insights of molecular biology, especially neurobiology and behavioral genetics, affect our regard for our neighbor, the question of ethics, and the public life? What then, could be said to be *de novo* questions in neuroethics? Below are notes toward an answer

## Memory and the truly perceived story

For narrative ethicists, the central possibility of the self in the world rests on the ability of the self to have memory, for the sense to carry about stories, as a person is a collection of narrative events that both are remembered and that have instantiated this by the growth of a plasticity of neurons (Zoloth 2000; E. Kandel, 'Learned fear responses', Childs Foundation Plenary Lecture, 2004).

> For many of us, myself included, the central question in philosophy at the beginning of the 21st century is how to give an account of ourselves as apparently conscious, mindful, free, rational, speaking, social and political agents in a world that science tell us consists entirely of mindless, meaningless, physical particles. Who are we and how do we fit into the rest of the world? How does human reality relate to the rest of reality? ... What does it mean to be human? (Searle 2004)

I would argue that there are also three central questions in bioethics, and in science. What does it mean to be human? What does it mean to be free? What must I do about the suffering of the other? Much of bioethics explores the third problem—but if one begins, as Searle argues, in 'first philosophy' the first two problems precede the last one. Edelman cogently raises another terrain for further ethical reflection: 'In addition to providing an analysis of causation and the phenomenal transform, theory of consciousness must account for subjectivity' (Edelman 2004). If the self has subjectivity it is possessive of both verticality (the simultaneous awareness of many states in the remembered present at once) and horizontality (the sense of being-in-time, the sense of having both long term memories and an ability to plan, the sense of memory being vital to the idea of being the subject of a life, being the 'witness' to the scenes that unfold) in thought.

But memory itself is at stake in much of brain research. If indeed memory and the ability to consider long- and short-term memory can be mapped and if the brain likewise is so well designed that it can create narratives over gaps, then the validity and veritude of the self can be called into serious question. Social behavior endures a certain deception in some regards; one can, for example, use make-up or hair dye to deceive. But ethical behavior is assumed to respect the boundaries of an authentic self, with a coherent and actual set of remembered and exchanged narratives. Will new research in memory change what we think of as the self? Is a portion of our selves the ability to forget as we move in chronological distance from events? If we are able to retain more of the remembered past, would the remembered present be fundamentally altered? We can look historically at this issue for some reassurance, for every technology—starting with writing, the most basic of all technologies—has indeed altered our ability to remember. Painting, and later photography, redefines our sense of what we can remember, and what we understand as remembered. To a large extent, I would argue that ethical issues may track the same routes. We will be altered (as anyone can tell you whose memory of an event in childhood is actually the photograph of the event), but we are still humans.

## Rational agency and the oddity of the unconscious

Ethics needs rational moral agents, or what is the point of a good argument? Some have raised fears that research in neuroscience, and especially the search for an NCC, threatens to undermine this concept, or replace it with a reductionist sense that the brain is a machine with parts that can be analyzed and described. In this, the underlying feat is an assault on the freedom of will, which is to say, the freedom to choose behavior. If we come to understand much of behavior as work of the social brain, and if we understand consciousness itself as how genes make proteins that drive cellular processes in a particular way that leads to behaviors, it appears that we have a thin account of being and agency.

Yet, we are caught in a paradox. Most reasonable participants in current academic debates would agree that there is such a concept as social brain activity, and that brains differ in behaviors and capacities. Further, all human primates have to express consciousness in chemical and biological processes—genes and proteins. Thus there is a particular power in the search for the places in the mind/brain that quite literally are the site of acts, for if we hope to study and research, even to describe the truth of action or moral gesture, much less if we hope to cure disabilities in that capacity, we must begin with a clear description of the structure and function therein.

Searle has noted the oddity of the fact that sometimes acts can occur without intent, and struggles with the problem of how the unconscious processes affect our behavior. For Hume, Freud, Gilligan, and the entire psychoanalytic tradition, the role of emotions, both overt and covert, are critical, and disorders of thought and emotion are the largely assumed subject of much of the medical research on the brain and its function. The human brain functions as an automatic, as a willed, and as a passion-filled entity. Ethics traditionally rests on the assumption of a rational argument as being critical to discerning, judging, and acting. Yet learning more about how the unconscious works may lead us to question this, leading to complex questions about our relationship to other non-human primates and the nature of our dominance over them. Hence we have our second ethical question. What is the nature of the unconscious motive, and can it be all made rational by the descriptive power of science? Here, we might thoughtfully turn to the new work in neuroimaging. In the weeks just before this chapter was written, a cascade of papers about fMRI was released, including one that described persons in permanently (as far as could be discerned clinically) unconscious states as having identical fMRI results to those of conscious persons when a relative spoke to them about visual memories. Such results raise the problem to one with higher stakes: should we regard the non-responsive non-awake person as unconscious if his brain activity is indistinguishable from that of conscious persons?

## What makes a right act right? Justificatory reflections

If Searle notes a category of acts for which there is no intent, Hegel notes that intentions without acts do not actually 'exist' in a moral sense, for they can never be made public, and hence real. For Hegel, and for much of moral philosophy and bioethics, the interesting question is how the intention leads to action—in this sense, why consciousness matters only in its negation, in that the action is the negation, or bringing into being, the being of being (Pippen, 'How to live a moral life', Northwestern University, Evanston, IL, 2005). Justificatory action is the measure of consciousness, and it is the combination of prior historical reality and practical reason that justify our intentions, only when they have reality in the nouminal world of object acted upon. For Hegel, human beings are not primarily ontological, which is not to say that they are not conscious, but that they are primarily historical–physical: 'true being is in deed, not in intention'. The deed or consciousness in the world, is also for itself—it is a display of one's ipsity in view of universality. Hence what makes conscious action important is that it creates a subject matter for others to witness and to discern and to judge (Pippen R, 'How to live a moral life', Northwestern University, Evanston, IL, 2005). Such an act is assented to, and if many such acts are committed, they become norms—yet each is particular for it is consciousness made visible, created into agency.

For philosophers, the problem of rational agency has long been linked to the study of phenomenology, and in particular the work of Edmund Husserl, father of the field. For Husserl, philosophy itself is a descriptive activity; the mind can only be described in terms of the gaze on that which is actually in the world. Yet, to describe consciousness, one must think about this without prior assumptions, or categories of a priori thought (Schmitt 1967).

All mental acts are intentional—they cannot include the existence of the object in their description. 'We discover that whatever is in the world is only as an object for our pure consciousness'. Husserl called this ability to bracket, or suspend one's sense of the physical world as having fixities and value, 'epoche'. Note that it was a suspension not a denial of the existence of the real, for the real world is not a fiction; it is only bracketed for the purpose of analysis, and this is most clearly the case when the object of study is one's own mind. Knowing means seeing (noesis)—not only seeing in the visual sense, but understanding the physical world in its actuality—in its daily ordinariness, in its facticity ['Back to the thing itself!' (Kohak 1978)]. Like the Pierce sense of being—all that is real and all that is illusion, all that is presented to the mind is nousminal—what is interesting for phenomenologists is not only the noumena but the noesis, the seeing and not only the seen object.

For Husserl (1913), what was at stake was the relationship between the noesis (his word for the perceiving itself) and the noema (that thing perceived). Hence the noesis, to the extent that it is a factor in neurobiology, recalls for us that the problem of correlation is a fundamental one with a long prior account in philosophy. Husserl also explores the problem of how meaning, and an analysis of 'sentiment and violation', might provide a way to understand the making of value in a relative sense (Schmitt 1967).

Here, we begin to grasp why I noted that the ethical issues of consciousness and the search for a neurobiological explanation of it was encumbered by the philosophical tradition. Here, too, is our third ethical problem: To what extent is consciousness a justificatory description of moral action?

## Good and evil in the NCC

In 1935, the young Emmanuel Levinas, the closest disciple of Martin Heidegger, whose *Being and Time* Levinas would bring to the French Academy, faced a time of growing crisis. Heidegger would join the Nazi Party. A year earlier, Levinas had published a political essay on the dangers of fascism. Neither politics nor Heidegger is mentioned in this work; it is an essay on the problem of being, and the inescapability of the facticity of the self in the body. There is a sense of being that is akin to being 'thrown-in' to the world—the term that Levinas uses is 'dereliction' or 'abandonment to imposed possibilities...that gives to human existence its character of a *fact* in the strongest and most dramatic sense of the term, in relation to which the empirical facts of the sciences are but derivative' (Levinas 1935). The essay *On Escape* first describes the problem of achieving a theory of consciousness.

> The revolt of traditional philosophy against the idea of being originates in the discord between human freedom and the brutal fact of being that assaults this freedom. The conflict from which the revolt arises opposes man to the world, not man to himself. The simplicity of the subject lies beyond the struggles that tear it apart, and that, within man, set the 'I' against the 'non-I' which—when purified of all of that is not authentically human in it—is given to peace with itself, completes itself, closes on and rests upon itself. . . . (Levinas 1935)

Yet this self-referential self is no longer possible in modernity, he argues, for to understand being now is to understand the immediacy and 'rivetedness' of qualia—to the very experience of 'pure being'. Such a realization brings about the yearning for an escape from being, yet there is no escape—not in pleasure, and not in death (it is, after all, 1935). To become aware of consciousness in the twentieth century was to understand the impossibility of German idealism or of transcendence—we are beings, in existence, rooted to the physical body.

In later works, after Levinas has been imprisoned in and liberated from the camps of the Second World War, he will write of how the yearning to escape can only be sought in the being-for-the-other that ethics, not ontology, will describe. For Levinas, the problem of the theory of consciousness will be the ethical gesture—ethics will be 'first philosophy'. Levinas will come to ask the third question first—what must I do about the suffering of the other—and come to understand this question as providing the ground for the essence of existence itself. To escape is to be 'otherwise than being', to be 'for the other'.

For bioethicists who watch neuroscience uncover the boundaries of the 'rivetedness' of the brain to mind, and who explore how to describe the quality of 'thrown into the middleness of things' that so destabilized modern philosophy, the ethical issue will be the most compelling. A theory of consciousness will have to carry the water for the usual work of much of religion and morality—it will have to describe the processes, structure, and function not only of first-order events (the ability to follow rapid movement selectively, the ability to create short- and long term memories) but also of second-order phenomena (the ability to make choices we understand as moral). For this, we will need complex theories of being that include how beings choose evil and how we choose to create good, and why it is the case that this ability is linked to what we think of as thinking itself. Can we study where, why, and how the choice for altruism, or fairness, or honesty is made? Could it be that we could learn enough to do that which all faiths and all moral philosophies aspire—to shape the virtues of the good moral life?

Much remains to be learned about the brain, and the theory of consciousness is perhaps the most elusive. The shaping of the research questions themselves will suggest new possibilities. Finding an NCC for beingness will help us to understand what is physically required for discernment, judgment, and moral action itself. This last question will be the most challenging for bioethics. When we can explain how it looks and how it operates, will the tasks of ethics be altered? Can we ask how to be good, or how am I justified, in new ways that are clear about what we have learned now and honest about what we still need to learn. Just as finding the DNA structure of life and the transmission of the chemical possibilities of the self marked the beginning of understanding how beings inherit such possibilities and inevitabilities, finding the NCC structure and functions may help us to understand what Levinas calls the 'pluralities' of being. It may be like a sort of sudden sight—a puzzling array of choices, calling for a new sort of training in the patterns of our acts. In this way, all of neuroscience's yearning for solutions is a sort of escape, and yet, for ethicists, it will be a false escape unless it is captive to the other— captive to the great task of attention to the suffering of the other and its healing. Neuroscience's search for consciousness is a quest close to ethics' search for the formulation of the moral agents, and this is fraught with peril and with risk, as Levinas notes.

However, to read philosophy historically, as I have done with you in this chapter, allows for optimism, for the history of philosophy of being is an ongoing renegotiation of speculation with science, states, and history. At each juncture, we are called upon, as moral philosophers, to provide caution and linguistic remapping—for thinking about being and choosing is to provide a witness to both the research and our concern about the research. Ultimately, this witnessing is our best stance. We can neither do the work, nor stop the work—we can insist/ promise only on our presence in the inescapably ethical venture of neuroscience itself.

# References

Armstrong D (1981). The nature of mind. In: *The Nature of Mind and Other Essays*. Ithaca, NY: Cornell University Press.

Dennett D (1992). *Consciousness Explained*. Back Bay Books.

Descartes R (1641) Second meditation. In: *Meditations on First Philosophy* (trans Lafleur L). New York: Bobbs-Merrill, 1964; 81–91.

Dewey J (1881). Art as experience. In: Capps J, Capps D (eds) *James and Dewey on Belief and Experience*. Chicago, IL: University of Illinois Press, 2005; 274.

Edelman G (2004). *Wider than the Sky*. New Haven, CT: Yale University Press.

Edelman G, Tononi G (2000). *A Universe of Consciousness*. New York: Basic Books.

James W (1881) Reflex action and theism. In: Capps J, Capps D (eds) *James and Dewey on Belief and Experience*. Chicago, IL: University of Illinois Press, 2005; 45–9.

Husserl E (1913) reprinted 1990). Ideas, general introduction to pure phenomenology. In: Magill F (ed) *Masterpieces of World Philosophy*, New York: HarperCollins, 1990; 502–5.

Kandel ER, Schwartz JH, Jessell TM (eds) (2000). *Principles of Neural Science* (4th edn). New York: McGraw-Hill.

Koch C (2004). *The Quest for Consciousness: A Neurobiological Approach*. Englewood, CO: Roberts.

Kohak E (1978). Idea and experience: Edmund Husserl's project of phenomenology in ideas I. In: Magill F (ed) *Masterpieces of World Philosophy*, New York: HarperCollins, 1990; 505–7.

Levinas E (1935) 2003). *On Escape* (trans B. Bergo). Stanford, CA: Stanford University Press, 2003.

Parfit D (1987). Divided minds and the nature of persons. In: Blakemore C, Greenfield S (eds) *Mindwaves*. New York: Blackwell, 19–26.

Pinker S (1997). *How the Mind Works*. New York: Norton.

Russell B (1957). Do we survive death? In: *Why I am not a Christian*. New York: Simon and Schuster, 88–93.

Schmitt R (1967). Edmund Husserl. In: Edwards P (ed) *Encyclopedia of Philosophy*. New York: Macmillan.

Schwartz J (2000). Consciousness and neurobiology of the twenty first century. In: Kandel ER, Schwartz JH, Jessell TM (eds) *Principles of Neural Science* (4th edn). New York: McGraw-Hill, 1317–20.

Searle J (1982). The myth of the computer. *New York Review of Books*, 29 April.

Searle J (1995). The mystery of consciousness. *New York Review of Books*, 2 November, 16 November.

Searle J (2002). *The Rediscovery of the Mind*. Cambridge, MA: MIT Press.
Searle J (2004). *Mind*. Oxford: Oxford University Press.
Skinner BF (1964). Behaviorism at fifty. In Wann TW (ed) *Behaviorism and Phenomenology: Contrasting Bases for Modern Psychology*. Chicago, IL: University of Chicago Press.
Zoloth L (2003). '13 ways of Looking at a Blackbird: Ethics and Consciousness'.

Chapter 6

# Creativity, gratitude, and the enhancement debate

Erik Parens

## Introduction

Roskies has helpfully distinguished between what she calls 'the ethics of neuroscience' and 'the neuroscience of ethics' (Roskies 2002, see also Chapter 2). The 'ethics of neuroscience' explores questions that are now familiar to bioethicists and neuroscientists. Among these are questions concerning the ethical conduct of neuroscientific research involving human subjects and questions concerning the ethical, social, and legal implications of the new products that such basic research will give rise to. What, for example, are the implications of neuroscience-based technologies aimed at enhancing human traits and capacities? Bioethicists have asked such 'ethics of neuroscience' questions since the inception of the field (Ramsey 1970; Fletcher 1974; Murray *et al.* 1984; Glover 1984). The enhancement issue in particular has enjoyed increasing attention over the last decade (Walters and Palmer 1997; Parens 1998; Buchanan *et al.* 2000; Elliott 2003; President's Council on Bioethics 2003).

'The neuroscience of ethics' asks questions that hitherto have largely been foreign to bioethicists. Most bioethicists have thought of themselves as engaging in the rational work of articulating the difference between strong and weak reasons for a given position or action. However, the 'neuroscience of ethics' takes that view of ethics to be at best incomplete. The neuroscientists and philosophers who now consider 'the neuroscience of ethics' are interested in what is happening at the level of the neuron when persons decide what counts as a strong or weak reason for a given moral position or action (Greene *et al.* 2001). They are interested in the pre-rational processes that gain expression in such decisions.

What I want to discuss in this chapter is by no means perfectly analogous to what those neuroscientists and philosophers are doing. However, in an important respect it is closer to what they are doing than it is to what bioethicists are doing when, for example, they argue for or against this or that enhancement technology. Like those neuroscientitsts and philosophers considering the neuroscience of ethics, I am also interested in what is at work when bioethicists take different positions when they debate about, for example, enhancement technologies. Specifically, I am interested in trying to describe what I will call the different ethical frameworks that many scholars tend to operate from when they engage in academic battle over the enhancement question.

When I say frameworks, I am talking about constellations of interlocking intuitions and reasons which support and shape our responses to questions about, among many other things, new enhancement technologies. When I refer to those different frameworks as ethical, I use that term in its broadest possible sense, as designating **habits** of thought and being. If it were a more felicitous neologism, I would use something like 'psycho-ethical framework' to emphasize that these frameworks have an important psychological dimension. We tend to feel more comfortable in one framework than in the other.

While I want to insist that reasons alone do not explain why we feel more comfortable in one framework than the other, I am also deeply interested in the different reasons and arguments that are offered from the different frameworks. Indeed, in most of this chapter I will explore the different reasons that tend to be articulated from the different frameworks. However, before I turn to those reasons, I want to offer a preliminary suggestion about how to think about the nature of and relationship between the two frameworks.

## Two intimately related frameworks

Elsewhere I have suggested that when we try to understand the nature of, and relationship between, the different frameworks out of which people tend to operate when they debate about enhancement technologies, it helps to bring to mind the image of a single figure in a well-known book (Parens 2005).

You may recall or heard mention of the passage in Genesis, when Jacob's wife Rachel, who was unable to bear children, enjoins him: 'Give me children, or I shall die' (Gen. 30: 1). Famously, Jacob responded to Rachel's injunction with a question: 'Am I in the place of God?' (Gen. 30: 2). With his question Jacob expresses one of the book's central and best-known ideas: that human beings are not the creators of life; that they are creatures, whose job is to remember that life is a gift. It is our responsibility to express our gratitude for the mysterious whole, which we have not made. Moreover, it is our job to be wary of efforts to transform that gift. We need to learn to let things be.

I hasten to add that this sort of attitude does not require a commitment to any particular religious tradition, or indeed to any religion at all. Many an environmentalist (like Bill McKibben) adopts such an attitude. Many a left-leaning critic of corporatization (like Richard Hayes) adopts it. Michael Sandel invokes the secular version of this idea when he writes: 'If bioengineering made the myth of the "self-made man" come true, it would be difficult to view our talents as gifts for which we are indebted, rather than as achievements for which we are responsible' (Sandel 2004). In Sandel's words we can discern the sort of view symbolized by Jacob's question: If we forget that life is a gift—albeit from an unknown giver—we will make a mistake about the sorts of creatures we really are and the way the world really is. Again, on this sort of view, it is our responsibility to affirm the given, to let things be.

However, this very same Jacob, who exhibits this gratitude that many today associate with religion, also exhibits a radically different stance, which the book also celebrates. After all, as has been remarked more than once, Jacob, the very one whose name would become Israel, was the first genetic engineer. He was the one with the creativity to fashion a device ['rods of poplar and almond, into which he peeled white streaks' (Gen. 30: 37)] to transform the generations of his uncle's sheep and goats.

According to Genesis, and it seems to me much of Judaism, it is not only our responsibility to be grateful, to remember that we are not the creators of the whole. It is also our responsibility to be creative, to use our creativity to mend and transform ourselves and the world. As far as I can tell, Genesis, and at least one of the traditions it helped to create, does not exhort us to choose between gratitude and creativity. Rather, or so it seems to this pagan, it is our job to figure out how to maintain that fertile tension, working to insure that neither pole exerts too great or too small a force.

When we observe scholars and others debating 'enhancement technologies', I am suggesting that we often see people who have, at least for the moment, settled into either the gratitude or creativity framework. As one side emphasizes our obligation to remember that life is a gift and that we need to learn to let things be, the other emphasizes our obligation to transform that gift and to exhibit our creativity. As one framework emphasizes the danger of allowing ourselves to become, in Heidegger's famous formulation, 'standing reserve', the other emphasizes the danger of failing to summon the courage to, as Nietzsche put it, 'create' ourselves, to 'become who we are'.

I would emphasize several things about this image of two frameworks. First, it is a crude heuristic but, as a veteran of a decade's worth of battle over the enhancement question, I think it can help us to get a purchase on at least one important feature of the debate. Different from the image of the public arena as a neutral space that each of us comes to from nowhere in particular, I am trying to emphasize the particularity of the ethical frameworks out of which we operate. Secondly, by finding both impulses in an influential religious book, I am trying to emphasize that neither side of the enhancement debate relies only on reasons; each of us tends to feel more comfortable in one framework than in the other. Thirdly, by finding the gratitude and creativity impulses in the one figure of Jacob, I am trying to emphasize that none of us feels comfortable in only one framework.

Finally, the difference between those who feel most comfortable in the gratitude framework and those who feel most comfortable in the creativity framework is not the same as the difference between political conservatives and political liberals, or between people who are religious and those who are secular. One can find both conservatives and liberals, and both religious people and secular people, working out of each framework.

Proceeding from the claim that skeptics about enhancement seem most comfortable in the gratitude framework and that proponents seem most comfortable in the creativity framework, I now want to describe some of the different reasons that are articulated from, and thus help to constitute, these two different frameworks.

## Different views about the nature of human interventions into 'Nature'

As the label is meant to suggest, those operating out of the 'gratitude framework' are predisposed to be grateful for, to express their affirmation of, 'the given'. (Again, one can be 'grateful' without claiming to have any knowledge of a 'Giver'!) The first impulse of those most comfortable in the gratitude framework is not to creatively transform what is given, but to let it be. They tend to be humble, if not wary, about the prospect of human interventions into the given, into Nature. Sometimes, if they are not speaking carefully, they even suggest that such interventions would be 'unnatural'.

Insofar as creatively transforming ourselves and the world entails interventions into Nature, and insofar as those most comfortable in what I am calling 'the creativity framework' feel a responsibility to give an ethical account of their actions, they often offer a critique of the sort of humility and/or wariness that is sometimes expressed from the gratitude framework. Sometimes the critique does not consist in much more than an assertion that the putative desire to let things be is really no more than a mask for fear of, or anxiety about, the new. More often, however, arguments are offered which are meant to establish that it is irrational to worry in a general sort of way about human interference into natural processes (Harris 1992).

We can glimpse one of the first such efforts in 1982 in *Splicing Life*, the report of the President's Commission for the Study of Ethical Problems in Medicine and Biomedical and Behavioral Research. Against concerns that genetic engineering represented an important new and worrisome example of human interference into natural processes, the authors of that report suggested the sense in which genetic engineering itself is natural. After all, they observed, 'in nature' one can observe viral DNA being spliced into bacterial genomes; thus 'The basic processes underlying genetic engineering are…natural and not revolutionary' (President's Commission 1982).

A corollary of the argument that interventions like genetic engineering are not unnatural is that, insofar as human beings are themselves part of Nature, it is not rational to say that they interfere with Nature. A third line of argument often offered by those most comfortable in the creativity framework is that, even if there is a sense in which human beings do interfere with Nature, that does not show that something is wrong with such interventions. After all, all of medicine is an intervention in Nature. Indeed, that is what human beings do; we intervene in Nature in ways that further our purposes. Just think of farming the land, damming rivers, getting airplanes off the ground.

Thus, to advance the case for letting things be, those operating out of the gratitude framework need to offer reasons to believe that some human interventions might pose genuine ethical questions. To begin with, they dispute the psychological observation that ethical questions about human interventions are no more than masks for fear and anxiety. They suggest that what is behind their ambition to let things be is a genuine desire to affirm a wide variety of ways of being in the world. If they are fearful, they say that it is only about the prospect of these technologies being used to narrow the range of acceptable ways to be human. They worry, for example, that so-called enhancement technologies will be used mostly to help individuals to live up to dominant conceptions of normality and or perfection (Little 1998).

However, those most comfortable in the gratitude framework offer more than an assertion. They also offer arguments to support their view that we ought to consider letting things be. One of the first of those arguments begins by acknowledging that, as those working out of the creativity framework suggest, human beings are indeed a part of Nature and thus it is not helpful to characterize human interventions as unnatural. However, those working out of the gratitude framework go on to insist that human beings play a special role in the drama of the natural world (Kaebnick 2000). The claim is that human beings and Nature are different sorts of agents. It is true, for example, that over the course of natural history, Nature has produced major extinction events. But, for example, the number of species that became extinct grew exponentially when human beings went from inhabiting the rain forests to harvesting them. Therefore, while large-scale extinctions created by humans may be perfectly natural, it seems that it may sometimes be useful to distinguish between the agency of human beings and the agency of Nature as a whole. Similarly, goes this line of argument from the gratitude framework, it might be useful to distinguish between Nature as the agent of genetic engineering (splicing viral DNA into bacteria) and human beings as the agent (splicing human DNA into human beings). According to this sort of argument, human interventions are all too natural. But, goes this line of argument, instead of pursuing our all too natural short-term interests, we should sometimes consider letting things be (Parens 1995).

Those working from the gratitude framework not only point out that human beings and Nature are different sorts of agents, they also point out that we can and should distinguish between the different purposes of human interventions. Again, if they are reasonable, they need to acknowledge that insofar as virtually all of medicine intervenes in natural processes, intervening in natural processes cannot in principle be ethically troubling. But they want to argue that, even if sometimes it is difficult, we can and should try to distinguish between interventions aimed at medical purposes (e.g. treating or preventing diseases rooted in the body) and interventions aimed at non-medical purposes (e.g. enhancing traits either to promote social success or to reduce suffering rooted in harmful social norms) (Sabin and Daniels 1994).

If they are reasonable, however, those working out of the gratitude framework must appreciate how exceedingly difficult it is to distinguish neatly between: medical and non-medical interventions, between treatment and enhancement, and between disorders rooted in the body and those rooted in the mind or social norms. Is reconstructive surgery after mastectomy a medical or non-medical intervention? Are reading glasses for 40-year-olds a treatment or an enhancement? Is depression rooted in the body or in the mind?

Indeed, many of those working out of the gratitude framework, especially if they are of the progressive critical variety, are not only willing but eager to acknowledge the fuzziness of those distinctions. Criticizing binaries, dichotomies, etc. is their bread and butter. Not only do they have to acknowledge the permeability of those distinctions, but they also have to acknowledge that trying to apply them will in some cases seem unfair. To use a famous example, imagine that you have two boys. One is very short because he has a growth-hormone deficiency disease and the other is very short because his parents are very short. If they are both the same short height, and both suffer the same amount from the discrimination that goes with being short in a 'heightist' culture, would it not be unfair to intervene to make one boy taller and leave the other to suffer (Daniels 1994)?

Reasonable people operating out of the gratitude framework feel the force of this point. They should be eager to say that it would be a mistake to sacrifice the well-being of any individual on the altar of an ideal (like the ideal of fighting discrimination based on height). However, they can say that and insist on calling attention to the possible consequences of using medical means to deal with a problem that is primarily social (Dreger 2004).

Again, those working from the gratitude framework are keen to point out that, were we to change the social norms, we could let the healthy body of the short boy be. And if they are reasonable, they will not want to ban such interventions (thereby making it impossible for the healthy but unusually short boy to access the intervention that promises to ameliorate his suffering). However, they also want to criticize what they take to be the problematic phenomenon that goes by the name of medicalization. Like Goethe, who worried that the world might one day turn 'into one huge hospital where everyone is everyone else's humane nurse', those operating out of the gratitude framework want to caution against letting body-transforming creativity gain the upper hand. They want to remind us that we can also use non-medical means to ameliorate the suffering that besets us. They want to say 'Yes' to modern medicine and they want to warn against letting medicine become, as it were, a cancer.

Those working out of the creativity framework make several objections to the sorts of concerns raised by those working out of the gratitude framework. Next I will focus on one of the most powerful of those objections: that it is incoherent to privilege social means over medical means, or non-technological means over technological ones.

## Different views about the nature of technology

Those working out of the creativity framework point out the respect in which it is a mistake to worry about technological means in general. After all, fire can be used to cook for the hungry or to burn down their shelters. Technology itself, goes this important line of argument, is morally neutral.

Moreover, in variations on the lines of argument above (about all interventions being natural), those operating out of the creativity framework make two further points. First, they observe that it is extremely difficult to distinguish between technological and non-technological means (Brock 1998). If technology is whatever human beings create to help further their purposes, then why, for example, should we not call education a form of technology? Moreover, even if it were possible to distinguish between technological and non-technological means, what would that achieve? Noticing that a means is 'technological' hardly shows that it is somehow ethically troubling! Unless of course we are troubled by eyeglasses that help us to see better, or shoes that help us to walk better, or hearing aids that help us to hear better.

This idea—noticing that a given means is technological cannot alone tell us whether to embrace a given intervention—that is eloquently articulated out of the creativity framework is absolutely correct. It would be a serious mistake for someone in the gratitude framework to miss it. (Unfortunately, missing it is a predictable problem if we are more committed to defending 'our framework' than we are to understanding the question at hand.)

While thoughtful persons in the gratitude framework will grant that core idea, they neither do nor should grant without qualification the argument that technology is morally neutral (Heidegger 1953; Edwards 1997, 2005). They point out the respect in which technology is morally loaded: whether we like it or not and whether we are aware of it or not, the means we use emphasize different values and different understandings of the nature of human beings.

Consider, for example, the debate about using Ritalin to improve classroom performance in children. Those working out of the creativity framework often make some version of the argument from precedent. The inexplicit structure of the argument goes something like this: we have always deemed it ethical to use some means A to achieve some end Z; means B also aims at end Z; therefore means B should not worry anyone. So, for example, we have always deemed it ethical to increase the ratio of teachers to students (means A) to improve student focus and performance (end Z); Ritalin (means B) also aims at improving focus and performance; therefore Ritalin should not worry anyone.

From the point of view of what I have been calling 'the gratitude framework', this form of argument has problems. First, it assumes rather than argues for the view that there is no ethical difference between means A (increasing the teacher–student ratio) and means B (Ritalin). While people working out of the creativity framework are rightly skeptical about the utility of the natural–artificial and non-technological–technological distinctions, their skepticism can obscure their appreciation of the point being advanced by those from the gratitude framework.

The point of the latter is that different means emphasize different values. If we increase the teacher–student ratio to improve the child's performance, we emphasize our commitment to the value of engagement. If we give the child Ritalin to improve his performance, we emphasize our commitment to the value of efficiency. Notice that engagement and efficiency are not mutually exclusive values. Both are important and estimable, but they are different.

Those operating out of the gratitude framework are quick to point out that different means also emphasize different understandings of what it is to be a person. Increasing the teacher–student ratio emphasizes our understanding of persons as dialogical relational creatures; Ritalin emphasizes our understanding of persons as mechanisms. Again, the mechanistic and relational understandings of persons are not mutually exclusive. They are both important and estimable, but they are different. Different means emphasize different understandings.

Those in the gratitude framework would point out that, while those two understandings of persons are not mutually exclusive, the mechanistic understanding seems to enjoy increasing prestige in our culture. As Luhrmann (2000) has pointed out in the context of the treatment of mental illness, everybody agrees that the most effective treatment approach uses a combination of drugs (which emphasize the mechanistic understanding) and talk (which emphasizes the relational understanding); on the ground, however, drugs, along with the value of efficiency and the mechanistic understanding, increasingly tend to crowd out talk, along with the value of engagement and the relational understanding.

The second problem with arguments from precedent is that they take for granted the goodness of our current practices. Those from the creativity framework are prone to argue: 'Look, we already let and even encourage kids to take Stanley Kaplan courses to improve their performance on SATs. What's the problem with kids who aren't sick using a drug like Ritalin to improve their performance?' (Caplan 2002). Thus, even though those operating out of the creativity framework often and for good reason take themselves to be enemies of the status quo (N. Bostrom, unpublished work), insofar as the argument from precedent does not question the goodness of our current practices, it is a friend of the status quo. Needless to say, to the extent that those in the gratitude framework are wary of new interventions, they can also be guilty of what Bostrom has called the 'status quo bias'.

## Different views about the nature of freedom

When people from the two frameworks make different predictions about the results of the proliferation of a given enhancement technology, it is at least in part because they are operating with different views about how free we are to choose our own purposes. Or, perhaps more precisely, they are emphasizing different dimensions of the phenomenon we call choosing.

To the extent that those working out of the creativity framework celebrate the capacity of individuals to create their own life projects as they see fit, they have to assume that humans are indeed free to choose those projects for themselves. Those working out of the creativity framework think that by pursuing their projects of self-creation, individuals will become who they really are—or authentic. According to this line of argument, so-called enhancement technologies are tools with which individuals can engage in their own authentic projects of self-creation (DeGrazia 2004).

Not only do those speaking out of the creativity framework assume that individuals are free to pursue such projects of self-creation, they also assume that if all individuals pursue their own projects, an ever-wider range of human life projects will flourish (Silver 1997; Stock 2002). That is, those who work out of the creativity framework value not only authenticity, but diversity; they think that the best way to promote a wide variety of life projects is to leave individuals to themselves to conceive of their own projects. Their greatest fear is that the state might interfere in such projects.

Those working out of the gratitude framework share a commitment to diversity, but they emphasize the respect in which the freedom of individuals is constrained. They emphasize the extent to which individual choices affect—and are affected by—the choices of others (Bordo 1995; Frank 2004). In other words, they tend to emphasize the extent to which individual choices are always shaped and even constrained by social and cultural forces. They are skeptical about the unqualified view that individuals simply choose for themselves.

For example, when someone reports that he has freely chosen cosmetic surgery, the person working out of the gratitude framework is prone to ask a suspicious question. Are individuals really free when they choose to pay money to put their bodies at risk to make themselves look different than they 'really are'? The person working out of the gratitude framework tends to think that we ought to let our bodies be; we ought to learn to affirm the way we are, not change it. Often, when such a person is moved to give a reason for his intuition that we should let people's bodies be, he will say that he worries that the intervention will separate us from who we really are. The worry is that the intervention will make us 'inauthentic'. To shore up this sort of claim, he will invoke terms like false consciousness, which suggest that, while people think they are free to choose, they are not. Or at least they are not as free as they assume when they avail themselves of the intervention that helps them to live up to some dominant norm. It is a worry about a narrowing of the acceptable ways to be a human being that motivates this sort of argument. At the root of that worry is the desire to affirm the wide variety of ways that humans are thrown into the world.

Thus those working out of the gratitude framework, like those working out of the creativity framework, are also committed to the value of diversity. However, whereas those working out of the creativity framework predict that enhancement technologies will facilitate a widening of the variety of life projects that will proliferate, those working out of the gratitude framework fear the contraction of the same. Just as both sides are committed to authenticity, but make different predictions about whether enhancement technologies will promote or thwart that value, so both sides are committed to diversity, but make different predictions about whether enhancement technologies will promote or thwart it.

## From general frameworks to particular questions

So far, I have tried to suggest that when it comes to reflecting on new enhancement technologies, we tend to feel more comfortable in speaking about them from one of two readily available frameworks. From the gratitude framework, the first impulse is speak on behalf of letting things be. The first worry is that the intervention compromises authenticity, that it might separate us from what is most our own. From the creativity framework, the first impulse is to speak on behalf of the liberating authenticity-promoting potential of the intervention. If we accept my earlier claim that each of those frameworks deserves respect, then we want to know the answer to the following question: Given a possible and particular intervention aimed at enhancement, which framework should carry the day?

I think the answer is: It depends. As lovely as it would be to have a good one-size-fits-all answer to the question, I do not see how we can. The hope of settling down and becoming comfortable in just one framework may be quintessentially human, but it is the foe of thinking. When we come to the discussion of a particular intervention aimed at enhancement, we need to become better at remembering that each framework has much to recommend it. If we could spend less time defending the framework in which we are most comfortable, and more time considering the particular case, we might find that we do not disagree with those from the other framework as much as we tend to assume.

Consider again the case of using a drug like Ritalin to enhance a child's focus in the classroom. When you ask people comfortable in the gratitude framework what they think about using Ritalin to enhance the performance of children, you will hear concerns about, for example, separating young boys from their natural rambunctious tendencies. You will be told that, instead of changing the minds of children with drugs, we should change our expectations of them, and so forth. However, when you ask people most comfortable in the creativity framework you are likely to be reminded about our responsibility to reduce the suffering of children who are not keeping up. They will remind you that improving the performance of children is an essential part of good parenting.

The problem with readily available responses is that, by definition, they do not require thinking. If I am most comfortable in the gratitude framework and trying to persuade you of the goodness of my framework and response, it is all too easy for me to forget, for example, that there are children who will not be able to thrive in any sort of school without the aid of the pharmacological intervention. Insofar as I believe that receiving an education is a crucially important part of being an authentic or flourishing person, I ought to be prepared to bracket my gratitude and remember the virtues of what I have called the creativity framework. It is after all our job to mend where we can, to reduce suffering and promote flourishing where we can. If, on the other hand, I am committed to the creativity framework, it is very easy for me to forget that children are thrown into the world with a huge range of temperaments and learning styles, and that perhaps some interventions will reduce rather than increase the variety of life projects.

If we were to recognize the virtue of the other framework, we might free ourselves up to go beyond readily available responses and begin to think. Indeed, as Jonathan Glover has recently observed, these new technologies force us to think anew about the oldest, most pressing, and most infuriatingly difficult question: What does genuine, as opposed to fake, human flourishing consist in? What sorts of enhancements should we pursue if we are to flourish?

After all, people in the gratitude framework are not against technologies that they think genuinely enhance the lives of children; they are against technologies that appear to enhance, but really impoverish. Similarly, people in the creativity framework are not for interventions that they think will make children worse off; they are for interventions that they think will genuinely enhance children's lives.

In other words, the debate is not really about whether enhancement (or enhancement technologies) is good or bad, but about whether a given intervention produces a genuine enhancement. Surely, reasonable people will disagree about the nature of the difference between genuine and fake enhancements. But what I want to insist is that, despite the fact that they might be more comfortable in one framework or the other, they might also sometimes agree.

Not long ago I was at a meeting which, as academic meetings are wont to do, pitted academics against each other. Critics of enhancement technologies were set against proponents. One of the most eloquent critics aimed some of his remarks at Ritalin, and cited, among other concerns, the possibility that its proliferation might ultimately increase stress on children. However, one of the speakers who spoke most eloquently on behalf of enhancement technologies mentioned in passing that he, too, was concerned about increasing stress on children. In his view, a technology that was used in ways that increased the stress on children would not be a real enhancement. Although he did not use the word, he was suggesting it would be a fake.

This is all to say that rather than spend our time debating whether enhancement technologies are good or bad in general, or whether this or that framework ought to prevail, we should be asking, as Eric Juengst recently has: Will this intervention promote or thwart ('hobble' or 'enable') the flourishing of an individual and those around him? (Juengst, 2004) (I believe that in addition to Juengst and Glover, Thomas Murray has been making the same point) (Murray, 2006.)

It is not that our conceptual problems would go away if we gave up the term enhancement! It is not as if distinguishing between interventions that promote and thwart human flourishing (or distinguishing between genuine and fake enhancements) is easy. Far from it. But perhaps putting the question in terms of whether the intervention will thwart or promote someone's genuine flourishing at least gets us away from the notion that the difference between what is good and what is bad is somehow written in some straightforward way into Nature (as friends of the treatment–enhancement distinction sometimes seem to hope). While those working out of the gratitude framework need to give up the hope of finding in Nature a firm ground for letting things be, those in the creativity framework need to become better at acknowledging that their view of what constitutes human flourishing is not as neutral as they sometimes suggest. The idea that to be fully a person is to have a life project of one's own is hardly a neutral conception of personhood (Parens, 2005). Those working out of the creativity framework do not know as little about what human flourishing consists in as they sometimes profess. That is, as those operating out of the gratitude framework can tend to exaggerate how much we know about what human flourishing consists in, those operating out of the creativity framework can tend to exaggerate how little we can know. Both sides remind us of important insights, but neither side alone is adequate for thinking well about particular interventions aimed at enhancement. If we are to think better about particular interventions aimed at enhancement, we need to become better at giving up the idea of one framework being adequate—and better at keeping in mind the insights of both.

## Coda

In this chapter I have tried to label and briefly describe two ethical frameworks out of which people seem to come to the academic debate about enhancement technologies. I have suggested that the impulse to creativity (or self-transformation) can be thought of as the organizing commitment for one framework, and that the impulse to gratitude (or letting things be) can be thought of as the organizing commitment of the other. I have also described some of the different sets of reasons that seem to cluster around each of those commitments. Different reasons seem most salient, depending on one's framework.

Given the respect in which the two frameworks are at odds, there are at least two pieces of good news for those who aspire to productive debate. First, even though people on two sides of the same question may be partial to different sets of reasons, they also share many values, including large values like authenticity and diversity, and also smaller values like shielding children from stress. Yes, those in the gratitude framework tend to argue that enhancement technologies will thwart authenticity and reduce diversity, and those in the creativity framework tend to argue that enhancement technologies will have the opposite effects, but we should not forget the values they share. If we were to remember that more, perhaps we would be better at recognizing the smaller shared values as well.

Secondly, even though we tend to settle into one framework for the sake of engaging in academic debates, if we are thoughtful, we do not feel comfortable in only one. I tried to emphasize that point by offering the image of the single figure, Jacob, in whom we can observe the impulses to gratitude and creativity. None of us is committed only to gratitude or creativity. None of us should hope for or expect an end to the deep and fertile tension between those two impulses and frameworks.

As those who consider neuroethics move forward, debating questions like those surrounding technologies aimed at enhancing human traits and capacities, perhaps it will be useful to remember that each of us comes to these questions from somewhere in particular. Perhaps some day the 'neuroscience of ethics' will help us to understand better why we tend to feel more comfortable in one framework than in the other. In the meantime, perhaps it will be useful just to notice that we come to these debates from different but equally estimable places.

Perhaps remembering that we ourselves are coming from somewhere in particular can help to make us more modest in the articulation of our views. Perhaps remembering that our interlocutors are also coming from somewhere in particular can help to make us more generous in our interpretations of their views. Our interlocutors do not just come from somewhere where they feel comfortable; they come from somewhere where we also sometimes feel comfortable, even if we are reluctant to admit as much in the heat of academic battle.

## References

Bordo S (1995). *Unbearable Weight: Feminism, Western Culture, and the Body.* Berkeley, CA: University of California Press.

Brock DW (1998). Enhancements of human function: some distinctions for policymakers. In: Parens E (ed.) *Enhancing Human Traits: Ethical and Social Implications.* Washington, DC: Georgetown University Press, 48–69.

Buchanan A, Brock DW, Daniels N, Wikler D (2000). *From Chance to Choice: Genetics and Justice.* Cambridge, UK: Cambridge University Press.

Caplan A (2002). No-brainer: can we cope with the ethical ramifications of new knowledge of the human brain? In: Marcus SJ (ed) *Neuroethics: Mapping the Field.* New York: Dana Press, 95–105.

Daniels N (1994). The Genome Project, individual differences, and just health care. In: Murphy T, Lappe V (eds) *Justice and the Human Genome Project.* Berkeley, CA: University of California Press, 110–32.

DeGrazia D (2004). Prozac, enhancement, and self-creation. In: Elliott C, Chambers T (eds) *Prozac as a Way of Life.* Chapel Hill, NC: University of North Carolina Press, 33–47.

Dreger A (2004). *One of Us: Conjoined Twins and the Future of Normal.* Cambridge, MA: Harvard University Press.

Edwards JC (1997). *The Plain Sense of Things.* University Park, PA: Pennsylvania State University Press.

Edwards JC (2006). Concepts of technology and their role in moral reflection. In Parens E (ed) *Surgically Shaping Children: Essays on Technology, Ethics, and the Pursuit of Normality.* Baltimore, MD: Johns Hopkins University Press.

Elliott C (2003). *Better than Well: American Medicine Meets the American Dream.* New York: Norton.

Frank A (2004) Emily's scars: surgical shaping, technoluxe, and bioethics. *Hastings Center Report* **34**, 18–29.

Fletcher J (1974). *The Ethics of Genetic Control: Ending Reproductive Roulette.* New York: Anchor–Doubleday.

Glover J (1984). *What Sort of People Should There Be? Genetic Engineering , Brain Control, and their Impact on our Future World.* Harmondsworth, Middlesex: Penguin Books.

Greene JD, Sommerville RB, Nystrom LE, Darley JM, Cohen JD (2001). An fMRI investigation of emotional engagement in moral judgment. *Science* **293**, 2105–8.

Harris J (1992). *Wonderwoman and Superman: The Ethics of Human Biotechnology.* Oxford, UK: Oxford University Press.

Heidegger M (1953). The question concerning technology. In: Krell D (ed) *Martin Heidegger: Basic Writings.* New York: Harper and Row, 1997.

Juengst J (2004). *Enhancement uses of medical technology.* In: Post S (ed.) *The Encyclopedia of Bioethics,* 3rd Edition. New York: MacMillan Pub Co: 753–57.

Kaebnick G (2000). On the sanctity of nature. *Hastings Center Report* **30**, 16–23.

Little M (1998). Cosmetic surgery, suspect norms, and the ethics of complicity. In: Parens E (ed.) *Enhancing Human Traits: Ethical and Social Implications.* Washington, DC: Georgetown University Press, 162–76.

Luhrmann TM (2000). *Of Two Minds: The Growing Disorder in American Psychiatry.* New York: Knopf.

Murray TH, Gaylin W, Macklin R (eds) (1984). *Feeling Good and Doing Better: The Ethics of Nontherapeutic Drug Use*. Garden City, NJ: Humana Press.

Murray TH (2006). *Enhancement*. In: Steinbeck B (ed.) *The Oxford Handbook of Bioethics*. Oxford: Oxford University Press.

Parens E (1995). Should we hold the (germ) line? *Journal of Law, Medicine and Ethics* **23**, 173–6.

Parens E (ed) (1998). *Enhancing Human Traits: Ethical and Social Implications*. Washington, DC: Georgetown University Press.

Parens E (2005). Authenticity and ambivalence: toward understanding the enhancement debate. *Hastings Center Report 35, 3: 34–41*.

President's Commission for the Study of Ethical Problems in Medicine and Biomedical and Behavioral Research (1982). *Splicing Life: A Report on the Social and Ethical Issues of Genetic Engineering with Human Beings*. Washington, DC: US Government Printing Office.

*President's Council on Bioethics* (2003). *Beyond Therapy: Biotechnology and the Pursuit of Happiness*. New York: Regan Books.

Ramsey P (1970). *Fabricated Man: The Ethics of Genetic Control*. New Haven, CT: Yale University Press.

Roskies A (2002). Neuroethics for the new millennium. *Neuron* **35**, 21–3.

Sabin JE, Daniels N (1994). Determining 'medical necessity' in mental health practice. *Hastings Center Report* **24**, 5–13.

Sandel M (2004). The case against perfection. *Atlantic Monthly* April 2004, 51–62.

Silver L (1997). *Remaking Eden: Cloning and Beyond in a Brave New World*. New York: Avon Books.

Stock G (2002). *Redesigning Humans: Our Inevitable Genetic Future*. Boston, MA: Houghton Mifflin.

Walters L, Palmer JG (1997). *The Ethics of Human Gene Therapy*. New York: Oxford University Press.

# Chapter 7

# Ethical dilemmas in neurodegenerative disease: respecting patients at the twilight of agency

Agnieszka Jaworska

[A] man does not consist of memory alone. He has feeling, will, sensibilities, moral being...And it is here...that you may find ways to touch him. (A.R. Luria, quoted by Sacks 1985, p. 32)

## Introduction

Neurodegenerative disease can significantly affect the requirements for an ethically appropriate treatment of an individual. The deterioration of the brain profoundly alters psychological functioning and capacities, and so profoundly alters the kind of being others are called upon to relate to and respond to from the point of view of ethics. Such transformations are easiest to see in cases in which the current preferences and interests of a patient in a degenerated state come into conflict with the values and choices the person professed before the neurodegeneration began. Which set of preferences should the caregiver follow? The answer will be different depending on the ethically relevant metaphysical and mental properties that the patient still possesses. Thus to resolve such dilemmas we must get the ethically relevant conceptual distinctions right, but we must also be true to empirical facts. To the extent that neuroscience has developed a detailed understanding of how various brain disorders undermine psychological functioning and capacity, it has increasingly become more pertinent to the untangling of such ethical puzzles. The following case study illustrates the interplay between ethical conceptual analysis and neuroscientific findings in the resolution of moral dilemmas that arise in Alzheimer's disease.

I defend the philosophical view that the immediate interests of an individual cannot be overridden as long as the individual possesses the capacity to value. In the context of each particular neurodegenerative disease, this recommendation must be guided by a scientifically informed assessment of when in the course of the disease the capacity to value could possibly be lost, and when it is likely to be retained. In the case of Alzheimer's disease, neuroscientific evidence indicates that the capacity to value is slowly and gradually weakened, and in some cases may not be completely lost until relatively far along in the disease's progression. Similar neuroethical analyses must be carried out for other diseases and disorders, and will probably yield different results.

# Respecting the margins of agency: Alzheimer's patients and the capacity to value

Mrs Rogoff was always an independent woman. Raised in an immigrant family, she was used to working hard for what she wanted. Most of her life she ran a successful business selling liquor. She also developed local fame as an outstanding cook and hostess. She was an introvert, liked living alone, and always carefully guarded the way she presented herself to others.

In her early eighties Mrs Rogoff developed severe motor impairments, which could only be corrected by a risky neurosurgery. She decided to undergo the procedure, insisting that she would rather die than be immobile. She prepared a living will, requesting not to have her life prolonged if she became a burden to her family or if she could no longer enjoy her current quality of life.

The surgery was successful, but shortly thereafter Mrs Rogoff developed early signs of dementia: memory and word-finding difficulties. As she became more and more disoriented, her daughter hired a live-in housekeeper, Fran. Fran takes care of Mrs Rogoff in the way one would take care of a child. Mrs Rogoff enjoys the long hours she spends with Fran, and with her grandchildren when they visit, telling them somewhat disjointed stories about her earlier ventures. She watches television a lot, and her stories often incorporate the more exciting episodes from television as if they pertained to her own life. In her more lucid moments, Mrs Rogoff tells her grandchildren that she is scared to die, that 'she doesn't want to go anywhere'.

Fran has to make day-to-day decisions for Mrs Rogoff: Should Mrs Rogoff get dressed if her family is coming to visit and she insists on wearing pajamas? Should she take a bath every day even if she is afraid of water? In general, should the current decisions reflect the care Mrs Rogoff used to take in how she presented herself to others? Mrs Rogoff's daughter faces the more weighty decisions: Should she use up Mrs Rogoff's savings to pay Fran's salary, allowing Mrs Rogoff to keep enjoying her companion, or should she place Mrs Rogoff in a nursing home, increasing the likelihood that, when the time comes, there will be some money left to execute Mrs Rogoff's will? What treatments should she authorize if Mrs Rogoff develops a dangerous but treatable infection?[1]

People who care for Alzheimer's patients—family members, nursing home providers, physicians, medical researchers—face such dilemmas routinely, and these dilemmas are likely to become more and more familiar as baby-boomers approach the age of high risk for Alzheimer's disease. The particulars of each dilemma may seem unique, but they typically have the same underlying structure. There is a conflict between the attitudes and values the patients espoused when they were still healthy and their later interests as people afflicted with dementia. The quandary, in a nutshell, is this: Should we, in our efforts to best respect a patient with dementia, give priority to the preferences and attitudes this person held before becoming demented, or should we follow the person's present interests?

## Competing theoretical perspectives

There are two dominant theoretical perspectives on how such dilemmas ought to be resolved, expressed most prominently by Rebecca Dresser and Ronald Dworkin. According to Dresser, decisions affecting a demented person at a given time must speak to the person's point of view as current at that time. Heeding values and wishes that the patient no longer espouses and that cannot be said to represent his present needs and interests can do no good for the patient (Dresser 1986).

Dworkin directly challenges this line of reasoning, adducing compelling reasons to adhere to the demented patients' earlier wishes and values (Dworkin 1993). In Dworkin's view, we fail to take seriously both the autonomy and the well-being of a demented patient unless we adhere strictly to the patient's earlier wishes, wishes that originated when he was still capable of acting autonomously and still able to judge what was required for his overall well-being.

In this chapter, I develop an alternative to both Dresser's and Dworkin's analyses. Like Dresser, I want to take seriously the current interests of demented patients, but for very different reasons: I believe that many of these patients may still be capable of autonomy to a significant degree and that they may still have authority concerning their well-being. Yet I emphasize very different aspects of both autonomy and well-being than Dworkin, who predicates autonomy on decision-making capacity and for whom well-being depends centrally on promoting one's own design for one's life as a whole. I associate potential for autonomy primarily with the capacity to value, and well-being with living in accordance with one's values (Jaworska 1997). Thus the central question for a caregiver attempting to best respect an Alzheimer's patient becomes not, 'Can this patient reason thoroughly and come to a rational decision?' or 'Does he grasp what's best for his life as a whole?' but 'Does this patient still value?' I will argue that the capacity to value is not completely lost in dementia, and, to the extent that it is not, respect for the immediate interests of a demented person is contrary neither to his well-being nor to the respect for his autonomy.

Dworkin's arguments are a fruitful point of departure because their kernel is very plausible. After someone loses his status as an agent—as a creature capable of guiding his actions—his earlier autonomously chosen values should continue to govern what happens to him, despite his current inability to appreciate these values. This accurately locates the central issue of our dilemmas: At what point in the course of dementia are the attributes essential to agency lost? While I consider most of the ideas in Dworkin's arguments well-founded, I challenge his two crucial premises. In the argument focused on the patient's well-being, I dispute the claim that demented patients are no longer capable of generating what Dworkin calls 'critical interests'. In the argument concerning autonomy, I question the premise that demented patients no longer possess the 'capacity for autonomy'. In each case, I will trace how the problematic premise arises within Dworkin's argument and then develop an alternative account of the relevant capacity.

# Reconceiving well-being

## Experiential interests versus critical interests

When we take enhancement of the demented patient's well-being as the caregiver's goal, we need to distinguish two types of prudential interest that the patient may have. Dworkin labels these two types of interest 'experiential' and 'critical'. Experiential interests concern the quality of the person's experience, his state of mind. We have an interest in experiencing pleasure, satisfaction, enjoyment, contentment, lack of pain, and so forth; what states of mind count here and how they can be brought about is determined fully by how these experiences feel to the person in question. But most of us also have critical interests—interests in doing or having in our lives the things we consider good and in avoiding the things we consider bad, no matter what sorts of experiences result from fulfilling these interests. For example, a person's critical interests may include being a successful soldier or securing contentment and harmony for his family, however much stress or anguish the pursuit of these goals may engender.

Experiential interests are inherently time specific—to satisfy them at a given time, the person must still espouse them at that time. For instance, it only makes sense to want to satisfy your experiential interest in having a good time with your guests if at the time they arrive you will still be interested in enjoying their company. Not so with critical interests; it may make sense to have your critical interest satisfied even if you are unaware of its being satisfied, even if you are dead at the time, or unconscious, or too demented to grasp what your critical interest has been all along. Fulfillment of a critical interest bears only on the object of that interest. It involves bringing about whatever state of affairs the person in question judged good; the fate of the person himself is not relevant to this, provided that the object of the interest is external to the person. Thus fulfilling a father's critical interest in the well-being of his family does not require his awareness of how well they are doing. This critical interest could be advanced, for example, by obeying a deathbed promise to take care of his wife and children after he passes away.

Dworkin readily grants that Alzheimer's patients, even at late stages of their illness, can experience pleasures as well as frustrations, and thus have the basis for contemporaneous experiential interests. He would interpret the dilemmas under discussion in this chapter as cases of conflict between these experiential interests and critical interests that the person professed when he was still healthy (e.g. a conflict between Mrs Rogoff's experiential interest in continuing the enjoyable storytelling sessions and her critical interest in not being dependent on her family). And here Dworkin assumes that, at least in the types of cases he wants to address, the demented patient is not capable of generating contemporaneous critical interests. From this point, there follows a very plausible analysis. The fact that the demented patient no longer affirms critical interests in no way implies that he does not have critical interests. Since such interests are not inherently time specific, the prudential importance of satisfying them may survive the person's unawareness of their satisfaction, whether due to unconsciousness, dementia, or even death. Thus a demented person who cannot generate contemporaneous critical interests may still have some of the same critical interests he professed when he was healthy. And this means that the conflict occurring in our dilemmas is best described as a conflict between the patient's *ongoing* experiential interests and his *ongoing* critical interests.

This description helps to clarify how the conflict ought to be resolved. In the case of an ordinary competent person, when his critical interests (his judgments and values) come into conflict with his experiential interests (what would lead to the optimal state of mind for him), we do not hesitate to give precedence to his well-considered values and judgments, and we concede that, overall, this is best for him. For example, we would accept that it is in the best interest of a devoted father to sacrifice his experiential interest in his current comfort for the sake of the future of his children, or that it is in the best interest of a patriotic soldier to forgo his experiential interest in a carefree life and sign up for demanding military training. The case of our demented person turns out to be no different: in *his* conflict between ongoing experiential and critical interests, it is also best to privilege the latter. We serve Mrs Rogoff best by satisfying her critical interest in not being a burden to her family, at the expense of her experiential interest in enjoying television and storytelling.

This analysis stands or falls with the assumption that demented patients no longer originate critical interests. For if they do—if the conflict in our dilemmas is between the patient's contemporarily professed critical interests and the critical interests he professed before becoming demented—Dworkin's framework would readily allow that contemporarily professed critical interests ought to take precedence. In this case, the demented person would be viewed as any other person whose values and commitments change over time and whose *currently* professed values are taken to have bearing on what is best for him.

It should be noted that the idea that a demented person can originate critical interests need not imply that the person generates brand new critical interests. What matters is whether the person still has an ongoing commitment to his critical interests. After all, the most likely scenario of a conflict between a demented person's current critical interests and his critical interests from the pre-dementia period is not one in which a person's demented mind generates completely new critical interests, but rather one in which dementia causes a person to lose some of his earlier more complex interests, so that in the new, simpler configuration the remaining interests gain import.

Dworkin defends the claim that the demented cannot generate critical interests as follows:

> [B]y the time the dementia has become advanced, Alzheimer's victims have lost the capacity to think about how to make their lives more successful on the whole. They are ignorant of self—not as an amnesiac is, not simply because they cannot identify their pasts—but more fundamentally, because they have no sense of a whole life, a past joined to a future, that could be the object of any evaluation or concern as a whole. They cannot have projects or plans of the kind that leading a critical life requires. They therefore have no contemporary opinion about their own critical interests. (Dworkin 1993 p. 230)

In contending that demented persons cannot have opinions about their critical interests, Dworkin presupposes that one needs to have a sense of one's life as a whole in order to originate critical interests, a sense that a person may begin to lose relatively early in the progression of dementia. Dworkin thinks of critical interests as stemming from 'convictions about what helps to make a life good on the whole' (Dworkin 1993 p. 201–2). But do critical interests have to reflect the person's comprehensive design for the progression of his life? An alternative view, tacitly embedded in Dworkin, is more plausible.

Critical interests may well be understood to issue from something less grand—simply from convictions about what is good to have, which do not require the ability to grasp or review one's whole life. Dworkin himself describes 'opinions about my critical interests' as 'opinions about what is good for me' (Dworkin 1993 p. 202), indicating that these are opinions about values, and that the ability to generate critical interests goes hand in hand with the ability to value. And it does seem possible for a person to value something at a given time, without referring this value to his conception of his life as a whole. This possibility is evident in patients with severe loss of memory and linguistic ability who are still aware of their decline and deeply regret it. I recently observed a patient who, in response to a simple question about what he did that day, had great difficulty keeping track of the sequence of his thoughts and of the sequence of words in the sentence he was composing, and after several starts and long pauses, said slowly, his voice trembling: 'Here you can see Alzheimer's at work'. There was no doubt that this man, who had little grip on 'his life as a whole', nevertheless valued the abilities he could no longer command and was expressing profound regret.

## Understanding values

Intuitively, it is easy to recognize when someone expresses a value—and not merely a simpler attitude such as a craving, a desire, or a wish. But to exhibit more clearly that valuing need not involve a grasp of one's life as a whole, let us characterize more systematically what valuing is and distinguish it from these simpler attitudes, which even Dworkin readily attributes to Alzheimer's patients.

The main difference between *mere* desiring and valuing is this: One way to deal with one's non-value-laden desires is to try to eliminate them—to try to bring it about that one does not feel them—but this would not be a satisfactory response to a valuing. A person could contemplate being free of a mere desire with a sense of relief, but one would always view the possibility of not valuing something one currently values as an impoverishment, loss, or mistake. We can all recognize clear cases when a strong desire is definitely not a value: Think of a priest eager to rid himself of his sexual desires, or a temporarily depressed person seeking relief from his persistent wish to hurt himself. Also, even if one's attitude toward a desire is more neutral—perhaps one views it only as a nuisance—as long as one would not mind lacking it, it is still a mere desire. Cravings for specific food items are paradigmatic cases here. In contrast, when one values something, say a particular friendship or a local community, one cannot be indifferent to whether one happens to value these things or not—a state in which one lacked one's feelings for one's friend or one's need for a sense of belonging would call for regret.[2] We can see this in our patient mourning the losses caused by Alzheimer's disease—he would view with horror the projected future in which he will no longer care about these losses.

Thus values have special attributes that do not apply to mere desires: We think that it would be a mistake to lose our current values—we hold our values to be correct, or at least correct for us. This means that we can typically give a rationale for why we consider something valuable or good, usually by situating this value in a larger normative framework. Also, since values are the sorts of attitudes that we allow could be correct or incorrect, they are open to criticism and revision. At minimum, there are consistency requirements on what one can consider good—if one values something and also values its opposite, one will be under rational pressure to resolve the conflict. For example, if you truly value a committed relationship, you cannot just as easily value the freedom of a lack of commitment; you may well see the merits of both, but you cannot be fully committed to your spouse unless you cease to care as deeply about your freedom. In contrast, as a matter of sheer desire, you may surely remain ambivalent without any rational impetus to settle the conflict—you may simply keep craving just as strongly the kind of intimacy possible only in an ongoing partnership as well as the excitement of always being able to walk out and entice a new partner.

Another mark of valuing as opposed to mere desiring is that a person's values are usually entangled with his sense of self-worth: A person values *himself* in terms of how well he lives up to his values. Some people pay little attention to their own value, so what I am now describing is not a necessary condition of having values. However, it is a sufficient condition: Anyone who has a conception of himself, a set of ideals that he wants to live up to and in virtue of which he assesses his own value, is no doubt a valuer.

I have isolated two features essential to, or strongly indicative of, valuing: the person thinks he is correct in wanting what he wants, and achieving what he wants is tied up with his sense of self-worth. Nothing here suggests that valuing would require a grasp of the narrative of one's whole life.

Furthermore, for the purposes of the argument I outlined earlier, Dworkin does not need to interpret the capacity to generate critical interests as anything more than the so-specified capacity to value. As we have seen, the backbone of Dworkin's justification for disregarding current wishes of patients who can no longer originate critical interests is the perception that, ordinarily, critical interests take precedence over experiential interests in determining what is best for a person. But, presumably, critical interests are of such overriding importance because they stem from the person's values—because they reflect the person's opinion of what is correct for him. And this standing of critical interests is independent of whether they encompass the person's design for his life as a whole. For instance, a devoted father's critical interest in the well-being of his children overrides his interest in having optimal experiences, no matter whether he came to value his children by reflecting on the narrative of his whole life. Thus, to endorse Dworkin's compelling argument that deference to current wishes of a demented patient ought to depend on whether the patient can still originate critical interests, we have no need to understand critical interests in terms of the person's grasp of what is good for his life as a whole; we can just trace critical interests to the person's convictions about what would be good and correct for him—to the person's values as understood in the above specifications.

## Values do not require assessments of one's life as a whole

Of the three claims I have made—that critical interests are values, that conceptually such values may be understood as quite independent of the agent's grasp of his life as a whole, and that this is the interpretation relevant to Dworkin's argument—the second is the most contentious. However, it is confirmed by many real-life Alzheimer's cases in which valuing becomes uncoupled from the person's grasp of the narrative of his whole life.

Consider, for example, Mrs D, a patient interviewed in a study by Sabat (1998), diagnosed with probable Alzheimer's for 5 years. As for her level of impairment:

> ...she was moderately to severely afflicted (stage 4, Global Deterioration Scale, score of 7 on the Mini-Mental State Test). She could not name the day of the week, the date, the month, the season, year, the city and county she was in...She underestimated her age...and had difficulty finding her way to the bathroom at the day care center she attended two days each week. (Sabat 1998 p.46)

Mrs D's memory deficiency was rather acute. Since she could not keep track of the passing time or of her own age, and had severe difficulties forming new memories, Dworkin could safely assume that she had lost grasp of the narrative of her whole life, that she lacked a sense of 'a past joined to a future'. However, Mrs D still conducted herself as a valuer. She often volunteered as a research subject for tests and experiments at the National Institutes of Health. Although she did not choose to do so through systematic reflection on the whole trajectory of her life, she clearly felt that this was, for her, the right choice: 'That was the nicety of it, cause I could have said, "no", but believe me, if I can help me and my [fellow] man, I would do it' (Sabat 1998 p. 46). Her conviction that it would have been a mistake to say 'no' comes across rather starkly here. And she had no need to review her life as a whole to affirm this conviction. What mattered for her was that this felt right to her, then and there. One has the sense that Mrs D was simply enacting a basic part of her personality, one that had remained relatively intact despite her other impairments.

For a less altruistic example, consider another of Sabat's interviewees, Dr B, an Alzheimer's patient who scored even lower than Mrs D on cognitive tests. Like Mrs D, he 'could not recall the day of the week, the month, or the year' (Sabat 1998 p. 41). His ability to evaluate his life as a whole could not have been better than that of Mrs D. Yet he too proved capable of valuing. He became very interested in Sabat's research project. Although his grasp of its design was rather rudimentary, he thought of the project as his 'salvation', as a way to engage, despite his impairments, in something other than 'filler' (Sabat 1998 p. 41), in something giving him a mark of distinction. He told Sabat more or less explicitly that he considered the project right and appropriate: 'And you know I feel a way is that, I feel that this is a *real good*, big project, and I'm sure you do too. This project is a sort of scientific thing' (Sabat 1998 pp. 41–2, emphasis mine). This assessment of the project went hand in hand with a boost to Dr B's sense of pride and self-worth that ensued from his participation. The impact on his self-esteem was most evident whenever he compared the project to various 'filler' group activities at the day care center: 'If I'm working with you, I can—look, I can work in here for 30 times and all that, but in this group, *I'm nothing*' (Sabat 1998 p. 41, emphasis mine). That his role in the project could so alter his self-image demonstrates most poignantly that he valued the project.

Mrs Rogoff's case also demonstrates that the ability to value may outlast the patient's grasp of her life as a whole. Her confusion between a television-generated world and events of her own life easily rules out her having an adequate grasp of her life's narrative. However, she does remain a valuer, most clearly when her former reputation as a great cook is at stake. She invariably becomes upset and agitated seeing Fran usurp the mastery of the kitchen. One day, after Fran made a particularly delicious chicken leg roast, Mrs Rogoff insisted that she would cook dinner herself, and asked her granddaughter, in secret, to buy 'a hen with five legs', clearly in the spirit of one-upmanship with Fran. At such times, Fran arranges small make-work kitchen tasks that appease Mrs Rogoff. Here, as before, the clearest indication of retained values comes from visible effects on the person's self-esteem: Mrs Rogoff's self-image suffers whenever she realizes that Fran has taken over as a culinary expert, and these effects can be mitigated, at least temporarily, by a semblance of participation in culinary affairs.

## Insights from neuroscience

My observations that valuing may be quite independent of grasping the narrative of one's life, and that this separation often occurs in Alzheimer's patients, are also supported by current findings in neurophysiology and in the neuropathology of Alzheimer's disease. The neuronal loss characteristic of Alzheimer's disease is not distributed evenly in the cerebral cortex. The disease affects most severely an area of the brain indispensable for maintaining the sense of one's life as a whole, but not particularly important for the ability to value.

In the early stages of Alzheimer's disease the neuronal damage affects primarily the hippocampus. As the damage spreads, the hippocampus continues to be affected much more severely than other regions of the brain (Geula 1998; Laakso *et al.* 2000). The hippocampus is of crucial importance in the acquisition and processing of long-term explicit memory for facts and events. Although it is not involved in short-term memory or in the eventual storage of long-term memories, the hippocampus nonetheless plays an essential role in transforming a fresh short-term memory into a lasting long-term memory (Squire and Zola-Morgan 1991; Riedel and Micheau 2001). Accordingly, while damage to the hippocampus affects neither a person's processing of his immediate experience nor his memories of events that occurred long before the damage, it causes him to lose track of ongoing events soon after they happen, so that he typically has no recollection of the previous day (Squire and Zola-Morgan 1988). Such damage impairs a person's ability to come back to a recent thought or memory after a shift of attention to something new (Squire and Zola-Morgan 1991). These very impairments are, of course, the typical first clinical indications of Alzheimer's disease. They are also central to Dworkin's assessment that Alzheimer's disease destroys one's sense of one's life as a whole. Damage to the hippocampus alone leaves the person unable to update his autobiographical narrative. As he continually forgets his immediate past, he loses the sense of 'a past joined to a future', which Dworkin deems necessary for the ability to formulate critical interests.

However, there is no reason to think that impairment of the hippocampus would obliterate one's ability to espouse critical interests when this ability is understood, following my recommendation, as the ability to value. While removal of the hippocampal formations leads to the memory defects described above, it does not otherwise compromise the patient's mental functions (Young and Young 1997). Moreover, there is neurophysiological evidence that other regions of the brain are primarily responsible for interactions of reasoning and decision-making processes, especially those concerning personal and social matters, with feelings and emotions (Damasio 1994). It is damage to these regions that is most likely to directly compromise a person's ability to value.

Thus consider Elliot, a patient with brain damage localized in the ventromedial prefrontal cortices. He performed normally or even superiorly on a full battery of psychological tests (including intelligence, knowledge base, memory, language, attention, and basic reasoning), and yet was a very poor decision-maker in everyday life (Damasio 1994). He showed no abnormalities in means–ends reasoning and problem-solving; he was perfectly able to come up with a full array of options for action in a particular situation as well as to work out the consequences of each option. As it turned out, his impairment concerned the ability to choose among the options he could reason through so well. After a full analysis of all the options he would comment, 'I still wouldn't know what to do!' (Damasio 1994 p. 49). His emotional responses and feelings were severely blunted and this 'prevented him from assigning different values to different options, and made his decision-making landscape hopelessly flat' (Damasio 1994 p. 51). He lacked the very starting points of the ability to value: he was no longer sufficiently invested in anything; he ceased to care.

The ability that Elliot lacked is the indispensable core of the capacity to value. When you value something—be it a particular friendship or a local community—your commitment to these things is first and foremost a form of emotional engagement. You would not call it 'valuing' or 'being committed' unless there is some confluence between thinking about and acting upon what you say you value and your emotional life. True enough, since the conviction that it is right for you to care about these things and that you would be mistaken if you did not care is open to criticism, sophisticated and varied cognitive abilities are required to develop a robust set of values, values most immune from such criticisms. But having such convictions in the first place amounts to attaching emotional significance to the object of value; it involves having the corresponding emotional attitudes and reactions, so that some things simply 'feel' important to you (Jaworska 1997). Elliot was unable to value because of the numbing of his affective response.

The neuronal destruction of Alzheimer's disease eventually reaches the regions of the brain most responsible for 'giving emotional quality to occurrences which renders them important to the person concerned' (Souren and Franssen 1994 p. 52). However, the destruction and the isolation of the hippocampus are always several steps ahead of the pathologies in the areas most likely to affect the capacity to value (Braak and Braak 1995). Therefore, on the basis of neuropathological findings, one would expect Alzheimer's patients to lose their sense of life as a whole even as the essence of their ability to value remains relatively robust.

On the neuropathological picture of full-blown Alzheimer's disease, the loss of the sense of one's life as a whole is typically acute, while the destruction of the areas implicated in valuing remains more selective. Thus we would expect a patient in the moderate stage to have lost some, but not all, of his former values. With his ability to form new long-term memories compromised, he is unlikely to develop any new values. But his selective loss of former values may well result in changes of values pertinent to our dilemmas: As I previously observed, once some of the earlier values drop out, the exact content and the importance of the remaining values are typically reconfigured.

In this section I have chiefly argued that the ability to value is independent of the ability to understand the narrative of one's whole life, and that demented people may well retain the former ability long after they lose the latter. We also saw that, at least when the well-being of the demented is the focus, Dworkin's recommendation to disregard the patient's current wishes derives from the loss of the former capacity, the capacity to value. Thus, for a Dworkinian, the threshold capacity level necessary to lend prudential authority to a person's current wishes should not be set at the ability to grasp one's life as a whole, but rather at the ability to value. As long as the demented person still espouses values, we have seen no reason to override these in the name of values he professed earlier—Dworkin's recommendations do not apply.

## Rethinking autonomy

Let us now turn to respect for the patient's autonomy as the primary goal of those caring for demented patients. How should we now approach our dilemmas? According to Dworkin, we need to consider whether the demented patient, in his current condition, still possesses the capacity for autonomy. The rationale here is that respecting people's autonomy is morally important only because a human being's very ability to act autonomously is morally important. If a person is not even capable of making autonomous decisions, allowing him to carry out his current wishes would do nothing to promote his autonomy. As Dworkin sees it, the only way to respect the autonomy of such patients is to respect their earlier ability to act autonomously; if their autonomous choices from that earlier time can still be satisfied now, these should be the focus of respect for autonomy. Of course, choices associated with critical interests are often still satisfiable, since, as we saw earlier, critical interests can be meaningfully fulfilled at a time when the person no longer espouses these interests. Thus, for Dworkin, the only way to respect the autonomy of patients who lost their capacity for autonomy is to adhere to the critical interests that they professed before this loss. He readily concludes that the types of demented patients he is interested in lack the capacity for autonomy, and hence that in order to respect their autonomy one must adhere to their earlier wishes, wishes that expressed this capacity.

The claim that demented patients no longer possess the capacity for autonomy is clearly pivotal to this part of Dworkin's analysis. But how plausible is the underlying interpretation of the capacity for autonomy?

## Fundamentals of autonomy

Dworkin describes the capacity for autonomy as 'the capacity to express one's own character—values, commitments, convictions, and critical as well as experiential interests—in the life one leads' (Dworkin 1993 p. 224). So understood, this is the capacity to be fully in charge of one's life—to enact one's own values and convictions in the life one leads. Demented people may easily lose this capacity, because as they lose the understanding of the world around them and become increasingly disoriented, they no longer know how to translate their values and convictions into appropriate activity in the world. But suppose that a demented person who still espoused values and convictions received some help in enacting those values in his environment. Imagine, for instance, a demented man who values his independence above all else, but who is confused about what he is still able to do on his own. Were he left to make his own decisions, his choices would not ultimately enhance his independence, and perhaps would even lead to his harm. But imagine further that his family makes living arrangements for him that allow a maximum degree of independence feasible in his predicament. There is an important sense in which this man is still capable of exercising his capacity for autonomy, of living according to his convictions and values, albeit with some help in translating ends into means. Thus a possibility opens up that the capacity for autonomy ought not to be thought of as the capacity to carry one's convictions into action without external help, a capacity that requires reasoning through complex sets of circumstances to reach the most appropriate autonomous decisions; rather, that the capacity for autonomy is first and foremost the capacity to espouse values and convictions whose translation into action may not always be fully within the agent's mastery.

In his own elaboration of why the demented lack the capacity for autonomy, Dworkin emphasizes the claim that they have 'no discernable even short-term aims' (Dworkin 1993 p. 225). Presumably, Dworkin thinks that Alzheimer's patients cannot have even short-term aims because as soon as they embark on a course of action they forget what it was they were doing and are forced to start anew. But he should distinguish between an inability to form and then remember a plan for fulfilling one's purposes, and a lack of a stable set of purposes and preferences. For we can imagine an Alzheimer's patient who always wants the same set of things—say, he wants to feel useful and appreciated—and yet is unable to set up and carry through a plan for achieving any of them, partly because he cannot figure out the means to his ends, and partly because he cannot keep track of the steps he is taking. These latter deficiencies seem to be at stake in Dworkin's claim that the demented lack the capacity for autonomy, despite his explicit focus on their lack of consistent purposes.

For Dworkin, Alzheimer's patients cannot be autonomous because, left to their own devices, they cannot lead their lives by their own lights. This is largely because they have lost the ability to reason from their preferences to the appropriate decisions and actions—they have lost the adeptness for means–ends reasoning and planning.

However, there is no good reason to restrict the right to autonomy only to people who possess these abilities. After all, as the case of Elliot and other patients with prefrontal brain damage powerfully brings home, the very idea of governing one's life autonomously is a complete nonstarter unless the person knows how he wants his life to be governed—unless he has his own substantive principles or directives for running his life. These principles constitute the foundation of autonomy; means–ends reasoning and planning are mere tools for implementing the principles. Moreover, while having one's own directives is indispensable for exercising autonomy, we can well imagine that the tools of means–ends reasoning and planning could be supplied for the autonomous person from the outside. Accordingly, the essence of the capacity for autonomy consists in the ability to lay down the principles that will govern one's actions, and not in the ability to devise and carry out the means and plans for following these principles.[3]

Dworkin's analysis, then, focuses on peripheral rather than essential aspects of the capacity for autonomy. However, to offer a convincing alternative, we must specify more precisely what the essence of the capacity for autonomy amounts to, and in particular what counts as one's own principle or guideline for running one's life. Presumably this cannot be just any run-of-the-mill wish or desire, because a person may distance himself from a mere desire and not recognize it as truly his own.[4] So, at the very least, a principle suitable as a basis for self-governance must be viewed by the person as correct for him.

## Values as starting points of autonomy

To explore this proposal, let us consider whether autonomy would be possible even for a hypothetical creature unable to judge the correctness or appropriateness of his desires.[5] Suppose that this creature can control whether or not he will act on a desire[6], and yet he experiences his desires simply as events in his body. There are two possibilities here. In one, the creature is ultimately indifferent to whether he will act on his desires—he finds himself inclined toward certain things, but upon reflection he never sees anything worthwhile in what he is inclined to do. In the other variant, although the creature finds himself inclined

toward certain choices, he is altogether incapable of reflecting on the merits of these incli-
nations. In both cases, the desires, precisely because they lack the approval of the one who feels
them, are too passive to be regarded as authentic directives for self-governance. Thus, indeed,
to qualify as such an authentic directive, a principle must be viewed by the person as correct for
him.

Following my earlier observations, this means that a principle qualifying as such an authentic
directive must have the status of a value. As I explained above, a person's values specify his own
sense of what is correct and appropriate for him; they are his guidelines for behavior. Values are
also directly connected to a person's sense of self, since the person measures his own worthiness
according to how well he lives up to his values. This connection further confirms that values are
genuinely the person's own principles of behavior, that they are the apt foundation for self-
governance.

We can now restate in a more familiar form our earlier finding that the mere laying down
of principles for one's conduct makes one capable of autonomy. Since such principles are
values, the very ability to value, even if more instrumental abilities are absent, supplies the
starting points for the exercise of autonomy, and thereby renders the person capable of
autonomy.

Of course, possessing the capacity to value does not guarantee that the person can exercise
autonomy to a full degree. Full-blown autonomy involves not only acting on one's own
principles and convictions, but also the ability to scrutinize these principles and to revise
them in light of critical evaluation, so that they are well articulated and robust. The capacity to
value merely makes possible the most minimal and basic level of autonomy; other capacities are
necessary to further develop and perfect autonomy. All the same, the capacity to value by itself
does, in a very important sense, render a person capable of autonomy.

## Autonomy of Alzheimer's patients

Alzheimer's patients usually retain their ability to value long after other capacities necessary for
making their own decisions and fully directing their lives are gone. For example, Mrs D's
conviction that she ought to help her fellow man in any way she could certainly comes across in
the interview as a truly self-given authentic principle of conduct. She talked of this conviction
just as any other person would ordinarily talk of her commitments to her principles. Yet, since
Mrs D struggled even to find her way to the bathroom in a relatively familiar place, she clearly
would have had trouble implementing her altruistic principles on her own; she would not
have been able to figure out, for instance, how to enroll in a research study to help her 'fellow
man'. However, with the assistance of others she was able to continue to lead a life informed by
her valued self-selected principles, and thereby to continue to exercise a measure of self-
government.

The paramount symptom of Alzheimer's disease, as we saw above, is the inability to form
new long-term memories. This does not significantly affect a person's ability to value, but it
does directly and severely hamper his efforts to implement his values, even more than it affects
his grasp of his life as a whole. Even a modest impairment of long-term memory limits the
person's access to information about the world around him and distorts his assessment of his
own competence, compromising his ability to select the course of action befitting his values.

In her account of her husband's battle with Alzheimer's disease, Ann Davidson provides
beautiful testimony that simultaneously illustrates Julian Davidson's relatively intact capacity
to value and his slipping ability to implement his values.

Julian insisted that he had to compose a 'Thank You' speech to be delivered at a banquet honoring his scientific contributions. On his own he was only able to produce phrases such as:

> ... it will be a pleasure and joy to come back with and me tu omar see and and attend to the evening of June and its and day... Although I have not in worked in the day most loved and I will be a persual... strangely I was finished re this important and pleasure. (Davidson 1997 p .210)

But when Ann patiently interviewed him about what he wanted to say, he 'spoke haltingly, but passionately, about leaving his career. In garbled phrases he described what he felt about science and why he was quitting. He needed his colleagues to know why he had left. He wanted them to know, too, that people with Alzheimer's are still "regular folks"' (Davidson 1997 p. 210).

Julian communicated his conviction that it was right for him to care deeply about science, and likewise that it was appropriate to give his colleagues an explanation. He was definitely conveying *values* here, his authentic ideals. At the same time, he needed Ann's help to translate these values into appropriate actions—he could not have figured out on his own that Ann needed to rewrite his speech and that it would be best if someone else delivered the speech on his behalf.

There are abundant variations of cases of Alzheimer's patients who remain valuers despite severe impairments in their decision-making capacity. On my analysis, these patients are still capable of fundamentals of autonomy. Accordingly, a caregiver committed to respect for autonomy must respect these patients' *contemporaneous* autonomy. This is a perfectly coherent goal, albeit respecting the autonomy of such patients usually requires much more active participation of the caregivers than what is required for ordinary competent patients. To properly respect the autonomy of many an Alzheimer's patient, one must do quite a bit to *enhance* his autonomy. One must help the person no longer able to do so on his own to lead his life according to his remaining values, to the extent that this is still feasible. This involves figuring out how his values would be best upheld in a reality he no longer fully understands, as well as helping him implement these solutions in practice. We saw this approach employed by Julian Davidson's wife, by Mrs Rogoff's caregiver Fran, and by the researcher working with Dr B. Sometimes enhancing a person's autonomy in this way may even involve going against his explicit choices. Ann Davidson did not simply allow Julian to try to deliver his jumbled speech, and Fran would not simply give in if Mrs Rogoff insisted on cooking a potholder for dinner. The caregiver must learn to pay attention to the person's values rather than to her concrete, yet perhaps ill-informed, selection of options. All the same, as long as the patient is still able to value, respect for autonomy does not license the caregiver to disregard the patient's immediate interests altogether.

In sum, contrary to Dworkin's assumptions, in the context of dementia, the capacity for autonomy is best understood not as the ability to lead one's life by one's lights when one is left to one's own devices, and not as a full capacity to make a decision from the beginning to end, but as the capacity to value—to originate the appropriate bases for one's decisions that can then be, if the need arises, partly taken over by others. An Alzheimer's patient may be too disoriented to form a life plan or to choose specific treatment preferences, but as long as he still holds values, he is, in the most basic sense, capable of self-governance, and this fact about him commands utmost respect. Autonomy-based recommendations to disregard his contemporaneous interests have no purchase.

## Conclusion

No matter whether we emphasize well-being or autonomy of Alzheimer's patients, we should approach our dilemmas mindful of Julian Davidson's insight that many people with Alzheimer's disease are still 'regular folks'. In some morally very important respects, many Alzheimer's patients remain, at least for a time, surprisingly similar to ourselves. As neuroscience allows us to corroborate, patients moderately afflicted with Alzheimer's disease may well remain valuers, and thus retain the essential characteristics by virtue of which persons and their interests enjoy an exalted moral status.

## Acknowledgments

A version of this article appeared in *Philosophy and Public Affairs* **28**, 105–38, 1999 (see that version for acknowledgements). The opinions expressed are those of the author and do not necessarily reflect the policies or positions of the National Institutes of Health, the Public Health Service, or the US Department of Health and Human Services.

## Notes

1. This case was reported to me by a family member. To protect the privacy of the patient, I use a fictitious name. I also do not list the name of my source, but I would like to thank her for her generous help.
2. In the case of some (often less central) values, one may anticipate a gradual transformation and loss of a value without thinking that it would be a mistake. This is not a counter-example to my characterization of valuing, because my claim concerns our attitudes to our present espousal of a value: It is part of valuing something that one would view the possibility of not caring about it *here and now* as an impoverishment, loss, or mistake. Imagining a future without the alleged value is a good test for this in many cases, but it does not work in every case because some values are dependent on context and are important only at a specific time in one's life.
3. None of what I say here should be taken to imply that, in a normal case, a person's own exercise of means–ends reasoning and planning could be ignored by those aiming to respect his autonomy. My point is that a person largely incapable of such reasoning may still be able to exercise autonomy, and not that such reasoning can be taken lightly in an ordinary person who exercises his autonomy through the use of such reasoning.
4. Some readers may think that this requirement is too stringent, and that the hypothetical individuals I go on to describe are still capable of autonomy. If so, it is only easier for me to claim that many Alzheimer's patients retain the capacity for autonomy.
5. I speak of a 'creature' rather than a 'person' here to allow for the view that the ability that my hypothetical creature lacks is essential to personhood.
6. Why this stipulation? If we imagined a creature who was also unable to control his response to a desire, it would have been easier to see him as lacking the capacity for autonomy. However, I want to show that our intuition that my imagined creature lacks the capacity for autonomy depends on something else; even a creature in control of his desires seems to lack the capacity for autonomy if he can never approve or disapprove of his desires.

# References

Braak E, Braak H (1995). Staging of Alzheimer's disease-related neurofibrillary changes. *Neurobiology of Aging* 16, 271–8.

Damasio AR (1994). *Descartes' Error: Emotion, Reason, and the Human Brain.* New York: Putnam.

Davidson A (1997). *Alzheimer's, a Love Story: One Year in my Husband's Journey.* Secaucus, NJ: Carol.

Dresser R (1986). Life, death, and incompetent patients: conceptual infirmities and hidden values in the law. *Arizona Law Review* 28, 373–405.

Dworkin R (1993). *Life's Dominion: An Argument about Abortion, Euthanasia, and Individual Freedom.* New York: Knopf.

Geula C (1998). Abnormalities of neural circuitry in Alzheimer's disease: hippocampus and cortical cholinergic innervation. *Neurology* 51, S18–29.

Jaworska A (1997). Rescuing Oblomov: a search for convincing justifications of value. Ph.D. Dissertation, Harvard University.

Laakso MP, Hallikainen M, Hänninen T, Partanen K, Soininen H (2000). Diagnosis of Alzheimer's disease: MRI of the hippocampus vs delayed recall. *Neuropsychologia* 38, 579–84.

Riedel G, Micheau J (2001). Function of the hippocampus in memory formation: desperately seeking resolution. *Progress in Neuro-Psychopharmacological and Biological Psychiatry* 25, 835–53.

Sabat SR (1998). Voices of Alzheimer's disease sufferers: a call for treatment based on personhood. *Journal of Clinical Ethics* 9, 38–51.

Sacks O (1995). *The Man Who Mistook His Wife for a Hat and Other Clinical Tales.* New York: Summit Books.

Souren L, Franssen E (1994). *Broken Connections: Alzheimer's Disease*, Part I (trans RMJ van der Wilden-Fall). Lisse, The Netherlands: Swets and Zeitlinger.

Squire LR, Zola-Morgan S (1988). Memory: brain systems and behavior. *Trends in Neurosciences* 11, 170–5.

Squire LR, Zola-Morgan S (1991). The medial temporal lobe memory system. *Science* 253, 1380–6.

Young PA, Young PH (1997). *Basic Clinical Neuroanatomy.* Baltimore, MD: Williams and Wilkins.

Part II

# Neuroethics in practice

Chapter 8

# From genome to brainome: charting the lessons learned

Ronald M. Green

## Introduction

It is 15 years since the start of the Ethical Legal and Social Implications (ELSI) program of the Human Genome Project (HGP). That program was an unprecedented effort to ensure that consideration of the ethical, legal, and social issues of an emerging field of science go hand in hand with research in that field (Clayton 2003; Cook-Deegan 1994).

Although neuroscientists and ethicists have already begun to confer and write about the emerging ethical issues in cognitive neuroscience research (Moreno 2003; Illes and Racine 2005), there has been nothing like the ELSI program in this field. One can speculate on why this is so. It may reflect the lesser degree of government involvement in neuroscience or fewer public fears about the misuses of cognitive neuroscience research. Modern molecular biology emerged in the wake of historic abuses in the field of eugenics (Kevles 1985; Garver and Garver 1991; Gallagher 1999; Carlson 2001). The ELSI program was a deliberate effort by scientists to allay fears generated by their research. (Watson 1997). Whatever the explanation, this difference in treatment is not justified. As other chapters in this book suggest, developments in neuroscience are as likely as those in genetics to have significant impacts on ethics, law, and society.

Those working in the field of neuroethics can learn from the Genome Project's ELSI program. This is partly because there are clear similarities between the two fields and the ethical issues that they share. At the same time, there are important differences between genetic and cognitive neuroscience research that caution us to respect the singularity of each field. In what follows I want to review some of these similarities and differences and indicate their implications for cognitive neuroscience research. With this as a background, I will then develop some of the broad lessons from the area of genetics that cognitive neuroscience researchers and ethicists should keep in mind as they move forward.

## Shared issues
### Issues of privacy, discrimination, and stigmatization

In different ways, molecular biology and neuroscience both afford penetrating insights into an individual's present or future health conditions. Genetics does this by developing the association between a person's genes and bodily states. To the extent that there is a genetic basis to behavior, it can also be diagnosed and predicted. Cognitive neuroscience focuses on brain structures and processes that can indicate normal and abnormal patterns. It can reveal patterns of thought or emotions that the individual wants to conceal from others. In genetics and neuroscience, disclosure of intimate private information can place the individual under study at risk. Bad health news or predictions of future disease can lead to stigmatization by others and even by oneself. Prediction becomes self-fulfilling prophecy when learning that one is predisposed to a disease makes one sick. Individuals found to have a genetic or cognitive predisposition to disease could also face discrimination in education, employment, or insurance. These considerations tell us that neuroscientists, like geneticists, must always consider the informational power and privacy implications of their research.

In both fields, informational dangers extend to incidental or inadvertent findings. Geneticists most commonly encounter this problem with regard to the issue of false paternity, when discrepancies in family linkage studies contradict assumed parent–child relationships (Lucassen and Parker 2001; Richards 2003). Neuroscientists encounter the problem when a study of cognitive structure or function turns up unrelated but potentially dangerous brain anomalies (Illes *et al.* 2004). In both fields, these events present researchers with difficult moral questions of who should be informed about these findings and how they should be informed.

In the early 1990s, when wide-scale genetic research was just beginning, it was not unusual for consent forms to come before institutional review boards with the only indicated risk of the study being a 'minor inflammation at the site of the blood draw'. Genetic researchers have come a long way since then. They now widely recognize the informational risks of their investigations. There is pervasive awareness of the need to include discussion of these risks in the consent process (Reilly *et al.* 1997). Many studies have been published on the specific risk of genetic research, including risks associated with the use of stored or anonymized samples (Clayton *et al.* 1995; Knoppers and Laberge 1995; Goulding *et al.* 2003). Because of what scanning technologies reveal, cognitive neuroscience researchers should also be aware of these privacy and informational risks. Nevertheless, researchers and institutional review boards, long accustomed to viewing biomedical research in terms of physical risks to the subject, will have to be constantly educated into the special informational risks of these emerging sciences. Both research and clinical activities in these fields must start from the premise that information gathered, if wrongly used, can be as toxic as a dangerous drug.

## Forensic applications

To an exceptional degree both genetics and neuroscience are fields that lend themselves to forensic applications. DNA analysis has furnished powerful new tools to crime investigators and has greatly impacted the legal process, leading to the conviction (or release) of people whose cases were previously beyond investigative reach (Dwyer *et al.* 2000). DNA databases have enhanced the powers of law enforcement and defense agencies, and are challenging assumptions about citizens' constitutional rights (Belluck 2005).

Compared with genetics, forensic neuroscience is in its infancy. But the promise—or threat—is obvious. Research on the use of neuroimaging for lie detection, drug abuse monitoring, or the diagnosis of insanity and other brain states relevant to criminal prosecutions is actively underway and, in some cases, is supported by interested governmental agencies (Langleben *et al.* 2002; Frith 2004). It is an irony of genetics and neuroscience, but a further consequence of their informational density, that research begun to provide means for improving human health may eventually come to be known best for its contributions to social control.

## The movement from curing diseases to enhancing traits

Biomedical research usually begins with the promise of providing new approaches to preventing or curing disease. Our nearly universal aversion to illness stimulates the interest of the researcher and patient communities and prompts the support of foundations and governments. But resources that can that used to remedy disease can also be used to alter human nature or 'improve' it beyond what is normal for the species. For better or worse, new biomedical approaches often have a way of moving out of the clinic and into the streets. Curing gives way to recreational or cosmetic use (and abuse).

The movement toward nonmedical utilizations already has a toehold in genetics in the area of prenatal diagnosis. Amniocentesis and preimplantation genetic diagnosis were originally developed to detect serious genetic or chromosomal disorders, but these technologies are now sometimes being used for sex selection or the identification of 'savior children'. The latter are embryos or fetuses produced so that their genotype matches that of a sick sibling. This permits their cord blood or bone marrow to be used for transplant purposes. Since neither sex nor HLA status are disease conditions, these uses of genetic technologies aim at satisfying parental desires rather than curing disease (although the case can reasonably made that HLA genotyping has an indirect relationship to medical therapy for the sick sibling). As our ability to identify the genetic bases of phenotypical traits grows, we can expect parental requests to move in the direction of enhancement. Qualities such as IQ, memory performance, stamina, eye color. and height are all likely candidates for genetic manipulation and selection (Juengst 1997; Parens 1998; Buchanan *et al.* 2000). Negatively, parents may seek to select such traits as skin color or sexual orientation in ways that confirm or reinforce social prejudices (Berkowitz and Snyder 1998; Stein 1998; Ten 1998).

In terms of the drift toward enhancement, neuroscience is already in some ways more advanced than genetics. This is especially true for neuropharmacology, where we have seen widespread use of selective serotonin-reuptake inhibitors like Prozac by people who have no recognized illness but are using the drug prophylactically or to enhance mood (Farah and Wolpe 2004; Farah *et al.* 2004). Writers like Kramer (1994) have even argued for the use of Prozac by individuals not experiencing depression but interested in attaining a state that is 'better than well'. In the future, emerging technologies like transcranial magnetic stimulation may permit the direct manipulation of brain states for pleasure, mood enhancement, or the achievement of competitive advantage (Green *et al.* 1997; see also Chapter 14).

This tells us that neuroscientists, like their counterparts in genetics, must anticipate the uses and abuses of their research. In ways appropriate to their special field, but informed by work in genetics, neuroethicists should identify likely enhancement technologies, their risks and benefits, and the morally and socially appropriate strategies for responding to them.

## Differences

Despite the similarities between neuroscience and genetics, there are interesting and important differences between the two fields. Acute ethical challenges in one field may be less important in the other and vice versa.

### Ease of access

A first difference pertains to the accessibility of genetic versus neurocognitive information. One of the striking features of genetics is that an individual's complete genome is present in virtually every cell in the body (red blood cells are an exception since they possess no nucleus.) Technologies like polymerase chain reaction (PCR) make it possible to amplify even the smallest trace of DNA. Because we potentially leave some of our DNA on almost everything we touch, it is relatively easy to obtain an extraordinary amount of genetic information about a person without their knowledge or consent. This opens the way to widespread use of DNA in even routine criminal investigations (Dewan 2004), by employers or insurers for purposes of applicant screening, and even by romantic partners. For example, in the genetic science fiction film *Gattaca*, a young woman submits a strand of hair from a lover to a genetic testing service in order to assess his prospects.

Such easy and unconsented access to DNA information currently has no counterpart in the neuroscience area. For the most part, neuroimaging requires the use of large installed machines and the voluntary participation of the subject—an abrupt movement in an MRI machine can alter results. These limitations may partly be overcome in the future as new technologies, such as infrared scanning, permit remote, noninvasive, or covert access to a person's brain states (see Chapters 11 and 17). Even now, it is possible to gather private information about an individual under the pretext of performing a routine medical test. Nevertheless, this relative difference in the accessibility of information between the fields suggests that some of the privacy implications of neuroimaging may be less extensive than is true for genetics.

## The scope and relevance of information

When we look more closely at the kind of information developed by genetics and neuroimaging, we see two very different pictures. Genetic information is far broader in scope. Access to a person's DNA can have direct implications for many other individuals, although the significance of that information for all involved may be unclear. In contrast, neurocognitive information can be highly relevant to the individual under study, but have limited implications for others.

The scope of DNA information is a result of its inherited nature. One shares one's DNA with parents, offspring, and other blood relatives. To the extent that we belong to communities and ethnicities characterized by relatively higher rates of intermarriage than surrounding groups, our DNA also has import for the genetic status of these groups.

In genetic ethics, the familial nature of DNA magnifies the implications of genetic research and compounds problems of informed consent. For example, tests that reveal an individual's increased risk of cancer or Alzheimer's disease expose him to employment or insurance discrimination and they can also expose his children and other relatives. Should his relatives be informed of his test results? This issue of the duty to warn is one of the most controversial legal implications of genetics for clinical practice (Geller *et al.* 1993; American Society of Human Genetics 1998; Clayton 1998; Boetzkes 1999; Sommerville and English 1999). Should relatives participate in the consent to testing when such testing unavoidably affects them? In the field of population genetic research, this question comes up whenever research can affect other members of the group, as can alcoholism genetic research in a Native American community (Reilly 1998). It also arises when research on some members of a group reveals lineage information that can impact on group membership criteria or the community's sacred origin myths (Greely 1997; Juengst 1998, 2000; Davis 2000, 2004; Sharp and Foster 2000; Weijer and Emanuel 2000; Foster 2001). In all these cases, the shared nature of genetic information challenges standard clinical and research assumptions about who is the patient or research subject and whose consent for research is needed.

There is currently no analogue to this issue in cognitive neuroscience research. It is true that the detection of brain anomalies in one subject may have implications for close blood relatives, but that connection depends on genetic factors. The ethical issues it raises belong to the sphere of neurogenetics.

However, if neuroscience and neuroethics lack this group issue, they more than make up for it in terms of the relevancy of the individual information that can be gathered. Genetic information is often highly probabilistic in nature. For example, if a woman is tested and shown to have one of the breast cancer gene mutations, she has a much higher likelihood than someone without the mutation of getting breast cancer (Guttmacher and Collins 2003; King *et al.* 2003). But because of the multiple causal pathways to disease and the important role of environmental factors, it is still possible that she may die of old age without ever having cancer.

In contrast, information gathered by neuroimaging usually has considerably more clinical or investigative relevance. True, neuroscience also has its probabilistic aspects. Those who employ neuroimaging technology to predict disease or identify mental states must always be aware of the fact that even dramatic cerebral anomalies or idiosyncrasies may not correspond to predictable behaviors, thoughts, or emotions. I will return to this point shortly when I discuss the risks of deterministic thinking. Nevertheless, because the information provided by neuroimaging and related brain technologies is closer to phenotypic expression in the individual under study, it usually has more relevance to understanding that individual's vulnerabilities and propensities. Thus the powers of genetic and neurocognitive research and the informational risks associated with each field tend to point in different directions.

A further consequence of the difference between genetic and neurocognitive information is that the most pressing issues of informed consent are different between the two fields. In genetics, the shared nature of genes raises the question of whether the individual is the appropriate locus of consent. When one person's genetic status affects others, should they be involved in the decision-making and should they be informed of test results? Who is the patient? The presenting individual? The family? Or is it the community or ethnicity as a whole? Nothing like these questions exists in neuroethics.

However, a different question arises in neuroscience because here the disease process may affect the very organ of consent, the individual's brain. As Roskies (2002) observes, 'neurodegenerative diseases and psychiatric disorders may impair cognition so that informed consent, as generally conceived, may be impossible'. How should investigators proceed in such cases? What guidelines can be developed to protect the individual while facilitating research on the disease condition?

A related problem concerns use of court-ordered or otherwise coercive cognitive neuroscience interventions to bring about cooperative behaviors in persons who are mentally impaired or prone to act in antisocial ways. This is already being practiced in connection with the use of anti-androgen treatment with convicted sex offenders. As cognitive neuroscience interventions and psychopharmacology grow in scope and power, we may see more use of them in the penal or psychiatric context (Farah 2002). Here, coercive methods are used without the consent of individuals to render them more tractable and cooperative. This ability to coerce 'free consent' reveals the special power of neurocognitive intervention and some of the unique questions presented to neuroethicists.

## Broad lessons

We should keep these similarities and differences in mind as we explore the broader lessons that genetic research may have for neuroethics. As I develop these lessons, the reader should keep in mind the ways that field differences reduce or intensify the issues for neuroethics.

## Hazards of the 'therapeutic gap'

A first lesson is one that has been reinforced time and again in the course of genetic research. While a new biomedical science may greatly enhance our diagnostic skills, it does not always increase our ability to prevent or cure disease. This means that there is often a gap between the onset of improved diagnostic capabilities and the availability of new treatments. In some cases this gap is rapidly closed; in others, it remains open for long periods of time.

Many disease conditions illustrate this problem but Huntington's disease (HD) is a particularly vivid example. HD is a severe neurodegenerative disorder with onset usually in the fourth or fifth decade of life that eventually leads to severe physical and mental problems and death. Its genetic basis—a genomic 'stutter' in the form of a series of triple nucleotide repeats—has been understood since 1993 and the relevant protein product has been identified (Wexler 1995). Yet little or no progress has been made in translating this knowledge into therapies or cures. An HD diagnosis is a death sentence. Small wonder that many people in the HD community have chosen not to undergo testing when the results would only increase their mental distress and their risks of stigmatization and discrimination (Decruyenaere *et al.* 1997; Mandich *et al.* 1998; Taylor 2004; see also Chapter 16).

For individuals in the HD community, it could reasonably be said that genetic research, to this point, in some respects has been more of a bane than a blessing. The same could be said for other genetic diseases like sickle cell disease and cystic fibrosis. It is true that, in some cases, knowledge of the genetic basis of the disease affords a form of prevention through the option of prenatal testing. But for religious or other reasons, many carriers of an inherited genetic disease regard this option as a source of anguish, a burden of knowledge that they sometimes choose to escape by refusing testing altogether (Rothman 1987).

As cognitive neuroscience advances and neuroimaging capabilities improve, it is likely that the therapeutic gap will become a problem here as well. Scanning technologies will improve our ability to detect and predict brain pathologies, but the tools for ameliorating or curing these conditions will probably advance more slowly. In many cases, this will create new ethical and emotional problems for patients and their caregivers. There is already discussion of the appropriateness of using neuroimaging as a diagnostic tool for Alzheimer's disease. Here, many of the issues reappear that that have occurred in connection with HD testing (Moreno 2003).

As neuroscience moves forward, it can benefit by learning from some of the bitter experience of genetics. Scientists and clinicians are well advised to avoid 'over-promising' beneficial results for their research. There is a powerful tendency in all biomedical areas to offer enticing therapeutic visions as a way to elicit public support or increase governmental funding for research. Yet the same public enthusiasm that leads to increased funding can turn into budget cuts, resentment, and even research restrictions, when, instead of cures, the actual payoff is burdensome knowledge and a host of new ethical quandaries produced by poor therapeutic options.

A related problem is the specific challenge of clinical implementation that accompanies new biomedical advances. Technologies that have value in a highly developed research setting often do not translate well into clinical practice. The result is misuse of these technologies and the creation of new risks and harms for patients.

Breast cancer genetics provides a good example of this problem and the 'therapeutic gap'. Discovery of the BRCA mutations initially provided hope that it would lead to new approaches to cancer prevention and cure. But more than a decade after these discoveries, the therapeutic options, such as bilateral mastectomy, remain limited or difficult. Despite this, those with a stake in the commercial exploitation of BRCA tests have promoted their use. Myriad Genetics, patent holder of the BRCA gene and gene test, developed a prototype direct-to-consumer television advertising campaign to increase women's awareness of the availability of the test. But breast cancer genetics is a complex matter, best handled by skilled genetics professionals. One independent study performed after the campaign revealed that the advertisements elicited interest from many women who were not appropriate targets for the information (Centers for Disease Control 2004). More worrisome, many of the physicians consulted by these women were unable to provide adequate guidance about cancer susceptibilities. The result was confusion, inappropriate utilization of testing, and the stimulation of unjustified hopes and fears among women in the cities where the advertisements were aired.

This shows that we must pay considerable attention to the clinical implementation of promising new biomedical technologies. Premature deployment of technologies not ready for prime time can not only lead to the waste of scarce medical resources, it can decrease the public's trust in medical professionals. Unfortunately, as the BRCA advertising experience shows, the difficulty of appropriate clinical implementation is increased when commercial interests drive developments. This tells us that those working in an emerging medical field must understand that many challenges lie between the first research successes with an advanced technology and the eventual widespread dissemination of effective diagnostic and therapeutic modalities. Furthermore, all those involved should understand that the improper handling of some of these innovations can delay or prevent proper clinical implementation.

## The allure of determinism

A much reprinted cartoon depicts a laboratory with a group of scientists in white coats. Posters on the wall announce the 'gene for intelligence, homosexuality, violence' and so on. One of the scientists proudly tells his colleagues, 'I discovered the gene that makes us believe that everything is in the genes'. We laugh, but the appeal of genetic determinism, the belief that all features of the self and all behaviors can be reduced to a genetic explanation, has been present in genetics from the start. On the basis of little or no scientific evidence, early eugenicists portrayed many complex social problems, such as poverty or criminal behavior, as resulting from people's inherited predispositions. More recently, genetic determinism has regained renewed attention in the behavioral area as a result of twin studies and some animal research (Bouchard 1994; Hur and Bouchard 1997; Pennisi 2005).

Although the allure of genetic determinism remains powerful, it should always be resisted. Genetics can greatly increase our understanding of causal pathways to disease, the molecular bases of human differences, and the inherited components of some human behaviors. It can enhance our powers of prediction. But it rarely permits certainty with regard to future states, and the belief that it does usually ensnares the field in serious ethical, legal, and social problems. This lesson also applies to neuroscience.

To understand the limits of genetic or neuroscience determinism one does not have to postulate a 'ghost in the machine', a hidden 'soul' or free human will, that confounds biochemical predictions. The underlying problem is scientifically understandable: human biology is enormously complex. Countless illustrations of this can be given from the field of genetics. The genomic era began with what has been called 'the central dogma' enunciated by Francis Crick that one gene begets one messenger RNA that in turn begets one protein. From this dogma, it naturally followed that if you understood a gene sequence, you could make substantial progress toward understanding the biological structures and processes to which it led.

Over the years, it became clear that there were many problems with this model. Similar genes often produced multiple effects (pleiotropy). Identical gene mutations did not always lead to the same phenotypical results, in ways not easily explained by different environmental factors. Cystic fibrosis (CF) is an example. Since the early 1990s when the array of CF mutations became known, it has been obvious that there are many uncharted links between mutations and phenotypical effects. The availability of testing for CF mutations has even revealed the existence of a population who bear known deleterious mutations but who experience little or no frank disease. Obviously many other genetic, developmental, and environmental factors are at work.

The full identification of the human genome sequence brought with it a surprising finding that helps to explain some of this complexity. Human beings have far fewer genes than was believed. Instead of the nearly 100,000 genes that had been predicted on the basis of protein products, only about 30,000 genes have been found. How can we explain the incredible biochemical productivity of this reduced number? The answer, now being developed, is that the human genome is highly modular in nature. Genes have many component parts spread physically across the genome and often separated by noncoding regions containing various transcription factors and promoter regions. Together with other regulatory components, this modular structure permits many different combinatorial events. As Venter *et al.* (2001) observed in their paper accompanying the publication of the human genome sequence, 'A single gene may give rise to multiple transcripts and thus multiple distinct proteins with multiple functions, by means of alternative splicing and alternative transcription initiation and termination sites'. Recent studies have consistently shown a high rate of alternative splicing in the human genome. Between 35 and 59 percent of human genes have at least one alternative splice form, and most of these appear to have functional significance because they change the protein product (Modrek and Lee 2002). Further accentuating this complexity, each component of the process is modulated through feedback loops involving various cellular and organismic environmental factors. All of this has led to a waning of the dogma that one gene equals one protein. Reflecting on these developments, Paul Silverman, one of the early leaders of the Human Genome Project, observes that in current thinking:

> The gene may not be central to the phenotype at all, or at least it shares the spotlight with other influences. Environmental, tissue and cytoplasmic factors clearly dominate the phenotypic expression processes, which may, in turn, be affected by a variety of unpredictable protein-interaction events. (Silverman 2004)

This complexity recommends a cautionary note in all approaches to disease or behavior prediction in the area of genetics. Genetic information is almost always, at best, probabilistic. Ethically, legally, and socially, this reduces the power of genetic information and significantly increases the risks of its misuse.

This caution against determinism should extend to the very terms we use to describe things. For example, it is now common for prosecutors, journalists, and others to speak of 'DNA fingerprinting'. But the term 'fingerprint' is misleading. As far as we know, fingerprints are unique; not even identical twins have the same ones. This is not true of DNA. Although the chance of DNA matching between two people at all the loci selected for forensic purposes is vanishingly small, there are many things that can distort probability estimates of DNA matches. These include common laboratory errors, the susceptibility of the PCR process to contamination, and poor information with regard to gene frequencies in relevant subgroups. Thus use of the term 'fingerprint' conveys a misleading impression of certainty that can cause wrongful convictions.

The problem of excessive determinism in conclusions is also acute in the health care area, where faulty diagnoses or predictions can lead to mistreatment, discrimination and stigmatization. The difficulty is compounded by the fact that, for many purposes, probabilistic information is useful. In the fields of insurance risk assessment or pre-employment testing, for example, one does not need certainty that any particular individual tested will succumb to disease or evidence a harmful trait. It is enough to know that the possession of a particular DNA sequence places that person at higher risk of doing so. When processing large numbers of applicants, an insurer or employer can significantly reduce costs by routinely denying coverage or employment to those whose tests show them to be at higher risk. Although error-prone testing may wrongly exclude some individuals, it can prove economically efficient.

As Nelkin and Tancredi (1989) have observed, this actuarial mindset sets the stage for multiple injustices. It can cause some individuals to be denied social protection or access to opportunities and create a burgeoning social underclass. Prophecy becomes self-fulfilling through its own destructive effects. If we are to avoid these outcomes, those who use genetic information must understand its scientific limits, and society as a whole must determine when actuarial information is appropriately used and when it is not.

An additional philosophical point is relevant here. Difference does not amount to disease. Many people hold the view that difference itself is pathological: left-handed persons or gay persons are 'abnormal' and must be cured of their 'disorder'. These attitudes have sometimes even been carried into the philosophical literature, where disease has been defined in terms of departures from 'normal functioning' (Boorse 1975). However, difference and abnormality are not sufficient to make something an illness or disease condition. The condition by its very nature must lead to an increased risk of suffering harm, such as death, pain, or disability (Gert et al. 1997). Difference without an increased risk of suffering harm is not a disease. Redheads are not sick!

Advances in genetic science make this point more important. The Human Genome Project has already revealed the existence of an enormous amount of variation in the human genome. A random pair of human haploid genomes differs on average at a rate of 1 in 1250 bp (Venter et al. 2001). However, very few of these differences have functional significance, and among those that do, even fewer result in increased risk of harm for the individual. If genetic difference or abnormality were the same thing as illness, all of us would be genetically diseased because at the sequence level we all differ in some ways from the human norm. Given the historic abuses of genetics and the powerful consequences that can follow from being diagnosed as carrying diseased genes, it is extremely important that we not confuse disease with difference or abnormality.

All these cautions pertain to cognitive neuroscience and associated neuroimaging technologies. Superficially, this field seems different from genetics, since the focus is not on underlying genetic mechanisms, which can often be remote from phenotypical expression, but on the phenotype itself in the form of observable brain structures and functioning. Nevertheless, there still remains an enormous gap between our ability to identify existing brain structures and processes and our understanding of their implications for an individual's thoughts, emotions, behaviors, and health. Again, part of the reason for this is the enormous complexity of the brain as a system and our relatively poor understanding of the interactions of its many parts. Neural pathways that function one way in one individual can produce entirely different outcomes in another. This has great relevance to disease diagnosis and behavior prediction. For example, Moll *et al.* (2003) note that damage to the ventromedial prefrontal region of the brain is sometimes associated with acquired sociopathy. Nevertheless, it is also true that there are individuals who have all the expected structural ingredients for sociopathy, including massive destruction of the polar and mediobasal parts of both frontal lobes, but who never exhibit it. Observations such as these indicate that specific behaviors only emerge when the destruction and sparing of specific neural structures occur in certain combinations. The brain, no less than the genome, is an extraordinarily complex combinatorial system. When we consider that almost undetectable microscopic alterations in neural pathways or cellular functioning might signify profound differences at the level of thought, emotion, or conduct, the need for caution in the use of scanning data becomes even more apparent. The tools here can simply be too blunt for the work they are called on to do.

Here too, however, the danger is that the actuarial mindset will take advantage of better (or worse) probabilistic information to form social policies. Insurers do not need certainty to economically justify excluding from coverage people with structural brain anomalies that may be highly associated with neurological disease. In a period of intense fear about terrorism, it is tempting to identify terrorist suspects on the basis of information gathered from functional imaging or infrared scanning that associates certain neural processes with deception or violence. In actuarial terms, such policies may even reduce the immediate risks of a terrorist incident. But they can do so by perpetrating grave injustices on individuals who may never have behaved in antisocial ways. In yet another self-fulfilling prophecy, these injustices may breed the very resentment and violence they hope to prevent. All these problems are greatly magnified if anomalous brain findings not clearly associated with disease are made the basis of exclusion. In that case just being different makes one a pariah. In the area of neuropharmacology, the assumption that all differences or abnormalities are pathogenic can lead to the overprescribing and overuse of medication. Current widespread use of Ritalin in the classroom may partly reflect this problem (Diller 1996).

Therefore neuroscientists and neuroethicists, no less than geneticists, should exercise caution in presenting their findings. They must appreciate the philosophical point that difference, however striking it may be, does not amount to disease unless the difference itself causes an increased likelihood of suffering harm. Even when anomalies cause harm, neuroscientists should be aware that biological systems usually prove to be very complicated. Brain states that underlie impairment in one person may not do so in another.

Neuroscientists must always guard against prematurely deterministic conclusions. They should avoid the use of deterministic language. It is probably just as unwise for neuroscientists to speak of brain architecture, brain maps, or brain fingerprints, as it is for geneticists to use the term DNA fingerprint or to describe the DNA sequence as a blueprint (Rose 2002). All these images present a static and concrete picture of complex systems; all overestimate the role of one informational component and obscure the dynamic, often self-constructing nature of the organism; and all omit the fact that many exogenous factors and feedback loops shape structure, development, and expression.

Finally, people working in the field of cognitive neuroscience should anticipate and plan for pressures toward the actuarial application of their findings. The fact that actuarial reasoning is sometimes justified makes it particularly dangerous because it is easy to extend its use to circumstances where it is unjust and counterproductive. Added to this is the problem that there are enormous pressures in the commercial sector, in schools, and even in medical institutions for the deployment of predictive tests that produce measurable and standardized results, even when these tests are less than completely sensitive, specific, or valid (Nelkin and Tancredi 1989). This means that neuroscientists must resist pressures to deploy their findings and technologies prematurely. Neuroethicists must also undertake the hard job of drawing lines between social policies that are warranted on the basis of probabilistic information and those that are not.

## The temptation of metaphysics

A final major lesson that neuroscientists and ethicists can learn from genetics is that there is a powerful tendency for a cutting-edge life science to become the basis of metaphysical excursions that go well beyond the knowledge that the science itself offers. By definition, metaphysics deals with issues that defy scientific explanation and that have to do with questions of meaning, value, and purpose. Metaphysics comes to replace and distort science when scientists or others insist that scientific findings by themselves provide definitive answers to ethical and philosophical questions.

Some of the problems here are related to determinism. On the basis of predictive capabilities in a life science field, it is easy to slide into a full-bodied theory of human nature. 'We are our genes' has become a slogan in popular media (Nelkin and Lindee 1995). Dawkins' theory of the 'the selfish gene' has been extrapolated to explain everything from marital infidelity to war. Often lost in this rush to explain are the many other biological, environmental, and cultural systems that play a role in shaping human behavior.

But the problem goes deeper than this. Over the centuries, human beings have speculated about a host of questions beyond the boundaries of observable experience. As Kant observed, it is the nature of reason to seek ultimate answers to its questions even when this goes beyond the domain of available knowledge (Kant 1781). Because of their prestige, the life sciences have often been used as a way of answering questions of this sort. However, almost always when this is done scientific information is extrapolated beyond its appropriate domain to support conclusions that may be wrong in scientific, ethical, or metaphysical terms.

Genetics furnishes a good example of this with regard to the issue of the human soul. In Western religion and philosophy, there has long been a belief in a nonphysical (spiritual) aspect of a person that endures throughout all the changing phases of life and that explains the person's uniqueness and sanctity. The metaphysical importance of the soul derives, in part, from how it helps to account for such things as the persistence of personal identify and the difference between life and death. In religious terms, the idea of the soul provides comfort in the face of death and the corruption of the body.

As Mauron points out, since the advent of genetics, there has been a strong tendency to identify the person's genes with the soul. The genome lends itself to such characterization. It is easily conceived as a 'command post installed at the very core of the individual and conditioning broad aspects of his or her behaviour' (Mauron 2002). It is 'the innermost locus of being, while all other characteristics are, in some sense, more peripheral'. Once this privileged connection with human nature is set up, genes are then utilized well beyond their role as a biological agent. They are invoked in moral and philosophical debates where their use may be seriously misleading.

The eugenics movement provides one illustration of this problem. If genes are viewed as the core of the person, and if those genes are viewed as bad or diseased, it follows that society should reduce the incidence of such genes and prevent their proliferation. Policies of restricted reproduction and sterilization have been a hallmark of the eugenics movement (Sofair and

Kaldjian 2000; Bachrach 2004). Nazi policies of sterilization and extermination were an extreme expression of this way of thinking. Nazi eugenics fused basic eugenic prejudices with older anti-Semitic views. It followed that if the soul resided in the genes and the Jewish soul was diabolical in nature, then 'the Jewish problem' could only be solved by the elimination of 'Jewish genes'. Programs of sterilization, forced abortion, confinement, and genocide followed.

Our current debates about abortion, embryo research, and stem cells provide another vivid example of the tendency to metaphysicalize genes. In trying to determine at what stage nascent human life becomes morally protectable, it is tempting to look for some quality that is associated with the individual's coming into being and that remains in place as long as the individual is alive. In traditional religious and metaphysical thinking, this feature is the soul. It is believed to come into being some time near the individual's conception and it departs at death, when the sanctity of the physical person comes to an end. Against this conceptual background, it is not surprising that genes have come to play a leading role in abortion debates. In the minds of many who oppose abortion, it makes sense to see life as beginning in a moral sense with the creation of a novel genome at conception. As long as the genes remain active, informing all the other functions of the body, the person is 'alive'. At death, genetic material ceases to activate bodily functions and personhood ends. In all these ways, the genome seems to be an effective surrogate for the soul.

Despite the attractiveness of this idea, it is misleading and capable of seriously distorting complex scientific and ethical realities. For one thing, we know that the unique diploid genome is not established at conception. Twinning and embryo fusion can occur during the first 2 weeks of embryonic development, resulting in one genome in two persons or two genomes in a single individual. Hence conception cannot logically be the starting point for the unique human individual (Ford 1998; Shannon and Wolter; Mauron 2002). As twins themselves reveal, the genome itself is not the sole basis of personal identity. At the end of life, gene functioning can persist at the cellular level even though the person, as a moral or legal entity, is gone. This tells us that the genome is not the same as the soul and should not be regarded as the unique person-making feature of the organism.

As natural and attractive as the equation of the genome with the person may be, it also obscures key ethical and philosophical questions. Do we really want to associate what is most valuable and most protectable in human beings with the genes? What are the implications of doing so? If ethics and law require 'bright lines' to facilitate social policy and decision, is the emergence of genetic identity the best bright line to select? Could other alternatives serve us better? The real problem with genetic metaphysics is that it tends to bypass these morally difficult questions. It falsely equates the genome and the soul, and then uses the power of this equation to replace reasoned argumentation and analysis.

Mauron (2003) points out that neuroscience may be even more susceptible to this meta-physical allure than genetics. In many respects, the brain is closer to the core of the self than are the genes. Understanding a person's brain involves a profound penetration of the self. Changing brain states can also alter one's destiny and one's self-conception. Neuroethicists have noted that, in addition to the ethics of neuroscience, there is an emerging field that has been called the 'neuroscience of ethics' (Roskies 2002; see also Chapter 2). This involves the study and understanding of the neural bases of moral reasoning and behaviors. Thus neuroscience promises greatly increased understanding of what it means to be a moral agent and how variations in neural functioning can affect our sense of self, our values, and our conduct.

Because of the proximity of neuroscience to so many basic ethical and metaphysical questions, a metaphysics drawing on cognitive neuroscience research can lead to many misconceptions. One problem is the tendency to equate brain structures or processes with metaphysical realities. Selfhood, free will, or moral responsibility might be identified with some associated brain state or function. The presence or absence of this structure or function in an individual could easily lead to extravagant moral and legal conclusions. We can understand a defense attorney seeking to persuade a jury that his client should not be convicted or punished because the client possesses neural structures associated with a tendency to uncontrollable violence or lacks the functional abilities necessary for free choice. This is already being attempted in some legal cases (Murphy 2005), and pseudo-colors have even been used in scans (a black lesion against a red and green background) to identify an alleged problem area (Illes *et al.* 2004; see also Chapters 3 and 17). But from here it is just a short and misleading step to the conclusion that there really is one locus for good or evil in the brain and that all people with the undesirable feature pose a risk to society. We can imagine such findings being used to promulgate racist notions. And we can imagine a repressive regime choosing to imprison or otherwise marginalize individuals with this feature. Here, deterministic and actuarial ways of thinking are magnified by becoming allied with older metaphysical notions of an indwelling good or evil soul, now identified with some neural structure.

Another example of what I would call metaphysicalized brain science comes from its use in the abortion/embryo research/stem cell debates. Again, the quest is for a defining biological feature that identifies our humanity—a feature whose presence marks the beginning of moral protectability and whose absence marks the end. But if genes will not do this work, perhaps neural activity will? Hence some bioethicists and cognitive neuroscientists have proposed a neural test for personhood (Gazzaniga 2002; Sass 1994; Veatch 1994; see also Chapter 10). If the cessation of brain activity is now widely recognized legally and morally as signifying death, why not regard the start of neural activity, sometime around the first trimester of a pregnancy, as the moral/legal beginning of life? Here, neural activity performs a similar role to that played by the rational soul in classical Thomist metaphysics, where it was seen as being infused some weeks after conception (Wallace 1995).

As attractive as this approach may seem to some pro-choice people or advocates of stem cell research, it is no less misleading than the genetic one. A brain-dead individual differs from an early embryo or fetus. Although the neural structures of an embryo have not yet begun to function, they will do so if development is allowed to proceed. The same cannot be said of a brain-dead individual. Furthermore, the absence of neural activity is a concept requiring much greater specification. How much 'absence' counts? Must the brain as a whole be nonfunctional, or are there special regions (e.g. the cerebral cortex) that are important? How long must nonfunctioning continue? Are individuals in a persistent vegetative state 'persons'?

Behind these questions are a host of further scientific and ethical determinations. We may conclude that the absence of neural activity in certain circumstances is a useful marker for the beginning or end of moral and legal protection, but if we do so, it is because a variety of considerations, including the social costs of maintaining brain-dead individuals, lead us in this direction (Green 2001). Those matters will be ignored if we short-circuit this reasoning process by a metaphysical leap that equates brain functioning with the soul.

The lesson here is that science is not metaphysics, and neuroscience is not neuroethics. Scientists provide insight into physical realities. They have no special expertise in answering our enduring metaphysical and ethical questions. Neuroscience and neuroscientists can provide important new information about the human brain. But, while that information can feed into ethical reasoning, it cannot itself replace the ethical judgment needed for individual and social decision-making. Those who engage in what might be called 'metaphysical neuroscience' ignore this and find it tempting to jump from physical and physiological observations to moral, religious, and philosophical conclusions. This is a temptation that should be avoided.

## Conclusion

Neuroscience and neuroethics can learn from the experience of genetics. Many of these lessons are quite specific and can be gleaned from the extensive literature produced by the ELSI program of the Human Genome Project. For example, when should a test move from the research context to widespread clinical implementation? The experience of those in genetics working with tests for disorders like sickle cell disease, cystic fibrosis, or Huntington's disease can help to provide answers to this question (Holtzman and Watson 1998).

In addition, however, neuroscientists can profit from the broad lessons of the Genome Project and ELSI research. These include awareness that there will almost always be a gap between improved diagnosis and our ability to intervene to prevent and cure disease. The existence of the therapeutic gap urges caution in making treatment predictions, and alerts clinicians and investigators to a host of ethical problems that would not exist if the understanding of the etiology of a disease condition led immediately to its treatment or cure.

Deterministic ways of thinking are always a danger in fields where predictions are probabilistic and where average findings have importance but there are also significant differences at the individual level. The lesson here for neuroscientists and neuroethicists is not to overemphasize the certainty of cognitive neuroscience findings and to be ready to consider how we should use information that has actuarial value but may not be relevant to each individual patient or subject.

Finally, neuroscientists must be careful not to succumb to the metaphysical employment of their findings in ways that lead to overly broad claims about human nature or that attempt direct support of ethical or legal conclusions. Neuroscientists make their best contribution when they convey the knowledge developed in their field and make clear the limits of that knowledge. It remains for those working in the fields of philosophy, religion, ethics, law, and the social sciences, as well as those working specifically in neuroethics, to collaborate with scientists to develop the implications of this field for these other areas. Geneticists have had to learn all these lessons by trial and error. Neuroscientists can minimize their own mistakes by learning from this experience.

## References

American Society of Human Genetics (1998). Professional disclosure of familial genetic information (statement). *American Journal of Human Genetics* 62, 474–83.

Bachrach S (2004). In the name of public health—Nazi racial hygiene. *New England Journal of Medicine* 351, 417–420.

Belluck P (2005). To try to net killer, police ask a small town's men for DNA. *New York Times*, 10 January.

Berkowitz JM, Snyder JM (1998). Racism and sexism in medically assisted conception. *Bioethics* 12, 25–44.

Boetzkes E (1999). Genetic knowledge and third-party interests. *Cambridge Quarterly of Healthcare Ethics* 8, 386–92.

Boorse C (1975). On the distinction between disease and illness. *Philosophy and Public Affairs* 5, 49–68.

Bouchard TJ (1994). The genetic basis of complex human behaviors. *Science* 264, 1700–1.

Buchanan A, Brock DW, Daniels N, Wikler D (2000). *From Chance to Choice: Genetics and Justice.* Cambridge, UK: Cambridge University Press.

Carlson EA (2001). *The Unfit: A History of a Bad Idea.* Cold Spring Harbor, NY: Cold Spring Harbor Laboratory.

Centers for Disease Control (2004). Genetic testing for breast and ovarian cancer susceptibility: evaluating direct-to-consumer marketing—Atlanta, Denver, Raleigh–Durham and Seattle, 2003. *Morbidity and Mortality Weekly Report* 53, 603–6.

Clayton EW (1998). What should the law say about disclosure of genetic information to relatives? *Journal of Health Care, Law and Policy* 1, 373–90.

Clayton EW (2003). Ethical, legal and social implications of genomic medicine. *New England Journal of Medicine* 349, 562–9.

Clayton EW, Steinberg KK, Khoury MJ, *et al.* (1995). Informed consent for genetic research on stored tissue samples. *JAMA* 274, 1786–92.

Cook-Deegan RM (1994). *The Gene Wars*. New York: Norton.

Davis DS (2000). Groups, communities, and contested identities in genetic research. *Hastings Center Report* 30, 38–45.

Davis DS (2004). Genetic research and communal narratives. *Hastings Center Report* 34, 40–9.

Decruyenaere M, Evers-Kiebooms G, Boogaerts A, *et al.* (1997). Non-participation in predictive testing for Huntington's disease: individual decision-making, personality and avoidant behaviour in the family. *European Journal of Human Genetics* 5, 351–63.

Dewan SK (2004). As police extend use of DNA, a smudge could trap a thief. *New York Times*, 26 May.

Diller LH (1996). The run on Ritalin: attention deficit disorder and stimulant treatment in the 1990s. *Hastings Center Report* 26, 12–14.

Dwyer J, Neufeld B, Scheck B (2000). *Actual Innocence*. New York: Random House.

Farah MJ (2002). Emerging ethical issues in neuroscience. *Nature Neuroscience* 5, 1123–29.

Farah MJ, Wolpe PR (2004). Monitoring and manipulating brain function: new neuroscience technologies and their ethical implications. *Hastings Center Report* 34, 35–45.

Farah MJ, Illes J, Cook-Deegan R, *et al.* (2004). Neurocognitive enhancement: what can we do and what should we do? *Nature Reviews Neuroscience* 5, 421–5.

Ford NM (1988). *When Did I Begin?* Cambridge, UK: Cambridge University Press.

Foster M (2001). Ethical issues in developing a haplotype map with socially defined populations. Available online at: http://www.genome.gov/page.cfm?pageID=10001683

Frith S (2004). Who's minding the brain. *Pennsylvania Gazette* 23–31.

Geller G, Tambor ES, Bernhardt BA, *et al.* (1993). Physicians' attitudes toward disclosure of genetic information to third parties. *Journal of Law, Medicine and Ethics* 21, 238–40.

Gallagher NL (1999). *Breeding Better Vermonters*. Hanover, NH: University Press of New England.

Garver KL, Garver B (1991). Eugenics: past, present, and the future. *American Journal of Human Genetics* 49, 1109–18.

Gazzaniga M (2002). Zygotes and people aren't quite the same. *New York Times*, 25 April, p.31.

Gert B, Culver CM, Clouser KD (1997). Malady. In: Gert B, Culver CM, Clouser KD (eds) *Bioethics: A Return to Fundamentals*. New York : Oxford University Press, Chapter 5.

Goulding NJ, Waddell HC, Doyal L (2003). Adherence to published ethical guidelines by the UK research community. *Nature Genetics* 34, 117–19.

Greely HT (1997). The control of genetic research: involving the 'groups between. *Houston Law Review* 33, 397–430.

Green RM (2001). *The Human Embryo Research Debates* New York: Oxford University Press.

Green RM, Leone AP, Wasserman EM (1997). Ethical guidelines for rTMS research. *IRB* 19, 1–6.

Guttmacher AE, Collins FS (2003). Breast and ovarian cancer. *New England Journal of Medicine* 348, 2339–47.

Holtzman NA, Watson MS (eds) (1998). *Promoting Safe and Effective Genetic Testing in the United States: Final Report of the Task Force on Genetic Testing*. Baltimore, MD: Johns Hopkins University Press.

Hur YM, Bouchard TJ (1997). The genetic correlation between impulsivity and sensation seeking traits. *Behavior Genetics* 27, 455–63.

Illes J and Racine E (2005). Target article: imaging or imagining? A neuroethics challenge informed by genetics *American Journal of Bioethics* 5, 1–14.

Illes J, Desmond JE, Huang LF, Raffin TA, Atlas SW (2004). Ethical consideration of incidental findings on adult brain MRI in research. *Neurology* 62, 849–50.

Juengst ET (1997). Can enhancement be distinguished from prevention in genetic medicine. *Journal of Medicine and Philosophy* 22, 125–142.

Juengst ET (1998). Groups as gatekeepers to genomic research: conceptually confusing, morally hazardous, and practically useless. *Kennedy Institute of Ethics Journal* 8, 183–200.

Juengst ET (2000). Commentary: what 'community review' can and cannot do. *Journal of Law, Medicine and Ethics* 28, 52–54.

Kant I (1781). *The Critique of Pure Reason* (trans Meiklejohn JMD). New York: Dover Publications, 2003.

Kevles DJ (1985). *In the Name of Eugenics*. New York: Knopf.

King MC, Marks JH, Mandell JB (2003). Breast and ovarian cancer risks due to inherited mutations in BRCA1 and BRCA2. *Science* 302, 643–6.

Knoppers BM, Laberge CM (1995). Research and stored tissues. Persons as sources, samples as persons? *JAMA* 274, 1806–7.

Kramer PD (1994). *Listening to Prozac*. New York: Penguin Books.

Langleben DD, Schroeder L, Maldjian JA, *et al.* (2002). Brain activity during simulated deception: an event-related functional magnetic resonance study. *NeuroImage* 15, 727–32.

Lucassen A, Parker M (2001). Revealing false paternity: some ethical considerations. *Lancet* 357, 1033–5.

Mandich P, Jacopini G, Di Maria E, *et al.* (1998). Predictive testing for Huntington's disease: ten years' experience in two Italian centres. *Italian Journal of Neurological Science* 19, 68–74.

Mauron A (2002). Genomic metaphysics. *Journal of Molecular Biology*, 319 957–62.

Mauron A (2003). Renovating the house of being: genomes, souls and selves. *Annals of the New York Academy of Sciences* 1001, 240–52.

Modrek B, Lee C (2002). A genomic view of alternative splicing. *Nature Genetics* 30, 13–19.

Moll J, de Oliveira-Souza R, Eslinger, PJ (2003). Morals and the human brain: a working model. *Neuroreport* 14, 299–305.

Moreno JD (2003). Neuroethics: an agenda for neuroscience and society. *Nature Reviews Neuroscience* 4, 149–153.

Murphy DE (2005). Lawyers cite killer's brain damage as execution nears. *New York Times*, 18 January.

Nelkin D, Lindee MS (1995). *The DNA Mystique: The Gene as a Cultural Icon*. New York: W.H. Freeman.

Nelkin D, Tancredi L (1989). *Dangerous Diagnostics: The Social Power of Biological Information*. New York: Basic Books.

Parens E (ed) (1998). *Enhancing Human Traits: Ethical and Social Implications*. Washington, DC: Georgetown University Press.

Pennisi E (2005). A genomic view of animal behavior. *Science* 307, 30–2.

Reilly PR (1998). Rethinking risks to human subjects in genetic research. *American Journal of Human Genetics* 63, 682–5.

Reilly PR, Boshar MF, Holtzman SH (1997). Ethical issues in genetic research: disclosure and informed consent. *Nature Genetics* 15, 16–20.

Richards JL (2003). Medical confidentiality and disclosure of paternity. *South Dakota Law Review* 48, 409–42.

Rose SPR (2002). The biology of the future and the future of biology. *Journal of Molecular Biology* 319, 877–84.

Roskies A (2002). Neuroethics for the new millennium. *Neuron* 35, 21–23.

Rothman BK (1987). *The Tentative Pregnancy: Prenatal Diagnosis and the Future of Motherhood*. New York: Penguin Books.

Sass H-M (1994). The moral significance of brain-life criteria. In: Beller FK, Weir RF (eds) *The Beginnings Of Human Life*. Dordrecht, The Netherlands: Kluwer Academic, 57–70.

Shannon T, Wolter AB (1990). Reflections on the moral status of the pre-embryo. *Theological Studies* 51, 603–26.

Sharp RR, Foster M (2000). Involving study populations in the review of genetic research. *Journal of Law, Medicine and Ethics* 28, 41–51.

Sofair A, Kaldjian LC (2000). Eugenic sterilization and a qualified Nazi analogy: the United States and Germany, 1930–1945. *Annals of Internal Medicine* 132, 312–19.

Silverman PH (2004). Rethinking genetic determinism. *Scientist* 18, 32–33.

Sommerville A, English V (1999). Genetic privacy: orthodoxy or oxymoron? *Journal of Medical Ethics* 25, 144–50.

Stein E (1998). Choosing the sexual orientation of children. *Bioethics* 12, 1–24.

Taylor SD (2004). Predictive genetic test decisions for Huntington's disease: context, appraisal and new moral imperatives. *Social Science and Medicine* 58, 137–49.

Ten CL (1998). The use of reproductive technologies in selecting the sexual orientation, the race and the sex of children. *Bioethics* 12, 45–8.

Veatch RM (1994). The beginning of full moral standing. In: Beller FK, Weir RF (eds) *The Beginnings Of Human Life*. Dordrecht, The Netherlands: Kluwer Academic, 19–33.

Venter JC, Adams MD, Myers EW, *et al.* (2001) The sequence of the human genome. *Science* 291, 1304–51.

Wallace WA (1995). St Thomas on the beginning and ending of life. Autori Vari Sanctus Thomas de Aquino Doctor Hodiernae Humanitatis. *Studi Tomistici* 58, 394–407.

Watson JD (1997). Genes and politics. *Journal of Molecular Medicine* 75, 624–36.

Weijer C, Emanuel EJ (2000). Protecting communities in biomedical research. *Science* 289, 1142–4.

Wexler A (1995). *Mapping Fate*. New York: Random House.

Chapter 9

# Protecting human subjects in brain research: a pragmatic perspective

Franklin G. Miller and Joseph J. Fins

## Introduction

Brain research involving human subjects encompasses a vast territory of neuroscience and biomedical investigation. It includes studies with healthy volunteers aimed at elucidating normal functioning in areas such as attention, perception, cognition, memory, judgment, and emotion; investigation of neurobiological processes underlying deviant and addictive behavior; clinical research aimed at understanding the pathophysiology of diseases and disorders of the brain and nervous system; and clinical trials evaluating novel treatments for these conditions. The development and refinement of powerful techniques of *in vivo* examination of brain functioning and treatment modalities that intervene directly in the brain hold great promise for scientific advance and therapeutic benefit. As in all human investigation, however, brain research evokes perplexing and troubling ethical concerns. Rather than attempting to examine the full range of ethical issues relating to brain research—an endeavor far beyond the scope of a single chapter—we will focus on the ethics of clinical research in brain disorders, based on an approach to research ethics deriving from American philosophical pragmatism. We apply this perspective specifically to placebo-controlled trials of pharmacological treatments and deep brain stimulation for psychiatric and neurological disorders.

## Pragmatism and research ethics

All approaches to the ethics of research involving human subjects, at least implicitly, appeal to or invoke philosophical assumptions regarding the moral life, the nature of moral principles, and methods of moral reasoning. The ethical perspective presented in this chapter is guided by American philosophical pragmatism, especially as developed systematically by John Dewey (1859–1952). We see the following pragmatic themes as relevant to the ethics of clinical research in general, and research on brain disorders in particular (Miller *et al.* 1996).

First, the moral life, in all its domains, is complex. Ethical analysis must reflect and do justice to the concrete practical contexts in which moral problems arise. In the case of the ethics of clinical research, methodological issues of experimental design and the clinical situations faced by patient-subjects must always receive due attention. On the one hand, the search for rigorous unbiased scientific data drives investigators to adopt experimental methods that may pose moral problems, as in the use of placebo and sham procedure controls and deceptive disclosures to research subjects about the nature of the research. On the other hand, clinical research takes place within a context of vulnerability of research subjects to exploitation, especially sick patients, and trust in clinical investigators and research institutions that the research is worthwhile and safe. Appreciation of methodological considerations is basic to sound ethical analysis, along with the search for adequate subject protections that can alleviate moral concerns while permitting valid experimental methods in the service of valuable research.

Secondly, moral values, rules, principles, standards, and virtues are apt to conflict when applied to contextually complex situations, calling for careful balancing of competing morally relevant considerations. Most broadly, clinical research is guided by two primary moral objectives: developing knowledge to improve public health or medical care, and protecting research subjects from harm or exploitation. These two moral considerations inevitably conflict in the design and conduct of clinical research. No simple formulas are available for resolving these moral conflicts. Careful ethical analysis is required to identify and appraise the specific moral considerations at stake in any challenging problem in the ethics of clinical research and to guide satisfactory resolutions.

Thirdly, moral norms should be understood logically as hypothetical guides to ethical judgment, rather than categorical or absolute rules. The test of the meaning and value of moral principles, rules, and standards, pragmatically understood, lies in the extent to which they provide, on critical reflection, satisfactory guidance in the resolution of challenging moral problems. From the pragmatic perspective, ethical guidance is fallible and tentative. In other words, it is contingent, never certain, and is always subject to reconsideration.

Regarding moral rules and principles as fallible and tentative hypotheses departs fundamentally from traditional ethics and moral philosophy. When norms and standards of research ethics are seen as working hypotheses, they are recognized as open to modification, in light of the consequences of adhering to them, rather than as fixed rules. This does not mean that they will be so changeable as to undermine any confidence in the direction that they afford. Pragmatists analogize general ethical rules and principles to scientific laws and theories, which have the status of hypotheses. Just as scientists are reluctant to jettison hypotheses that have proved fruitful in inquiry, so treating ethical norms as hypotheses means that, other things being equal, they can be relied on for sound guidance. However, they have no claim to permanent validity.

Fourthly, in any controversial case the likely consequences for human well-being of competing positions need to be assessed along with the value of giving due recognition to basic principles governing human conduct in a liberal-democratic society. Accordingly, in the definition of moral problems and the assessment of consequences, pragmatic ethical analysis is informed by relevant empirical inquiry. Finally, proposals or recommended policies for resolving moral problems should be considered experimentally, subject to evaluation and modification in light of how well they work in practice. Given its commitment to the hypothetical status of moral guidance, fallibilism, and the relevance of empirical consequences, the pragmatic orientation to bioethics promotes skepticism about the conventional wisdom—dogmatic commitment to allegedly settled bioethical positions.

As this discussion of pragmatic themes suggests, pragmatism provides an orientation to thinking about moral issues in any given domain rather than a system of discrete moral principles and rules. The spirit of pragmatism in ethics is nicely captured by William James:

> A pragmatist turns his back resolutely once and for all upon a lot of inveterate habits dear to professional philosophers. He turns away from abstraction and insufficiency, from verbal solutions, from bad *a priori* reasons, from fixed principles, closed systems, and pretended absolutes and origins. He turns toward concreteness and adequacy, toward facts, toward actions, and toward power. (James 1907)

As a gloss on this quote, Joseph Fletcher, one of the pioneers of bioethics who is identified with pragmatism, notes: 'By power he meant effectiveness, desirable consequences; the "acting out" of our ideas as the only way to judge what they mean and whether they are valid' (Fletcher 1987). Ethical inquiry leads to guidance understood pragmatically as working hypotheses, which are valid insofar as they meet the experimental test of leading to satisfactory resolution of concrete moral problems. In sum, the pragmatic perspective to research ethics adopts methods of moral reasoning that are analogous to those used in clinical and scientific disciplines.

Arras (2002), the most thoughtful and systematic critic of pragmatism in bioethics, has recently argued that appeal to pragmatism is neither necessary nor fruitful, primarily because mainstream bioethics is already saturated with the tenets of pragmatism. Although implicit allegiance to pragmatism may characterize much scholarship and practical guidance in contemporary bioethics, we submit that it remains helpful to formulate the elements of a pragmatic orientation to bioethics in general, and research ethics in particular. If nothing else, it functions as a reminder of how to think, and how not to think, about ethical analysis in this domain. More significantly, there remains important work for pragmatic critique of various views espousing the conventional wisdom of bioethics. In research ethics some prominent doctrines (indicated below) reflect a simplistic and absolutistic moral stance, insufficient attention to concrete practical contexts, and lack of due concern for the consequences of adhering to these positions. Accordingly, pragmatism continues to have cash value in guiding ethical thinking, especially with respect to challenging moral controversies relating to the design and conduct of human subject research.

Detailed theoretical justification of the pragmatic approach to ethics lies outside the scope of this chapter. However, we invite readers to judge whether our ethical analyses of selected issues relating to brain research, inspired by a pragmatic perspective, provide accurate and sound guidance.

## Pragmatic critique of moral absolutism

Complex situations that call for balancing competing norms often provoke moral discomfort. In such cases of moral complexity, it is natural to search for ethical formulas that give us the right guidance without facing the burdens of moral uncertainty and fallible judgment. Thus bioethicists not infrequently appeal to absolute categorical pronouncements aimed at settling moral conflicts. A notable example is the principle of clinical equipoise, widely believed to be an unassailable axiom governing the ethics of clinical trials. This principle requires as a condition for ethical clinical trials the existence of a state of uncertainty in the expert medical community concerning the therapeutic merits of the treatments under investigation and other clinically available treatments, if any (Freedman 1987).

Clinical equipoise is often invoked to rule out randomized placebo-controlled trials whenever proven effective treatment exists for the disorder under investigation (Freedman *et al.* 1996). Behind this principle lies the seemingly compelling idea that patients seeking treatment in the context of a clinical trial should not have their medical care compromised by being randomized to interventions known to be inferior to the standard of care. Apart from conflating the ethics of clinical research with the ethics of medical care (discussed in the next section), clinical equipoise pre-empts ethical reflection aimed at balancing considerations of scientific validity in the design of clinical trials with adequate protection of subjects from undue risk of harm (Miller and Brody 2003).

To be sure, in many cases the implications of clinical equipoise would be endorsed by all morally serious commentators. Virtually no one advocates randomizing patient-volunteers to placebo controls when withholding clinically available treatment would pose substantial risks of death or irreversible serious morbidity. But a wide range of cases exist in which placebo-controlled trials are methodologically indicated and the risks to subjects from withholding proven effective treatment are relatively minor or are not excessive as long as adequate safeguards are in place (Emanuel and Miller 2001). Is it clear that use of placebo controls is always unethical in such situations? If not, how do we decide what level of risk to subjects is morally acceptable and what criteria must be met for these trials to be ethically justifiable, all things considered? We discuss these issues in detail in the next section.

Clinical equipoise is by no means the only example of this strategy of evading moral conflict by issuing categorical pronouncements. Consider the debate over invasive placebo controls in randomized trials of surgical interventions. Faced with the complex and controversial case of a sham-controlled trial evaluating fetal neural tissue transplantation to treat refractory Parkinson's disease, several bioethical commentators went far beyond the facts of the case at hand to claim that sham surgery is always unethical (Macklin 1999; Dekkers and Boer 2001; Clark 2002; Weijer 2002a). They argued that it violates the therapeutic obligation of physician-investigators to promote the medical best interests of patients enrolled in surgical trials and/or that it necessarily violates the ethical requirement to minimize risks. Ethical analysis of sham-controlled surgery trials that pose considerably less risks to subjects than the fetal tissue transplantation research demonstrates that the categorical prohibition is erroneous (Horng and Miller 2002; Miller 2003). In both these examples, prevailing bioethics positions are unsatisfactory because they rely on 'bad a priori reasons', invoke 'fixed principles', and lack due attention to methodological issues and concrete factual contexts.

Such absolutistic positions in research ethics short-circuit the challenging task of ethical analysis when competing moral considerations are at stake. We speculate that these positions become entrenched because they promote the comforting illusion of moral certainty, *in the face of the uncertainty of clinical investigation*, which obviates the anxiety provoked by moral conflict and the hard work of seeking morally satisfactory, but uncertain, compromises aimed at doing justice to competing morally relevant considerations. The first chapter of John Dewey 's masterpiece *The Quest for Certainty* is entitled 'Escape from peril'(Dewey 1929) The search for and appeal to categorical absolute principles manifests an escape from the peril of uncertainty inherent in the task of examining and balancing conflicting values and norms. Pragmatists relish the challenge of making fallible but reasoned judgments, knowing that reasonable people might differ.

Once we take to heart the recognition that research ethics inescapably involves balancing the competing moral objectives of promoting valuable science and protecting subjects, it becomes apparent that, in general, there are two ways that we can go wrong in the effort to find morally satisfactory resolutions. First, we can err by failing to provide adequate protection for human subjects. The severe abuses of the past have largely been avoided, particularly because of the innovation of prior independent review and approval of research protocols. Nonetheless, complex issues of trial design continue to raise difficult challenges for subject protection, as we discuss below. Secondly, we can err by unduly constraining valuable research. Overprotection of human subjects may prevent or severely hamper the conduct of important studies with significant potential for improving medical care, when such studies might be designed in a way that provides adequate subject protection. Striking the right balance in protecting human subjects without unduly constraining valuable research is particularly challenging in research on brain disorders, as subjects may lack the capacity to give informed consent. This calls for creative thinking, honest debate, and responsible judgment.

In the next section we will apply the pragmatic perspective to an ethical analysis of placebo-controlled trials in neuropsychiatric research involving pharmaceuticals and the use of an experimental device for clinical brain research, the deep brain stimulator. By considering these differing investigational modalities that operate within the same clinical domain, we illustrate the importance of contextual details and pragmatic principles when making ethical judgments about the propriety of research.

## Placebo-controlled trials

Randomized controlled trials (RCTs) are considered to be the most rigorous method of evaluating treatment efficacy. They test the efficacy of investigational or existing treatments by comparing them experimentally with a control intervention. The control group may receive a placebo disguised to appear indistinguishable from the treatment under investigation or standard treatment. Placebo-controlled trials are frequently used to evaluate new and existing treatments for psychiatric and neurological disorders (e.g. depression, anxiety, Parkinson's disease, and migraine headaches).

Placebo-controlled trials have generated considerable ethical controversy and debate when they are conducted despite the availability of proven effective treatment. Critics have argued that the use of placebos rather than proven effective treatment in the control group is unethical (Rothman and Michels 1994; Freedman *et al.* 1996). It is alleged to violate the therapeutic obligation of physicians by randomizing patients to an intervention known to be inferior to standard treatment. These placebo-controlled trials contravene the principle of clinical equipoise, which is widely held to be an ethical foundation for the design and conduct of randomized clinical trials (Freedman 1987, 1990). Defenders of placebo-controlled trials have contended that placebo controls are ethically justifiable in these circumstances provided that sound methodological reasons support their use, and that they do not expose research participants to excessive risk of harm (Ellenberg and Temple 2000; Temple and Ellenberg 2000; Emanuel and Miller 2001). At the heart of the debate are fundamental issues concerning the nature and ethical justification of clinical research.

Whether placebo-controlled trials can be ethically justified in research on brain disorders with proven effective treatments depends on an understanding of the strengths and weakness of alternative scientific methods for evaluating treatments (Miller 2000). Accordingly, we examine briefly the methodological difficulties associated with active-controlled trials, especially those designed to test equivalence or noninferiority. The ethical debate is joined by undertaking a critique of clinical equipoise. This critique paves the way for developing a pragmatic ethical framework for determining when placebo-controlled trials are justified despite the existence of proven effective treatment.

## Methodological limitations of active-controlled trials

When proven effective treatment already exists for a given disorder, it is natural to think that any new treatment should be tested exclusively against the standard treatment. Apart from ethical concerns of protecting subjects, the use of placebo-controlled trials in this circumstance would seem to lack scientific or clinical value. Clinicians want to know whether an experimental treatment is as good as or better than existing treatment, not whether it is better than 'nothing' (Rothman and Michels 1994). Whereas first-generation investigational treatments should be tested against placebo, second- and subsequent-generation treatments should be evaluated exclusively in comparison with existing treatments in active-controlled trials (Freedman *et al.* 1996). However, this perspective can be challenged on methodological grounds.

Several methodological reasons support the use of placebo-controlled trials despite the existence of proven effective treatment. As a rule, placebo-controlled trials require fewer subjects than active-controlled trials, making them more efficient, i.e. they can be completed more quickly and at less cost (Leon 2000). This makes it advantageous to demonstrate the absolute efficacy of experimental treatments in placebo-controlled trials before planning larger-scale active-controlled trials.

Compared with active-controlled trials, placebo-controlled trials to evaluate treatments for a given disorder afford a more accurate determination of whether adverse events observed during a trial are caused by the pharmacological properties of the investigational drug or reflect the symptomatic expression of the disorder (Spilker 1991). A notable example is the question of whether antidepressants contribute to suicidal behavior, which is known to be associated with depression. The lack of a control group not receiving pharmacological treatment makes active-controlled trials less advantageous in this respect.

Active-controlled trials may not be feasible for testing unvalidated treatments used in clinical practice, such as alternative therapies. A recent example is a randomized trial comparing St John's wort with a standard antidepressant (sertraline) and placebo in the treatment of major depression (Hypericum Depression Trial Study Group 2002). This widely used herbal remedy was not expected to be superior, or even equivalent, to a standard drug. Hence the trial was powered to determine superiority to placebo. Whether St John's wort is effective in treating major depression was a clinically valuable question. When existing standard treatment is only partially effective, providing measurable relief of symptoms for some but not all patients, and causes distressing side effects, the availability of new or alternative treatments can expand the range of therapeutic options, even though they are no better on the whole, and possibly less effective, than the standard treatment but are more easily tolerated (Ellenberg and Temple 2000).

Placebo-controlled trials are also methodologically indicated for evaluating deep brain stimulation (DBS) (see also Chapter 15). DBS is a technique that utilizes stereotactic neurosurgical techniques to place small electrodes into the brain for the purpose of neuromodulation (Greenberg 2002; Fins 2004). Using an external frame that serves as a reference point for the localization of brain targets, electrodes can be placed precisely using imaging techniques such as CT or MRI. Unlike ablative surgery, in DBS electrodes can be inserted without injury to surrounding areas. Once in place, the electrodes are connected to a stimulator, much like a cardiac pacemaker, which provides a current. Effects are reversible and electrodes can be removed if there are complications (Beric *et al.* 2001; Oh *et al.* 2002). Currently, DBS is an approved modality for drug-resistant Parkinson's disease and essential tremor (Blank 1999). It is under active investigation for a range of neuropsychiatric disorders including obsessive–compulsive disorder, depression, and disorders of consciousness (Rapoport and Inoff-Germain 1997; Schiff and Pulver 1999; Koppell and Rezai 2000; Roth *et al.* 2001; Schiff *et al.* 2002).

Active-controlled trials comparing DBS with pharmacological treatment cannot be conducted by a double-blind method. This is problematic in trials of psychiatric and neurological disorders, which commonly have subjective outcomes based on patient reports. Placebo-controlled trials of DBS, in contrast, are designed to control for biased outcome assessments and the placebo effect, which may be pronounced in the case of dramatic invasive interventions

(Kaptchuk *et al.* 2000). The need for the double-blind placebo-controlled methods is demonstrated by the improved motor performance of subjects with Parkinson's disease who were led to believe that they were being stimulated (Pollo *et al.* 2002). This methodological consideration is confirmed by the results of trials of pacemaker treatment of patients with recurrent vasovagal syncope. Although positive results were obtained in randomized unblinded trials of pacemaker therapy compared with no treatment and medical therapy, two recent placebo-controlled trials (pacemaker on versus pacemaker off) failed to show any positive effects of pacing (Connolly *et al.* 2003; Raviele *et al.* 2004). Demonstrating actual efficacy by means of placebo-controlled assessment of invasive devices is also especially important because their risk profile may cause investigators to be biased toward classifying a borderline result as therapeutic when it is comparable only to a placebo effect (Miller *et al.* 1998).

Active-controlled trials of new drugs are often designed to test the equivalence or noninferiority of an experimental and a standard treatment. In the case of psychiatric and neurological disorders, these trials are subject to serious methodological difficulties (Makuch and Johnson 1989; Ellenberg and Temple 2000; Temple and Ellenberg 2000). A finding of no significant difference between the two treatments does not imply that the new treatment is effective. It is possible that in this particular trial neither the experimental drug nor the active comparator was effective. Many standard drugs which have been proven to be effective drugs, especially in the case of psychiatric and neurological disorders, are not uniformly effective in clinical trials (Laughren 2001). Without a placebo control to validate efficacy, active-controlled equivalence trials may not be capable of discriminating between apparent and real equivalence. This difficulty can be surmounted when standard drugs are consistently and robustly effective, making it probable that the lack of observed difference amounts to equivalence. Otherwise, active-controlled equivalence trials, in contrast with superiority trials, do not permit valid inferences about treatment efficacy, i.e. they lack 'assay sensitivity' (Temple and Ellenberg 2000).

These methodological considerations are ethically significant. The greater efficiency of placebo-controlled trials means that rigorous initial tests of efficacy can be conducted without exposing large numbers of subjects to potentially ineffective agents (Leon 2000). These trials also provide clinically useful information on the side effects of new treatments compared with an untreated control group. Moreover, there are serious problems with the use of active-controlled equivalence trials as evidence for licensing or validating psychiatric and neurological treatments when active-controlled superiority trials would not be feasible. These studies could lead to licensing new treatments, or validating available treatments that have not previously been proven effective for a given disorder, when these treatments in fact are no better than a placebo intervention. Since most drugs and devices cause unwanted and potentially harmful side effects, interventions that lack specific efficacy—therapeutic benefit beyond a placebo response—do not have an acceptable risk–benefit ratio.

However, these methodological considerations, although ethically relevant, are not sufficient to justify the use of placebo-controlled trials to test treatments for a disorder when proven effective therapy exists (Emanuel and Miller 2001). Ethical analysis must evaluate whether it can be acceptable to employ placebo controls that withhold proven effective treatment, and whether the risks from placebo assignment are not excessive and are justifiable by the value of the knowledge to be gained from the research. Although placebo-controlled trials might seem excessively risky when considering an invasive intervention such as DBS, these trials may have an acceptable risk–benefit ratio because the stimulator can be turned on and off (placebo control) without additional invasive procedures to allow for double-blind studies. This methodological approach to the assessment of DBS permits cross-over trials or the opportunity of patients randomized to placebo to receive the active intervention at the conclusion of the trial. This placebo-controlled double-blind design has been used to demonstrate that DBS is effective in advanced Parkinson's disease (Kumar *et al.* 1998; Deep-Brain Stimulation for Parkinson's Disease Study Group 2001). This level of rigorous validation is especially important given the incremental risks of an invasive procedure.

## Clinical equipoise

The principle of 'clinical equipoise', first articulated by Freedman (1987), is widely regarded as central to the ethical justification of RCTs. In order for an RCT to be ethical there must be a state of uncertainty in the expert medical community between the treatment under investigation and the existing standard of care. A placebo control is justifiable if no effective treatments are available or existing treatments have not been proven effective. However, when proven effective treatment exists, use of placebo controls is considered unethical, according to this principle, because it involves randomizing patients in need of treatment to interventions known to be inferior to the standard of care. Freedman and his colleagues described clinical equipoise, and its implications for placebo-controlled trials, in the following way:

> That principle can be put into normative or scientific language. As a normative matter, it defines ethical trial design as prohibiting any compromise of a patient's right to medical treatment by enrolling in a study. The same concern is often stated scientifically when we assert that a study must start with an honest null hypothesis, genuine medical uncertainty concerning the relative merits of the various treatment arms included in the trial's design. These principles allow for testing new agents when sufficient information has accumulated to create a state of clinical equipoise *vis-à-vis* established methods of treatment. At the same time they foreclose the use of placebos in the face of established treatment, because enrolling in a trial would imply that a proportion of enrollees will receive medical attention currently considered inferior by the expert community.' (Freedman *et al.* 1996)

To evaluate critically the principle of clinical equipoise it is important to appreciate the ethically significant differences between clinical research and medical care (Miller and Brody 2002, 2003). In routine medical care, physicians are obligated to offer personalized therapy to particular patients consistent with the professional standard of care. Risks of diagnostic and treatment interventions are justified exclusively by the prospect of medical benefits to the patient. In contrast, clinical trials differ from medical care in their purpose, characteristic methods, and justification of risks. The RCT is an experiment designed to answer a scientific question, not a form of personal therapy. Clinical trials aim to develop knowledge that can lead to improving the medical care of future patients, not at promoting the medical best interests of enrolled patient-subjects. Unlike routine medical care, RCTs assign patient-subjects treatment (or placebo) by a random method, they are often conducted under double-blind conditions, and they typically restrict the dosing of study treatments and the use of concomitant treatments in accordance with the research protocol. These trials often contain a drug 'washout' phase prior to randomization, designed to avoid confounding the evaluation of the treatments under investigation with the effects of medication that patients were receiving prior to trial partici-pation. Additionally, clinical trials include procedures, such as blood draws, biopsies, lumbar punctures, and imaging procedures, designed to measure trial outcomes, which carry some degree of risk of harm or discomfort to participants without compensatory benefits. In sum,

RCTs routinely incorporate features of study design that are not justifiable within the ethical framework of medical care.

These key differences between medical care and clinical trials are ethically significant. In view of these differences, the ethical principles that guide medical care are not the same as those that guide clinical trials. To be sure, in the abstract the leading principles of beneficence and nonmaleficence (as well as autonomy and justice) apply to both activities (Beauchamp and Childress 2001). However, the meaning of these principles differs importantly in the case of clinical research and medical care. Beneficence and nonmaleficence in medical care are patient-centered norms that guide physicians in the treatment of their particular patients. Together, they prescribe optimal medical attention or, at least, conformity to the professional standard of care. In clinical research, beneficence primarily concerns promoting the social good of improving health by means of producing generalizable knowledge; nonmaleficence limits the risks to which research subjects can be exposed for the sake of this goal. The investigator conducting clinical trials typically does not function primarily as the personal physician of enrolled patient-subjects, and therefore is not subject to the same therapeutic obligations that govern medical care.

Although intuitively appealing, clinical equipoise is fundamentally mistaken (Miller and Brody 2003). This principle conflates the ethics of clinical trials with the ethics of medical care. Clinical equipoise makes sense as a normative requirement for clinical trials only on the presumption that physician-investigators who conduct these trials have a therapeutic obligation to the research participants enrolled in them. However, the 'therapeutic obligation' of investigators constitutes a misconception about the ethics of clinical trials. The presumption that RCTs must be compatible with the ethics of the physician–patient relationship assumes erroneously that the RCT is a form of therapy, thus misapplying the principles of therapeutic beneficence and nonmaleficence that govern clinical medicine to the fundamentally different practice of clinical research. It is impossible to maintain strict fidelity to doing what is best medically for individual patients in the context of ethical RCTs, because they are not designed for, and may conflict with, personalized care.

Furthermore, clinical equipoise provides mistaken guidance about the ethics of placebo-controlled trials. Control groups in clinical trials that depart from a validated standard of medical care require justification but they are not inherently unethical. Placebo controls should be understood as no different in principle from any research procedures that pose risks to subjects without a prospect of compensating medical benefits (Miller and Brody 2002). Placebo controls are unethical if they are not necessary to answer a clinically valuable scientific question, or if they pose excessive risks. However, the normative assumptions behind clinical equipoise that evaluate clinical trials with respect to the duty of care owed by physicians to patients in need of treatment are ethically irrelevant to the situation of clinical research.

Clinical equipoise is also misguided because it confuses a valid methodological principle with a dubious stance on the ethics of selecting appropriate control groups for RCTs (Miller and Brody 2003). As the passage quoted above indicates, Freedman and his colleagues have equated the questionable thesis that physician-investigators have a therapeutic obligation to patient-subjects, such that it is unethical to randomize them to known inferior treatment, with the methodological, and ethical, requirement of RCTs stipulating that these studies have 'an honest null hypothesis'. These two components of clinical equipoise are not equivalent. To have scientific and potential clinical value, all RCTs require an honest null hypothesis (Emanuel *et al.* 2000). There must be sufficient uncertainty about the hypothesis being tested in a clinical trial to make it worth conducting. RCTs comparing an experimental treatment with placebo are instituted to test an honest null hypothesis. It is not known whether the experimental treatment being evaluated would be superior to a placebo control with respect to study outcomes. Yet when proven effective treatment exists for the disorder under investigation, these placebo-controlled trials violate clinical equipoise because randomization to placebo involves treatment that is known to be inferior to available therapy (Freedman 1990; Freedman *et al.* 1996). The critical assessment of clinical equipoise must detach the sound principle of scientific merit enjoining an honest null hypothesis from the erroneous ethical principle that control groups must always conform to the scientifically validated standard of medical care.

Weijer, a leading advocate of clinical equipoise, has recently claimed that 'Placebo-controlled trials in the context of serious illnesses such as depression or schizophrenia are ethically egregious precisely because no competent physician would fail to offer therapy to a patient with the condition' (Weijer 2002b). In view of the critique of clinical equipoise, drawing on the differences between the ethics of clinical research and of medical care, appeal to what competent physicians would do in medical practice has no inherent ethical bearing on what is justifiable in the context of clinical trials. Instead, we should be concerned about the methodological rationale for using placebo controls and the level of risks to patient-subjects of placebo assignment.

In our introductory discussion of pragmatism and research ethics we criticized clinical equipoise as exemplifying a stance of moral absolutism that evades the challenging task of balancing conflicting moral norms. We suggest that there is a deeper pragmatic critique of this and related positions on the ethics of clinical trials. Underlying the conflation between the ethics of medical care and the ethics of clinical trials is an effort to dispel the moral disquiet associated with clinical research, which derives from the use of current patients to gain knowledge for the benefit of future patients and society. Insisting that the ethics of clinical trials must be fundamentally compatible with the ethical framework of the physician–patient relationship obscures, rather than honestly faces, the ways in which clinical research necessarily and appropriately departs from the ethics of medical care. Accurate understanding of the nature of a given domain is a prerequisite to a pragmatic ethical perspective on that domain. The working hypotheses that guide ethical inquiry concerning clinical research must reflect the nature of clinical research. It would be convenient if physicians could preserve intact their therapeutic obligations to patients at the same time that they enroll them in RCTs aimed at generating clinically valuable knowledge. But the reality of clinical research does not permit such moral comfort, with the possible exception of RCTs where the objective is to determine whether one standard treatment is as good as or better than another. Pragmatism in ethics eschews the false moral comfort that comes from a distorted vision of the world which elides the tensions and conflicts that are difficult to face.

## Ethical framework for placebo-controlled trials

Ethical evaluation of placebo controls as a scientific tool for testing the efficacy of psychiatric and neurological treatments requires attention to four issues: methodological rationale, assessment of risks from placebo assignment, safeguards to minimize risks, and informed consent (Miller 2000; Emanuel and Miller 2001).

### Methodological rationale

The use of placebo controls must be methodologically necessary or desirable to achieve valid trial results. For the reasons indicated above, initial efficacy evaluation of experimental treatments for psychiatric and neurological disorders in comparison with placebo controls is often desirable, notwithstanding the fact that proven effective treatment exists, provided that the risks from receiving placebo are not excessive. Additionally, in comparing new treatments with standard treatments, including placebo controls will often be necessary to assure the internal validity of trials designed to evaluate equivalence. This holds for chronic disorders with waxing and waning symptoms, such as depression, anxiety, migraine headaches, and Parkinson's disease, when existing treatments are often only partially effective. RCTs of these disorders evaluate treatments on subjective outcomes of symptom relief and have high rates of placebo response. Without placebo controls, trials indicating lack of significant differences between experimental and standard treatments will not permit valid inferences regarding treatment efficacy.

## Assessment of risks

The risks of placebo controls derive from the placebo intervention itself and from withholding proven effective treatment. When placebos consist of inert substances, ingested by mouth, the risks of the placebo itself generally are nonexistent or minor. Unlike sham surgery, which we do not consider here, the use of a placebo condition in DBS trials does not add risk from the placebo itself.

It is important to recognize that a wide range of therapeutic benefits fall within the category of proven effective treatment. Therapeutic benefits include complete cures, more or less effective prophylaxis or symptom control, slowing progression of disease, and varying extent of symptom relief. Treatments may work in these ways for varying proportions of patients. Accordingly, the risks from withholding effective treatment will depend on the degree and probability of efficacy for patients with a given disorder and the severity of consequences for the health and well-being of these patients from lack of standard treatment during the course of trial participation. Side effects of standard treatment, which will not be experienced by those randomized to placebo, are also relevant to risk assessment. When existing treatments are only partially effective, placebo response rates are substantial, or the benefit–risk ratio of standard treatment is marginal owing to relatively severe side effects, patients may not be disadvantaged by receiving placebo. Indeed, much of the activity in new drug development is focused on reducing the side-effect profile while maintaining efficacy. Such work is assisted by the use of placebo controls.

Assessing the risks of harm from receiving placebo in clinical trials requires attention to three dimensions of risk: severity, probability, and duration of harm. At one end of the severity spectrum is the experience of mild symptoms with minimal threat to health, resulting from receiving placebo in trials of new treatments for conditions such as allergic rhinitis, heartburn, or headaches. At the other end of the spectrum, such as trials of cancer chemotherapy and antibiotics for a life-threatening infection, assignment to placebo would pose substantial risks of serious irreversible harm in view of illness severity and effectiveness of standard treatment. The use of placebo controls at the mild end of the severity spectrum is unlikely to evoke ethical concern, except for those who take a categorical stance that placebo controls are unethical whenever proven effective treatments exist. On the other hand, everyone agrees that placebo controls are unethical if withholding available treatment would be likely to expose research subjects to avoidable death or irreversible serious morbidity. The more difficult cases lie in the middle range between the two ends of the severity spectrum.

What, then, counts as excessive risk? Who decides? There is no reasonable way to formulate exactly the probability, severity, and duration of potential harm that would make the risks of placebo controls excessive. It calls for careful assessment and judgment. Such risk–benefit assessments are made by research sponsors, investigators, and most importantly by ethics review boards and research participants.

Ethics review boards, charged with prospective approval of research protocols, must carefully assess the risks to subjects from placebo assignment, when this involves withholding proven effective treatment, and determine that these risks have been minimized, that they are not intolerable or excessive, and that they are justifiable by the value of the knowledge to be gained by the study. Once placebo-controlled trials have been reviewed and approved by ethics review boards, patients make their own judgments about whether they are prepared to accept the risks of trial participation. In the case of chronic conditions where placebo-controlled trials are common, patients are familiar with the symptoms of their disorder; for example, they know what it is like to experience symptoms of depression, anxiety, multiple sclerosis, or migraine attacks. Therefore they are well placed to decide whether the risks of nontreatment are acceptable to them.

Some systematic data are available to inform risk assessments of placebo-controlled trials of treatments for brain disorders. A meta-analysis of antidepressant trials in the US Food and Drugs Administration database, encompassing thousands of patients, found that those de-pressed patients receiving placebo were not at significantly greater risk of suicide or attempted suicide (Khan *et al.* 2000). In addition, they experienced a mean 31 percent symptom reduction during trial participation, compared with a 41 percent symptom reduction for patients who received investigational or active comparator drugs. Thus it appears that, in the aggregate, depressed patients receiving placebo controls in short-term trials are not made worse off, or disproportionately disadvantaged, compared with those receiving pharmacological treatment. On the other hand, the negative results from placebo-controlled trials of pacemakers for vasovagal syncope (Raviele *et al.* 2004) indicate the need for caution in assessing the scientific rationale and risk–benefit ratio of novel uses of invasive devices for treating brain and nervous system disorders before initiating clinical trials.

## Safeguards to minimize risks

Careful screening of prospective patient volunteers for placebo-controlled trials is required to minimize risks. Severely ill patients at heightened risk of deterioration or severe suffering from lack of treatment should be excluded from participation. The duration of the placebo period should be limited to the shortest time required for adequate efficacy testing. During the conduct of the clinical trial, monitoring procedures are necessary to protect patient volunteers (Quitkin 1999). For severely ill patients, consideration should be given to limiting placebo-controlled trials to inpatient settings with constant monitoring and the ready availability of 'rescue' medications in case of significant deterioration. In outpatient trials investigators should maintain frequent contact with patient volunteers to assess symptomatic worsening and intervene appropriately. Consideration should be given to requiring research protocols to specify criteria for removing patient volunteers from clinical trials because of symptom severity or other adverse consequences. In any case, clinical judgment will be necessary and investiga-tors should err on the side of patient safety.

## Informed consent

Elements of informed consent do not differ essentially in placebo-controlled trials from other forms of clinical research. However, some points deserve emphasis. It is imperative that patient volunteers understand the nature of the study under consideration and how it differs from standard clinical practice, the meaning of placebo and the rationale for placebo use, random assignment, the probability of receiving a placebo, blinding of patient volunteers and investigators, alternatives for potentially effective treatment outside the research setting, and other pertinent aspects of study design. Among the risks that must be disclosed and understood are lack of improvement that patient volunteers randomized to placebo might have experienced if they had received standard treatment and the chance of symptomatic worsening during the placebo phase.

A variety of evidence indicates that many patients enrolled in RCTs are confused about, or fail to appreciate, the differences between routine therapy in medical practice and trial participation (Lidz and Appelbaum 2002). The invitation to enroll in RCTs at medical institutions may foster therapeutic misconceptions that lead patients to believe, despite disclosure about randomization, that they are being assigned treatment according to clinical judgments about what is in their best medical interests (Appelbaum *et al.* 1987). Consequently, special efforts are desirable to educate patient volunteers about the differences between clinical trials and personalized medical care. Educational aids may be helpful as part of the informed consent process for a particular study, such as computerized tutorials that explain the key elements of randomized placebo-controlled trials.

In the context of trials of DBS, it is especially critical that prospective subjects appreciate whether the procedure has demonstrated therapeutic value or is investigational, with a prospect of benefit that is speculative or based on weak evidence. Although DBS is approved therapy for drug-resistant Parkinson's disease and some other motor disorders, it is investigational in a host of disorders including obsessive–compulsive disorder, depression, and disorders of consciousness. Beyond the difficulty of distinguishing a therapeutic versus investigational application of the same technology, potential enrollees in trials are vulnerable to the desperation that comes from suffering from chronic and debilitating disease. They may be willing to consent to any treatment that offers the prospect of relief (Fins 2004). In this situation, a thorough process of patient education is indicated, and a safeguard such as consent monitoring by a clinician independent of the research may be desirable.

## Subjects who lack the capacity to give informed consent

Incompetent adults should not be enrolled in clinical trials unless their participation is scientifically necessary to test hypotheses about treatment efficacy (Wendler 2000). Since incompetent adults should not be enrolled in trials when subjects who can give informed consent are available, some process of assessing capability to give informed consent is needed to determine whether or not cognitively impaired adults lack competence (Chen *et al.* 2002). For example, patients with schizophrenia on the whole score below normal controls on standard evaluations of capacity to give informed consent (Grisso and Appelbaum 1998). However, most, but not all, are capable of giving informed consent to research participation, especially when intensive educational efforts are employed (Carpenter *et al.* 2000). The National Bioethics Advisory Commission (1998) recommended assessment of the capacity to give informed consent by professionals independent of the research team for all research with more than minimal risk involving individuals with mental disorders that affect decision-making capacity. When sound scientific reasons exist for enrolling incapacitated subjects, their participation must be authorized by surrogate decision-makers who are adequately informed about all the material elements of the study.

Can placebo-controlled trials be justified for incompetent subjects? Because the placebo control is a research procedure that does not offer the prospect of therapeutic benefit, the risks associated with placebo use must be deemed acceptable for subjects who are not capable of giving informed consent. Minor risks from withholding effective treatment or the placebo intervention itself might be reasonable for incompetent adult subjects. It is conceivable that higher risks from placebo assignment might be acceptable if the enrolled subjects have formulated clear research advance directives authorizing their participation in research with greater than minimal risk (Wendler and Prasad 2001). In this case, the potential clinical value of the research and the methodological rationale for use of placebo would need to be compelling.

An even more challenging proposition is Phase I studies with more than minimal risk in subjects who are unable to provide consent because of decisional incapacity. Subject enrollment becomes problematic because such early trials are primarily geared to the assessment of toxicity. They promise only a slim prospect of medical benefit.

This scenario might be encountered when a new intervention is first used in human subjects or when a device like a deep brain stimulator, approved for use to treat Parkinson's disease, is applied to a new condition (see also Chapter 13). In most cases, the challenges posed by enrolling incapacitated subjects with surrogate consent could be met by first performing Phase I studies on subjects who retained decision-making capacity. When this is possible, research should first proceed with this population.

This may not always be possible. First, a shift in study population may be untenable because it exposes a more cognitively intact population to unknown risks while offering only the prospect of a low likelihood of medical benefit. Secondly, the object of study might be a disorder that is marked by decisional incapacity such as advanced Alzheimer's disease or the newly characterized minimally conscious state that is characterized, in part, by a lack of reliable communication (Giacino *et al.* 2002).

In these scenarios it is important to be clear about the delineation between research and therapy so as to allow informed authorization by surrogates and avoid the possibility of therapeutic misconception. This will be difficult because investigators may be disposed to justify such early phase research by appeal to their 'therapeutic intent' (Lipsett 1982). Consequently, the aim of the research to evaluate the safety of an essentially investigational intervention may be obscured. Although the *prospect* of benefit is necessary, and may be viewed as a *sine qua non* for ethical justification of early phase research in incapacitated patient-subjects, it is important for investigators to communicate clearly the purpose of the research (to assess safety and not efficacy) and the lack of solid evidence supporting therapeutic benefit. Finally, this tendency to emphasize therapeutic intent may lead to a failure to place an adequate focus on the assessment of risks.

How might Phase I research with more than minimal risk proceed in neuropsychiatric disorders that impair the ability to provide consent? There is ambiguity at the interface of research and therapy, and transparency is not well served by the false moral comfort of an appeal to therapeutic intent, which obscures the differences between investigational work and clinical care. It is only by attending to the contextual differences between research and therapy that we can hope to pursue promising research while protecting the interests of subjects. Making these concerns explicit can help to address the challenges of surrogate authorization as well as the management of risk involved in Phase I studies. In the case of subjects who cannot provide consent, and do not have a research advance directive, alternative mechanisms are desirable to protect subjects while permitting important research (see also Chapter 16). We have previously proposed a consensus model for enrolling incapacitated subjects using a panel composed of the subject's next of kin authorized to consent to medical therapy, the attending physician, the investigator, and a trained subject advocate (Fins and Miller 2000).

Assessment of risk can also be made through analogical reasoning. In the case of the use of DBS, research involving subjects who cannot provide consent might be justified by the experience of DBS in subjects who were themselves able to assess the risks and benefits of study participation. Here the experience with advanced Parkinson's disease, using DBS with similarly deep nuclei, might support a favorable risk–benefit ratio for assessing the toxicity of the intervention in subjects whose neuropsychiatric condition precluded consent (Fins 2000). In sum, this experience rating from another disease might make the risk–benefit ratio more tenable because of more precise knowledge of expected risks.

## Coda: pragmatism and ethical analysis of clinical trials in brain disorders

Our ethical analysis of placebo-controlled trials in brain disorders and the use of deep brain stimulation is pragmatic in several respects. First, it is realistic about the nature of clinical research as an activity primarily aimed at generating knowledge with the aim of improving medical care. By exposing research subjects to risks for the benefit of future patients and society, the ethical climate of clinical research differs fundamentally from that of medical care, which is aimed at promoting optimal medical outcomes for individual patients. Accordingly, the ethical analysis challenges the conventional position that use of placebo controls is unethical when proven effective treatment exists, which derives from a misguided presumption that clinical trials should be governed by the ethics of the physician–patient relationship in medical care. In assessing the conditions under which placebo-controlled trials may be ethically justified, despite the existence of proven effective treatment, and the use of DBS in early-phase trials with incapacitated subjects, the pragmatic perspective pays close attention to relevant methodological, clinical, and risk–benefit considerations. These contextual considerations inform the positing of ethical guidelines that are understood as open to refinement and revision in light of changing circumstances and further reflection. This pragmatic perspective contrasts sharply with the doctrine of clinical equipoise which invokes an absolute and fixed principle concerning the ethics of placebo-controlled trials, regardless of the assessment of consequences to research subjects and to society. It faces squarely the need to balance the conflicting obligations to promote research with potential clinical and social value and to protect research subjects from exploitation and harm. Finally, and most importantly, the pragmatic perspective on research ethics helps to bring the potential of neuroscience to a historically underserved population struggling with the malignancy of neuropsychiatric disorders (Fins 2003).

## Acknowledgments

The opinions expressed are those of the authors and do not necessarily reflect the position or policy of the National Institutes of Health, the Public Health Service, the Department of Health and Human Services, the Department of the Army or the Department of Defense. JJF acknowledges the support of the Charles A. Dana Foundation and the Buster Foundation.

# References

Appelbaum PS, Roth LH, Lidz CW, Benson P, Winslade W (1987). False hopes and best data: consent to research and the therapeutic misconception. *Hastings Center Report* 17, 20–4.

Arras J (2002). Pragmatism in bioethics: been there, done that. *Social Philosophy and Policy* 19, 29–58.

Beauchamp TL, Childress JF (2001). *Principles of Biomedical Ethics* (5th edn). New York: Oxford University Press.

Beric A, Kelly PJ, Rezai A, *et al.* (2001). Complications of deep brain stimulation. *Stereotactic Functional Neurosurgery* 77, 73–8.

Blank RH (1999). *Brain Policy.* Washington, DC: Georgetown University Press.

Carpenter WT Jr, Gold JM, Lahti AC, *et al.* (2000). Decisional capacity for informed consent for schizophrenia research. *Archives of General Psychiatry* 57, 533–8.

Chen DT, Miller FG, Rosenstein DL (2002). Enrolling decisionally impaired adults in clinical research. *Medical Care*, 40 (Suppl), V20–9.

Clark PA (2002). Placebo surgery for Parkinson's disease: Do the benefits outweigh the risks? *Journal of Law, Medicine and Ethics* 30, 58–68.

Connolly SJ, Sheldon R, Thorpe KE, *et al.* (2003). Pacemaker therapy for prevention of syncope in patients with recurrent severe vasovagal syncope: second vasovagal pacemaker study (VPS II). A randomized trial. *JAMA* 289, 2224–9.

Deep-Brain Stimulation for Parkinson's Disease Study Group (2001). Deep-brain stimulation of the subthalamic nucleus or the pars interna of the globus pallidus in Parkinson's disease. *New England Journal of Medicine* 345, 956–63.

Dekkers W, Boer GB (2001). Sham neurosurgery in patients with Parkinson's disease: Is it morally acceptable? *Journal of Medical Ethics* 27, 151–6.

Dewey J (1929). The quest for certainty. In: Boydston JA (ed) *John Dewey: The Later Works, 1925–1953.* Vol 4: *1929.* Carbondale, IL: Southern Illinois University Press, 1984.

Ellenberg SE, Temple R (2000). Placebo-controlled trials and active-control trials in the evaluation of new treatments. Part 2: Practical issues and specific cases. *Annals of Internal Medicine* 133, 455–63.

Emanuel EJ, Miller FG (2001). The ethics of placebo-controlled trials—a middle ground. *New England Journal of Medicine* 345, 915–19.

Emanuel EJ, Wendler D, Grady C (2000). What makes clinical research ethical? *JAMA* 283, 2701–11.

Fins JJ (2000). A proposed ethical framework for interventional cognitive neuroscience: a consideration of deep brain stimulation in impaired consciousness. *Neurological Research* 22, 273–8.

Fins JJ (2003). Constructing an ethical stereotaxy for severe brain injury: balancing risks, benefits and access. *Nature Reviews Neuroscience* 4, 323–7.

Fins JJ (2004). Deep brain stimulation. In: Post SG (ed) *Encyclopedia of Bioethics* (3rd edn), Vol 2. New York: MacMillan Reference, 629–34.

Fins JJ, Miller FG (2000). Enrolling decisionally incapacitated subjects in neuropsychiatric research. *CNS Spectrums* 5, 32–42

Fletcher J (1987). Humanism and theism in biomedical ethics. *Perspectives in Biology and Medicine* 31, 110.

Freedman B (1987). Equipoise and the ethics of clinical research. *New England Journal of Medicine* 317, 141–5.

Freedman B (1990). Placebo-controlled trials and the logic of clinical purpose. *IRB* 12, 1–6.

Freedman B, Glass KC, Weijer C (1996). Placebo orthodoxy in clinical research: ethical, legal, and regulatory myths. *Journal of Law, Medicine and Ethics* 24, 252–9.

Giacino JT, Ashwal S, Childs N, *et al.* (2002). The minimally conscious state: definition and diagnostic criteria. *Neurology*, 58, 349–53.

Greenberg BD (2002). Update on deep brain stimulation. *Journal of ECT* 18, 193–6.

Grisso T, Appelbaum PS (1998). *Assessing Competence to Consent to Treatment.* New York: Oxford University Press.

Horng S and Miller FG (2002). Is placebo surgery unethical? *New England Journal of Medicine* 347, 137–9.

Hypericum Depression Trial Study Group (2002). Effect of *Hypericum perforatum* (St John's Wort) in major depressive disorder: a randomized controlled trial. *JAMA* 287, 1807–14.

James W (1907). Pragmatism: a new name for some old ways of thinking. In: *William James: Writings 1902–1910*. New York: Library of America, 1987; 508–9

Kaptchuk TJ, Goldman P, Stone DA, Stason WB (2000). Do medical devices have enhanced placebo effect? *Journal of Clinical Epidemiology* 53, 786–92.

Khan A, Warner HA, Brown WA (2000). Symptom reduction and suicide risk in patients treated with placebo in antidepressant clinical trials: an analysis of the Food and Drug Administration database. *Archives of General Psychiatry* 57, 311–17.

Koppell BH, Rezai AR (2000). The continuing evolution of psychiatric neurosurgery. *CNS Spectrums* 5, 20–31.

Kumar R, Lozano AM, Kim YJ, *et al.* (1998). Double-blind evaluation of subthalamic nucles deep brain stimulation in advanced Parkinson's disease. *Neurology* 51, 850–5.

Laughren TP (2001). The scientific and ethical basis for placebo-controlled trials in depression and schizophrenia: an FDA perspective. *European Psychiatry* 16, 418–23.

Leon AC (2000). Placebo protects subjects from nonresponse: a paradox of power. *Archives of General Psychiatry* 57, 329–30.

Lidz CW, Appelbaum PS (2002). The therapeutic misconception: problems and solutions. *Medical Care* 40 (Suppl), V55–63.

Lipsett MB (1982). On the nature and ethics of phase I clinical trials of cancer chemotherapies. *JAMA* 248, 941–2.

Macklin R (1999). The ethical problem with sham surgery in clinical research. *New England Journal of Medicine* 341, 992–6.

Makuch RW, Johnson MF (1989). Dilemmas in the use of active control groups in clinical research. *IRB* 11, 1–5.

Miller FG (2000). Placebo-controlled trials in psychiatric research: an ethical perspective. *Biological Psychiatry*, 47, 707–16.

Miller FG (2003). Sham surgery: an ethical analysis. *American Journal of Bioethics* 3, 41–8.

Miller FG and Brody H (2002). What makes placebo-controlled trials unethical? *American Journal of Bioethics* 2, 3–9.

Miller FG, Brody H (2003). A critique of clinical equipoise: therapeutic misconception in the ethics of clinical trials. *Hastings Center Report* 33, 19–28.

Miller FG, Fins JJ, Bacchetta MD (1996). Clinical pragmatism: John Dewey and clinical ethics. *Journal of Contemporary Health Law and Policy* 13, 27–51.

Miller FG, Rosenstein DL, DeRenzo EG (1998). Professional integrity in clinical research. *JAMA* 280, 1449–54.

National Bioethics Advisory Commission (1998). *Research Involving Persons with Mental Disorders that May Affect Decisionmaking Capacity*. Rockville, MD: National Bioethics Advisory Commission.

Oh MY, Abosch A, Kim SH, Lang AE, Lozano AM. Long-term hardware related complications of deep brain stimulation. *Neurosurgery* 50, 1268–74.

Pollo A, Torre E, Lopiano L, *et al.* (2002). Expectation modulates the response to subthalamic nucleus stimulation in Parkinsonian patients. *Neuroreport* 13, 1383–6.

Quitkin FM (1999). Placebos, drug effects, and study design: a clinician's guide. *American Journal of Psychiatry* 156, 829–36.

Rapoport JL, Inoff-Germain G (1997). Medical and surgical treatment of obsessive-compulsive disorder. *Neurological Clinics* 15, 421–8.

Raviele A, Giada F, Menozzi C, *et al.* (2004). A randomized double-blind, placebo-controlled study of permanent cardiac pacing for the treatment of recurrent tile-induced vasovagal syncope. The vasovagal syncope and pacing trial (SYNPACE). *European Heart Journal* 25, 1741–8.

Roth RM, Flashman LA, Saykin AJ, Roberts DW (2001). Deep brain stimulation in neuropsychiatric disorders. *Current Psychiatric Reports* 3, 366–72.

Rothman KJ, Michels B (1994). The continuing unethical use of placebo controls. *New England Journal of Medicine* 331, 394–8.

Schiff ND, Pulver M (1999). Does vestibular stimulation activate thalamocortical mechanisms that reintegrate impaired cortical regions? *Proceedings of the Royal Society of London, Series B Bioogical Sciences* 266, 421–3.

Schiff ND, Plum F, Rezai AR (2002). Developing prosthetics to treat cognitive disabilities resulting from acquired brain injuries. *Neurological Research* 24, 116–24.

Spilker B (1991). *Guide to Clinical Trials.* Philadelphia, PA: Lippincott–Williams & Wilkins, 62.

Temple R, Ellenberg SE (2000). Placebo-controlled trials and active-control trials in the evaluation of new treatments. Part 1: Ethical and scientific issues. *Annals of Internal Medicine* 133, 455–63.

Weijer C (2002a). I need a placebo like I need a hole in the head. *Journal of Law, Medicine and Ethics* 30, 69–72.

Weijer C (2002b). When argument fails. *American Journal of Bioethics* 2, 10.

Wendler D (2000). Informed consent, exploitation and whether it is possible to conduct human subjects research without either one. *Bioethics* 14, 310–39.

Wendler D, Prasad BS (2001). Core safeguards for clinical research with adults who are unable to consent. *Annals of Internal Medicine* 135, 514–23.

## Chapter 10

# Facts, fictions and the future of neuroethics

Michael S. Gazzaniga

## Introduction

Cognitive neuroscience, I will argue, has three main issues with respect to the current field of neuroethics. First, cognitive neuroscience can help with some current ethical dilemmas such as whether the embryo has the moral status of a human being. Secondly, there are important ethical areas to which neuroscientists are being asked to contribute when, in fact, they should not be. For instance, neuroscience has nothing to say about concepts such as free will and personal responsibility, and it probably also has nothing to say about such things as antisocial thoughts. Finally, and perhaps most importantly, cognitive neuroscience is building an understanding of how brain research will instruct us on ideas like universal morals possessed by all members of our species. This fundamental development will find cognitive neuroscience becoming central to the modern world's view of ethical universals. I have explored these three areas of concern in detail elsewhere (Gazzaniga 2005).

The term 'neuroethics' was coined by William Safire to refer to 'the field of philosophy that discusses the rights and wrongs of the treatment of, or enhancement of, the human brain'. I would argue that it goes further. Neuroethics should not simply be bioethics for the brain. I define neuroethics as the examination of the following (see also Chapter 2):

> ... how we want to deal with the social issues of disease, normality, mortality, lifestyle, and the philosophy of living, informed by our understanding of underlying brain mechanisms. It is not a discipline that seeks resources for medical cure, but one that rests personal responsibility in the broadest social context. It is—or should be—an effort to come up with a brain-based philosophy of life. (Gazzaniga 2005)

## Neuroscience influencing ethical issues: the case of the developing central nervous system and the moral status of the embryo

Taking the first part of the definition given above, cognitive neuroscience has valuable information to contribute to the discussion of certain topics that have traditionally been taken up by bioethicists, namely those issues in which brain science has relevant knowledge that should affect the ethical questions being debated. There are several issues in the area of enhancement, including possible selection of genes for intelligence, enhancing the brain to improve certain skill areas such as athletic or musical ability, or using 'smart drugs' to enhance brain performance. For the purposes of this chapter I will review one notable issue: when to confer moral status on an embryo.

The brain, specifically the frontal lobe of the cerebral cortex, is the part of the body that differentiates us from other species. The brain enables our body, our mind, our personality, and, many argue, our personhood. Thus, being able to identify when the brain develops in the human embryo should have a significant impact on the question of when to confer the moral status of being human on an embryo. Conferring moral status is a different issue than 'when life begins' and it is an important distinction—one that the neuroscientists suggest should be made.

Biological life and growth of the human organism begins at the moment of conception. But when does *human* life begin? The answer to this question has important implications for debates on abortion, *in vitro* fertilization (IVF), and biomedical cloning for stem cell research. Many neuroscientists and some bioethicists believe that human life begins when the brain starts functioning—we cannot have consciousness before the brain can operate. Consciousness is the critical function needed to determine humanness because it is a quality that, in its fullness with all its implications for self-identity, personal narrative, and other mental constructs, is uniquely human. Following this argument, it would seem that neuroscience would establish the beginning of human life as the point of development when the embryo has a nervous system and brain that is able to support consciousness.

However, as with many ethical issues, once the brain is involved, things tend not to be so black and white. Our grey matter creates many grey areas, and in the case of the embryo I would argue that there are different answers on this issue. The context of the question is everything when it comes to neuroethical questions. And there are several relevant contexts for this topic. First, for instance, if we ask when Sally's life began, the answer is at conception. But, again, when a specific human life began and when life begins are subtly but substantially different questions.

If fetal development alone is considered, the facts are as follows (Nolte 2002). The first signs of the brain begin to form around week 4 when part of the embryo called the neural tube starts to develop three bulges that will eventually become the forebrain, the midbrain and the hindbrain. The first sign of electrical brain activity occurs at the end of week 5 and the beginning of week 6 (Brody 1975). This is far from the beginning of conscious brain activity; it is primitive neural activity. (It is also worth noting that there is also neural activity in brain-dead patients, yet throughout the world and across cultures there is no problem in declaring such brain states as no longer human.) It is not until weeks 8–10 that the cerebrum truly begins to develop, with neuron proliferation, anterior commissure development, and a small first interhemispheric connection. Development continues: in weeks 12–16 the frontal and temporal poles begin to grow, and in week 16 the corpus callosum, which is responsible for communication between the two hemispheres, begins to develop; synapses start forming during week 17 and multiply rapidly around week 28, continuing at a rapid pace up until 3–4 months after birth. However, despite all this amazing and rapid growth and development, it is not until week 23 that the fetus can survive, with major medical support, outside the womb. Before this, the fetus is simply laying the foundations for a brain—a very different thing from having a sustainable human brain.

## Life beginning

Now take all of these facts about early fetal development and look at the arguments that are made for drawing a line regarding when life begins. The fact that the fertilized egg does not start the processes that begin to generate a nervous system until day 14 is one of the reasons why those engaging in biomedical cloning for stem cell research use the fertilized embryos only up until day 14. We have to jump all the way down the development time line to 23 weeks to reach the point where the fetus can survive outside the womb, and then only with the help of advanced medical technology. Thus one could argue that from the neuroscience perspective the embryo is not a human being, or deserving of the moral status of a human being, until week 23. Indeed, this is when the Supreme Court has ruled that the fetus has the rights of a human being. But here is where the fully-formed adult brain kicks in with its own opinions, sometimes drowning out the rational, purely scientific analysis. For instance, there is something about the look of a sonogram at week 9, or stage 23 of the Carnegie development stages of fetal development, where I have a personal reaction as a father to the image of the fetus—when it starts to look human. Despite what I know, this triggers a perceptual reaction that this forming ball of sensory–motor processes is one of us.

But before considering what to do with these different reactions, let us consider the main arguments on this question: continuity and potentiality.

The continuity argument that life begins at conception views a fertilized egg as the point at which one's life begins, and where it should be granted the same rights as a human being. There is no consideration of any of the developmental stages for those who adopt this view. And there is no rational arguing with those who see it this way. The potentiality argument is similar, in that it views having the potential to develop into a human being as conferring equal status to that of a human being. I have made the point elsewhere (Gazzaniga 2005) that this is akin to saying that a Home Depot do-it-yourself store is the same as 100 houses because it holds that potential. The main problem, and one that neuroscience cannot ignore, is that this belief makes no sense. How can a biological entity that has no nervous system be a moral agent?

This all leads into a third argument that most often comes into play with stem cell research: intention. Two kinds of embryos are used for stem cell research, unused IVF embryos and those created using biomedical cloning specifically for stem cell harvesting. In the case of IVF embryos, the argument is that the intention of creating several embryos using IVF is to create one or two viable ones for implantation. In natural sexual intercourse and selection, up to 80 percent of embryos spontaneously abort. Thus IVF is simply a high-tech version of what happens naturally. There was never an intention for each embryo created to be implanted; therefore those that are not deemed viable should be able to be used for research. In the case of biomedical cloning, the intention is solely the creation of an embryo for research purposes only.

This brings us back to my sense that there are different answers to the question of when life begins, depending on the context. The markers I identified happen to be similar to those of the 'discontinuity arguments' that some ethicists make. Discontinuity arguments take the view that an embryo is not due the equal moral status of a human being, and look for stages at which to grant it intermediate status. The stages tend to be 14 days (in these arguments, because this is the date after which twinning can no longer occur and so the zygote is cemented) and the formation of the nervous system. However, it is immediately apparent that there can be many different arguments made for when the nervous system starts to develop, ranging from the 14-day marker up to 23 weeks. And if you start to look at when consciousness begins, the parameters are even harder to pin down: the 23-week mark, or when you leave home for college?

## Why context is everything

Context is everything—and this, quite simply, is the lesson of neuroscience. It is our brains, enabling our decision-making processes, that allow us to reason, interpret, and contextualize. Indeed, as we shall we, we are wired to do this. Looking at the facts I see the contextual answers thus. A specific human life begins at conception. A 14-day-old embryo, a clump of cells created for research, has no moral status. An embryo is not a person. And yet parents may see the sonogram of a 9-week old fetus and see their future baby. What is worth noting on the question of the embryo is that, like many issues, despite what science presents us with, we still have a 'gut reaction' even though neuroscience tells us that a fetus cannot survive *ex utero* until week 23. Is this gut reaction an indication of a sense of moral instinct that our brains seek to make sense of with these various arguments? Cognitive neuroscientific research seems to be pointing towards this, as we shall see.

## Defining practical boundaries for real-world neuroscience

The second area of importance is where cognitive neuroscience should not be commenting because of its limitations. Ironically, this tends to be the exact area where our counsel is most often sought: namely, the court of law. With new neuroimaging techniques, lawyers and investigators are excited by the possibilities of being able to identify areas of the brain responsible for everything from violent behavior to lying. If we can put someone in a scanner and see if they are lying, or identify brains that are angrier than others, cannot this information be used to prove or defend against guilt in a court of law? In fact, the answer should be an emphatic 'No'. While the advances in neuroimaging techniques are exciting, they are not reductive in this way. Being able to see an area of the brain light up in response to certain questions or to pictures of terrorist training camps, say, may reveal some fascinating things about how certain cognitive states may work, but it is dangerous and simply wrong to use such data as irrefutable evidence about such cognitive states. What we know about brain function and brain responses is not always interpretable in a single way and therefore should not be used as infallible evidence in the way that DNA evidence is infallible (Illes 2004).

For instance, take the example of recent work on whether there is a brain mechanism for prejudice. Phelps and her colleagues have used functional MRI (fMRI) studies to examine responses of black and white undergraduates to pictures of known and unknown black and white faces. The results are that the amygdala (an area of the brain associated with emotion) is responsive in white undergraduates when they are shown pictures of unknown black faces, while the amagdyla is not activated when whites are shown famous black faces such as Martin Luther King Jr, Michael Jordan, or Will Smith. They concluded from their study that 'amygdala and behavioral responses to black-versus-white faces in white subjects reflect cultural evaluations of social groups modified by individual experience' (Phelps *et al.* 2000).

What we have to be wary of is how we interpret such data. It seems that we do tend to categorize people on the basis of race. But this does not mean that racism is built into the brain. The tricky idea here is that the brain allows us to concoct stories and theories about sets of circumstances or data—indeed it is bound and determined to do so. But the stories, even when based on data, are not always incontrovertible. They are not fingerprints or DNA. For instance, we could say: 'Well the fact that the amygdala lights up when whites see unfamiliar black faces shows that they are afraid of unfamiliar black faces'. Therefore someone who stabs a black man who approaches him, as in the well-known case of Bernard Goetz, are only reacting to a built-in brain mechanism. And it is supposed that Blacks become angry when they see famous white faces. Thus the 'black rage' defense—a black man who shoots a famous white person is only responding to his brain wiring. This is a leap that one could easily see happening in the court of law where we love to weave stories. But it is clearly a dangerous—and more importantly, inaccurate—leap to make.

This example of how a cognitive neuroscience finding can be interpreted and used to draw unreliable conclusions brings up another crucial area where the law and neuroscience should be kept apart: the 'my brain made me do it' defense (see also Chapters 1, 3, 4, and 17). Neuroscience simply does not have as much to say on the issue of personal responsibility or free will as people would think or hope. Cognitive neuroscience is identifying mechanisms that help us to understand how changes in the brain create changes in the mind. The concern arises, then, that if the brain determines the mind and our actions, independent of our knowing about it until after the fact, what becomes of free will? Free will is still alive and well. As I have argued, even if an action can be explained by a brain mechanism or function or malfunction 'this does not mean that the person who carries out the act is exculpable' (Gazzaniga 2005). Personal responsibility is something that arises out of interacting with human beings. In other words, our actions and reactions are still guided by social rules of behavior in addition to any determined brain mechanisms that we may all have.

To understand this idea more fully, let us first look at an example of research in the cognitive neurosciences that illustrates the automatic brain. The work of Libet, in the 1980s, first brought this issue to the fore (reviewed by Libet 1999). Libet conducted experiments in which he had subjects make voluntary hand movements while he measured their brain activity using event-related potentials. He noted that 500–1000 ms before they moved their hands, there was a 'readiness potential', a wave of brain activity that seemed to indicate a time lag between receiving and executing a command. He performed a series of experiments to try to pinpoint the time in that 500–1000 ms window in which we make a conscious decision to move our hand (Libet 1991; Dennet 2003). He devised an experiment in which a subject was told to look at a black dot that was slowly moving. After moving his hand, the subject reported what position the dot was in at the moment he made the conscious decision to move his hand. Then Libet compared that moment with the time that a readiness potential was recorded from the subject's brain waves.

What he found was that the brain was active even before the subject was aware of having made the conscious decision to move his hand. About 300 ms elapsed between the brain activity and the conscious decision. Thus it seems that the brain knows our decisions before we do—or before we become conscious of them. Such data seem to imply that free will may be an illusion. However, Libet himself noted that there is still a 100 ms window for the conscious mind to allow the decision, or to veto it, calculating that it is 500 ms from the beginning of the readiness potential to the actual hand movement and that it takes approximately 50–100 ms for the neural signal to travel from brain to hand to initiate the movement. Thus he argued that free will is in the vetoing power (Libet 1999).

Such research (and there is much more) indicating that our brains may be responding automatically is gold to defense lawyers looking for a biological basis for defective reasoning that could explain myriad criminal behaviors. But this is not the lesson of neuroscience. Neuroscience seeks to determine how the nervous system functions. The brain is a highly complex system that interacts constantly with the environment. It works automatically, but it also adapts and learns as it goes along, responding to learned rules and social rules, as well as its own built-in rules. As I have argued in an earlier work:

> 'But', some might say, 'aren't you saying that people are basically robots? That the brain is a clock, and you can't hold people responsible for criminal behavior any more than you can blame a clock for not working?' In a word, no. The comparison is inappropriate; the issue (indeed, the very notion) of responsibility has not emerged. The neuroscientists cannot talk about the brain's

culpability any more than the watchmaker can blame the clock. Responsibility has not been denied; it is simply absent from the neuroscientific description of human behavior. Its absence is a direct result of treating the brain as an automatic machine. We do not call clocks responsible precisely because they are, to us, automatic machines. But we do have other ways of treating people that admit judgments of responsibility—we can call them practical reasoners. Just because responsibility cannot assigned to clocks does not mean it cannot be ascribed to people. In this sense human beings are special and different from clocks and robots. (Waldbauer and Gazzaniga 2001)

Although cognitive neuroscience continues to show us how the brain is an automatic machine, that many of our actions are predetermined by our brains, and that our mind often concocts the rationale for the action after the fact, that does not mean that human behavior is predetermined and automatic. We still have personal responsibility. Not all schizophrenics are violent and not all people raised by bad parents are criminals. 'My brain made me do it' is not an excuse.

## Cognitive neuroscience: building towards the future

The single most important insight that the cognitive neurosciences can offer neuroethics is the understanding of how the brain forms beliefs. When you begins to understand how the brain works, how it forms beliefs and moral judgments, you must begin to question how certain long-held beliefs may be influencing our ethical and moral judgments, and often wrongly so.

In my own research, a powerful example of the brain's drive to form beliefs comes from observing 'split-brain' patients as they struggle to form an explanation for actions that their non-verbal right side has been told to execute. These are patients who have had their corpus callosum severed for treatment of epilepsy, which prevents information from being easily communicated between the left and right hemispheres. If a person fixates on a point in space, everything to the right of the point is projected to the visual areas in the left side of the brain and everything to the left of the fixation point is projected to the visual areas on the right side of the brain. This is true of everyone, but in split-brain patients that information is now isolated in the two halves of the brain—in other words, the left brain does not know what the right brain sees and vice versa.

Years of testing such patients has revealed that there is a brain mechanism, which I call 'the interpreter', residing in the verbal, or left, brain that crafts stories or beliefs to interpret actions. For instance, because of the ability to isolate the verbal and non-verbal hemispheres, when the word 'walk' is projected to the right hemisphere of a split-brain patient, he will get up and start walking. When the patient is asked why he is doing this, the left hemisphere, which is the site of language for most people, and which did not see the command 'walk', starts to create a response, such as, 'I wanted to go get a Coke'.

Such examples abound in split-brain research, and also in studies of neurological disorders. For instance patients who have suffered a stroke of the parietal cortex can suffer from anosognosia for hemiplegia, a state in which they do not recognize the fact that they have become paralyzed. The interpreter takes the information that it sees—that their limb is there, but not moving—and tries to reconcile it with the fact that the brain is receiving no message that the limb is damaged. (This is because the paralysis is caused not by damage to the limb, but by damage to the part of the brain that is responsible for operating the limb and so, in effect, the brain is receiving no information at all about this limb that it sees but cannot feel or move.) The interpreter goes to work to find an explanation when the patient is asked why he cannot move his arm, and patients will answer 'It's not mine', or 'I just don't feel like moving it'.

Another exciting area of research in cognitive neuroscience is Rizzolatti's work with mirror neurons. These are neurons that Rizzolatti and his colleagues have identified in monkeys that point to is a built-in mechanism for 'mind reading' or empathy. When a monkey sees another monkey reach for something, the neuron responsible for the movement fires in the reaching monkey—and that same neuron fires in the monkey that is only watching, but not moving (Rizzolatti *et al.* 2001). In other words, it may be that when we see another person do something, the same neurons are triggered in our brains, creating the same feeling or response in us. It could be a brain correlate for empathy, or understanding another's state of mind.

These are just a few powerful examples of how cognitive neuroscience is finding brain mechanisms that guide aspects of mind. Add to this observations about how we form beliefs and recent findings on how we make moral judgments, and the implications become even more interesting. Recent research indicates that moral reasoning may, in fact, be brain based. Greene has used fMRI to look at moral reasoning questions and what parts of the brain they trigger. One important observation is that we choose to act on a moral judgment (rather than just have it or assert it) when the emotion centers of the brain are activated (Greene *et al.* 2001). Hauser and his colleagues have been surveying people from around the world on standardized moral reasoning questions which show that they all have the same response patterns. Basically, we respond in similar ways to similar issues—the only thing that is different is our explanations about why we respond the way we do (Hauser, in press) The theory is that these similar responses are due to common brain networks, or reward systems in our own brains—moral reasoning is built in to our brains.

This growing understanding in the cognitive neurosciences of the brain mechanisms under-lying the formation of beliefs makes it difficult to accept an absolutist view about any and all belief systems. Belief formation is one of the most important areas where cognitive neuroscience needs to teach something to ethicists and the world: the brain forms beliefs based on contextual information, and those beliefs are hard to change. If you know that, it is hard to accept the wars that rage and lives that are lost due to differences in belief systems. At another level, however, it should come as no surprise that people behave as they do. We are wired to form beliefs, to form theories (using the interpreter); religious beliefs are basically a meta-narrative that explain why we should behave in a certain way in society (see also Chapter 20).

Cognitive neuroscience is revealing that the rationales we give for our actions are basically a social construct. Over time, people living in social groups develop a set of beliefs or practices—be they a form of government, religion, cultural practices, or all of these and the explanation for the way of living together becomes institutionalized. If we could come to understand and accept that the different theories or interpretations of our actions are the true source of different belief systems, then it seems to me we could go a long way toward accepting differences as a difference of narrative, not a universal difference in how all humans exist in the world.

## Summary

The cognitive neurosciences have three important messages for neuroethics. First, there are many traditional bioethical issues to which cognitive neuroscience should contribute. These include conferring moral status on an embryo and issues of aging, enhancement, and training. Any issue in which the brain or nervous system is involved should now be taking the latest cognitive neuroscience findings into account. But it is time to accept that such ethical questions will never have black-and-white answers. Context is everything when it comes to neuroethics, and an understanding of how our brain forms beliefs and makes decisions can and should inform how we contextualize these important questions. Taking the embryo example, we can see that there are different answers to when to confer moral status depending on the question being asked. When life begins, when *a* life begins, and the date by which an embryo created for research must be used are all very different questions and deserve different answers.

Secondly, there are many issues where ethicists long for neuroscience to provide answers. Everyone would love us to be able to point to an fMRI image and be able to identify a pixel that determines guilt or innocence, or answer definitively questions as to whether an individual's brain chemistry caused him to act in a certain way. Despite a growing body of research that suggests that the brain does indeed determine the mind, this does not mean that there is no such thing as personal responsibility or that brain imaging will be able to deliver the same incontrovertible evidence that a DNA match does. Neuroscience has its limitations and it is crucial to understand these.

Finally, the most important lesson of cognitive neuroscience is one that is still unfolding: that human beings may have a built in sense of moral ethics. Brain mechanisms for 'mind reading', or empathy—neurons and mechanisms that help us understand others' actions and react accordingly, that help us to develop a theory of mind about others—are rapidly being identified. As we continue to uncover and understand the ways in which the brain enables belief formation and moral reasoning, we must work to identify what this intrinsic set of universal ethics might be. It is a revolutionary idea, to be sure, but looking at how the modern world clings to outmoded belief systems, fighting wars over them in light of this knowledge is, in a word, unethical.

# References

Brody B (1975). *Abortion and the Sanctity of Human Life: A Philosophical View.* Cambridge, MA: MIT Press.

Dennett DC (2003). *Freedom Evolves.* New York: Viking Press, 228.

Gazzaniga MS (2005). *The Ethical Brain.* New York: Dana Press.

Greene JD, Sommerville RB, Nysstrom LE, Darley JM, Cohen JD (2001). An fMRI investigation of emotional engagement in moral judgment. *Science* 293, 2105–8.

Hauser M. *Moral Minds: The Unconscious Voice of Reason.* New York: Harper Collins, in press.

Illes J (2004). A fish story? Brain maps, lie detection, and personhood. *Cerebrum* 6, 73–80.

Libet B (1991). Conscious vs. neural time. *Nature* 352, 27–8.

Libet B (1999). Do we have free will? *Journal of Consciousness Studies* 6, 45.

Nolte J (2002). Development of the nervous system. *The Human Brain: An Introduction to its Functional Anatomy* (5th edn). St. Louis, MO: Mosby 37–41.

Phelps EA, O'Connor KJ, Cunningham WA, *et al.* (2000). Performance on indirect measures of race evaluation predicts amygdala activation. *Journal of Cognitive Neuroscience* 12, 729–38.

Rizzolatti G, Fogassi L, Gallese V (2001). Neurophysiological mechanisms underlying the understanding and imitation of action. *Nature Reviews Neuroscience* 2, 661–70.

Waldbauer JR, Gazzaniga MS (2001). The divergence of neuroscience and law. *Jurimetrics* 41, 357–64.

Chapter 11

# A picture is worth 1000 words, but which 1000?

Judy Illes, Eric Racine, and Matthew P. Kirschen

## Introduction

Throughout the ages, images have served as powerful mediators of thought and distinctive expressions of culture. From prehistoric drawings to the time of the Ancients when the Egyptians used hieroglyphics to communicate, and throughout the course of the history of science, the creation of images has paralleled human cultural activity. Graphical notations of numbers, Ancient Greek mythology, elaborate visual demonstrations of man and machines during the Renaissance (Lefèvre *et al.* 2003), and even analysis of the imagery of dreams and archetypes that have given us a glimpse of inner consciousness (Jung 1964) are all milestones along the path of how imagery has propelled our scientific understanding of the world. Images give us a depth of understanding of our experiences and increased appreciation of the complexity of natural phenomena.

Images transformed the face of medicine when, in 1895, Wilhem Roentgen made his great discovery of the X-ray. With the chance observation that he could acquire images, the first of one of his wife's hand, Roentgen provided a vital tool for visualizing the structure of the human body and revealing disease in ways that went far beyond traditional anatomical drawings. Only three decades later, in 1929, Hans Berger produced the first functional images of the human brain from electrical signals emitted at the human scalp (Borck 2001). The cascade of increasingly sophisticated technology for improving on these measurements of brain function, ultimately yielding colorful and appealing images in the form of spectra or activation patterns, has been unrelenting. Underlying many of the claims concerning the power of modern neuroimaging is the belief, real or desired, that functional imaging offers a direct picture of the human brain at work (Stufflebaum and Bechtel 1997). However, such belief brings both promise and apprehension.

In this chapter we provide a brief review of technological capabilities for imaging the brain with an emphasis on functional methods, and explore the range of applications for which they have been used. We then examine the epistemological issues associated with this research. We end by proposing a set of new dimensions for responsibility to accompany the still-emerging field as it realizes increasingly greater potential, continues to grapple with the technology, and faces unprecedented ethical and social challenges.

## From molecules to mind

The modern evolution of regional and whole-brain visualization techniques of brain structure and function has yielded bridges between molecules and mind. These advances have been possible in part because of new investigative paradigms and methods. While the earliest reliable non-invasive measures used electrical signals [electroencephalography (EEG)] to localize and quantify brain activity, measures of metabolic activity using positron emission tomography (PET) and single-photon emission computed tomography (SPECT) followed a few decades later in the 1960s (Mallard 2003). EEG studies had exceptional benefit for revealing cognitive processing on the subsecond level, localizing epileptogenic foci, and monitoring patients with epilepsy [Penfield's corticography work enabled even more accurate measurements from recordings made directly from the cortex during neurosurgery (Penfield and Boldray 1937)]. PET and SPECT have been used widely in basic research studies of neurotransmission and protein synthesis, further advancing our knowledge of neurodegenerative disorders, affective disorders, and ischemic states (Mazziotta 2000).

In the early 1970s, improved detection of weak magnetic fields produced by ion currents within the body enabled the recording of brain signals in the form of extracranial electromagnetic activity for the first time using the technique of magnetoencephalography (MEG) (Cohen 1972). While not as popular or available as EEG, PET or SPECT, MEG has still yielded fundamental knowledge about human language and cognition, in addition to important information about epilepsy and various psychiatric diseases (Mazziotta 2000).

The early 1990s witnessed the discovery of a yet more powerful method and technique for measuring brain activity using magnetic resonance imaging (MRI) principles. Using functional MRI (fMRI), brain function can be assessed in a rapid non-invasive manner with a high degree of both spatial and temporal accuracy. Even newer imaging techniques, such as near-infrared optimal imaging (NIR) are on the horizon, with a growing body of promising results from the visual, auditory, and somatosensory cortex, speech and language, and psychiatry (Coyle *et al.* 2004; Horovitz and Gore 2004).

In Table 11.1 we provide a brief comparison of the mainstream imaging capabilities today. However, we will use fMRI as the model for our discussion here, given its excellent spatial and temporal resolution, its adaptability to experimental paradigms and, most importantly for our purposes here, the increasing rate and range of studies for which it is being used. We have previously examined these increases in a comprehensive study of the peer-reviewed literature of fMRI alone or in combination with other imaging modalities (Illes *et al.* 2003). We showed an increase in the number of papers, from a handful in 1991, a year after initial proof of concept, to 865 in 2001. The average increase in this time period was 61 percent per year. Also vital to our interest was the multiplication of studies with evident social and policy implications, such as those relating to race judgments, competition or cooperation with others, and lying or truth-telling—all with real-world implications and practical possibilities. Table 11.2 provides a compendium of representative studies of this nature for easy reference.

We updated this database at the end of 2004, and showed that in the 3 years since the original study, another 3824 papers had been published. It was no surprise when we found a similar trend of increasing coverage reflected in print media (Racine *et al.* 2005).

With increases such as these, confidentiality and the protection of privacy in research—classic research ethics issues—are ubiquitous concerns. Those cautious of studies that appear to touch on our personal values and identity, or critics who are outright opposed to them, challenge their merit on a number of additional criteria. These include the perceived danger of identifying biological loci for personality, revealing an organic basis for hatred and racial discrimination, and demystifying spirituality. There are other concrete fears as well, such as the practical extension of the use of functional neuroimaging results in courtrooms—following in the gnarly footsteps of polygraphy and PET where judges and juries may become subject to reduced explanations of highly complex images. In the past, forensic neuroimaging has been

**Table 11.1** Some characteristics and trade-offs of major functional neuroimaging technologies[a]

| | Measurement | Technology | Strengths | Limitations | Notes |
|---|---|---|---|---|---|
| EEG | Electrical activity measured at scalp | Electroencephalogram; 8 to >200 scalp electrodes | Non-invasive, well tolerated, low cost, subsecond temporal resolution | Limited spatial resolution compared with other techniques | Tens of thousands of EEG/ERP reports in the literature |
| MEG | Magnetic fields measured at scalp; computed from source-localized electrical current data | Superconducting quantum interference device (SQUID); ~80–150 sensors surrounding the head | Non-invasive, well tolerated, good temporal resolution | Cost, extremely limited market and availability | |
| PET | Regional absorption of radioactive contrast agents yielding measures of metabolic activity and blood flow | Ring-shaped PET scanner; several hundred radiation detectors surrounding the head | Highly evolved for staging of cancers, measuring cognitive function, and evolving to a reimbursable imaging tool for predicting disease involving neurocognition such as Alzheimer's | Requires injection or inhalation of contrast agent such as glucose or oxygen; lag time of up to 30 min between stimulation and data acquisition, limited availability (<100 PET scanners in the USA today) given short half-life of isotopes and few locations with cyclotrons to produce them; cost | |

(Continued)

**Table 11.1** (continued) Some characteristics and trade-offs of major functional neuroimaging technologies[a]

| | Measurement | Technology | Strengths | Limitations | Notes |
|---|---|---|---|---|---|
| SPECT | Like PET, another nuclear medicine technique that relies on regional absorption of radioactive contrast to yield measures of metabolic activity and blood flow | Multidetector or rotating gamma camera systems; data can be reconstructed at any angle, including the axial, coronal, and sagittal planes, or at the same angle of imaging obtained with CT or MRI to facilitate image comparisons | Documented uses: mapping psychiatric and neurological disease including head trauma, dementia, atypical or unresponsive mood disorders, strokes, seizures, impact of drug abuse on brain function, and atypical or unresponsive aggressive behavior | Requires injection of contrast agent through intravenous line; cost | Currently available in two states (California and Colorado) for purchase without physician referral; emphasis is on attention deficit–hyperactivity disorder and Alzheimer's disease (out-of-pocket cost: ~$3000 per study) |
| FMRI | Surplus of oxygenated blood recruited to regionally activated brain | MRI scanner at 1–7 T and higher; 1.5 T most common because of its wide clinical availability | Non-invasive, study repeatability, no known risks; new applications of MR in imaging diffusion tensor maps (DTI), i.e. microstructural orientation of white matter fibers, has recently been shown to have good correlation with IQ, reading ability, personality, and other trait measures (Klingberg et al. 2000) | Cost of equipment and engineering expertise to run and maintain | Rapid proliferation of research studies using fMRI alone or in combination with other modalities, growing from 15 papers in 13 journals in 1991 to 2224 papers in 335 journals in 2003, representing an average increase of 61% per year |

[a]Combined modality systems such as EEG and fMRI are becoming increasingly common. PET and SPECT are forerunners to frontier technology in molecular imaging.
Reproduced with permission from *The American Journal of Bioethics*

**Table 11.2** Compendium of representative studies involving functional MRI (2000 to mid-2004) that have potential ethical, legal, and social implications

**Altruism, empathy, decision-making, cooperation, and competition**

Bartels A, Zeki S (2004). The neural correlates of maternal and romantic love. *NeuroImage* **21**, 1155–66.

Canli T, Amin Z, Haas B, Omura K, Constable RT (2004). A double dissociation between mood states and personality traits in the anterior cingulate. *Behavioral Neuroscience* **118**, 897–904.

Canli T, Zhao Z, Desmond JE, Kang E, Gross J, Gabrieli JDE (2001). An fMRI study of personality influences on brain reactivity to emotional stimuli. *Behavioral Neuroscience*, **114,** 33–42.

Decety J, Jackson PL, Sommerville JA, Chaminade T, Meltzoff AN (2004). The neural bases of cooperation and competition: an fMRI investigation. *NeuroImage* **23**, 744–51.

Farrow TF, Zheng Y, Wilkinson JD, *et al.* (2001).Investigating the functional anatomy of empathy and forgiveness. *Neuroreport* **12**, 2433–8.

Greene JD, Nystrom LE, Engell AD, Darley JM, Cohen JD (2004). The neural bases of cognitive conflict and control in moral judgment. *Neuron* **44**, 389–400.

Greene JD, Sommerville RB, Nystrom LE, Darley JM, Cohen JD (2001). An fMRI investigation of emotional engagement in moral judgment. *Science* **293**, 2105–8.

Hariri AR, Mattay VS, Tessitore A, *et al.* (2002). Serotonin transporter genetic variation and the response of the human amygdala. *Science* **297**, 400–3.

Heekeren HR, Wartenburger I, Schmidt H, Schwintowski HP, Villringer A (2003). An fMRI study of simple ethical decision-making. *Neuroreport* **14**, 1215–19.

Jackson JL, Meltzoff AN, Decety J (2005). How do we perceive the pain of others? A window into the neural processes involved in empathy. *NeuroImage* **24**, 771–9.

Knutson B, Momenan R, Rawlings RR, Fong GW, Hommer D (2001). Negative association of neuroticism with brain volume ratio in healthy humans. *Biological Psychiatry* **50**, 685–90.

Kumari V, ffytche DH, Williams SC, Gray JA (2004). Personality predicts brain responses to cognitive demands. *Journal of Neuroscience* **24**, 10636–41.

McClure SM, Laibson DI, Loewenstein G, Cohen JD (2004). Separate neural systems value immediate and delayed monetary rewards. *Science* **306**, 503–7.

Mitchell RL, Elliott R, Barry M, Cruttenden A, Woodruff PW (2004). Neural response to emotional prosody in schizophrenia and in bipolar affective disorder. *British Journal of Psychiatry* **184**, 223–30.

Moll J, de Oliveira-Souza R, Bramati IE, Grafman J (2002). Functional networks in emotional and non-moral social judgments. *NeuroImage* **26,** 696–703.

Moll J, de Oliveira-Souza R, Eslinger PJ, *et al.* (2002). The neural correlates of moral sensitivity: A functional magnetic resonance imaging investigation of basic and moral emotions. *Journal of Neuroscience* **22,** 2730–6.

Montague PR, Berns GS, Cohen JD, *et al.* (2002). Hyperscanning: simultaneous fMRI during linked social interactions. *NeuroImage* **16**, 1159–64.

Morrison I, Lloyd D, di Pellegrino G, Roberts N (2004). Vicarious responses to pain in anterior cingulate cortex. Is empathy a multisensory issue? *Cognitive, Affective and Behavioral Neuroscience* **4**, 270–8.

Paulus MP, Rogalsky C, Simmons A, Feinstein JS, Stein MB (2003). Increased activation in the right insula during risk-taking decision making is related to harm avoidance and neuroticism. *NeuroImage* **19**, 1439–48.

Rilling J, Gutman D, Zeh T, Pagnoni G, Berns G, Kilts C (2002). A neural basis for social cooperation. *Neuron* **35**, 395–405.

(Continued)

**Table 11.2** (continued) Compendium of representative studies involving functional MRI (2000 to mid-2004) that have ethical, legal, and social implications

**Altruism, empathy, decision-making, cooperation, and competition**

Rilling JK, Sanfey AG, Aronson JA, Nystrom LE, Cohen JD (2004). Opposing BOLD responses to reciprocated and unreciprocated altruism in putative reward pathways. *Neuroreport* **15**, 2539–43.

Sanfey AG, Rilling JK, Aronson JA, Nystrom LE, Cohen JD (2003). The neural basis of economic decision-making in the ultimatum game. *Science* **300**, 1755–8.

Shamay-Tsoory SG, Tomer R, Goldsher D, Berger BD, Aharon-Peretz J (2004). Impairment in cognitive and affective empathy in patients with brain lesions: anatomical and cognitive correlates. *Journal of Clinical and Experimental Neuropsychology* **26**, 1113–27.

Singer T, Seymour B, O'Doherty J, Kaube H, Dolan RJ, Frith CD (2004). Empathy for pain involves the affective but not sensory components of pain. *Science* **303**, 1157–62.

Takahashi H, Yahata N, Koeda M, Matsuda T, Asai K, Okubo Y (2004). Brain activation associated with evaluative processes of guilt and embarrassment: an fMRI study. *NeuroImage* **23**, 967–74.

Vollm B, Richardson P, Stirling J, *et al.* (2004). Neurobiological substrates of antisocial and borderline personality disorder: preliminary results of a functional fMRI study. *Criminal Behaviour and Mental Health* **14**, 39–54.

**Judging faces and races**

Cunningham WA, Johnson MK, Raye CL, Gatenby CJ, Gore JC, Banaji MR (2004). Separable neural components in the processing of black and white faces. *Psychological Science* **15**, 806–13.

Hariri AR, Tessitore A, Mattay VS, Fera F, Weinberger DR (2002). The amygdala response to emotional stimuli: a comparison of faces and scenes. *NeuroImage* **17**, 317–27.

Hart AJ, Whalen PJ, Shin LM, McInerney SC, Fischer H, Rauch SL (2000). Differential response in the human amygdala to racial outgroup vs ingroup face stimuli. *Neuroreport* **11**, 2351–5.

Golby AJ, Gabrieli JD, Chiao JY, Eberhardt JL (2001). Differential responses in the fusiform region to same-race and other-race faces. *Nature Neuroscience* **4**, 845–50.

Phelps EA, O'Connor KJ, Cunningham WA, *et al.* (2000). Performance on indirect measures of race evaluation predicts amygdala activation. *Journal of Cognitive Neuroscience* **12**, 729–38.

Richeson JA, Baird AA, Gordon HL, *et al.* (2003). An fMRI investigation of the impact of interracial contact on executive function. *Nature Neuroscience* **6**, 1323–8.

Singer T, Kiebel SJ, Winston JS, Dolan RJ, Frith CD (2004). Brain responses to the acquired moral status of faces. *Neuron* **41**, 653–62.

Winston JS, Strange BA, O'Doherty J, Dolan RJ (2002). Automatic and intentional brain responses during evaluation of trustworthiness of faces. *Nature Neuroscience* **5**, 277–83.

**Lying and deception**

Kozel FA, Revell LJ, Lorberbaum JP *et al.* (2004). A pilot study of functional magnetic resonance imaging brain correlates in healthy young men. *Journal of Neuropsychiatry and Clinical Neurosciences* **16**, 295–305.

Kozel FA, Padgett TM, George MS (2004). A replication study of the neural correlates of deception. *Behavioral Neuroscience* **118**, 852–6.

Langleben DD, Schroeder L, Maldjian JA, *et al.* (2002). Brain activity during simulated deception: An event-related functional magnetic resonance study. *NeuroImage* **15**, 727–32.

Lee TM, Liu HL, Tan LH, *et al.* (2002). Lie detection by functional magnetic resonance imaging. *Human Brain Mapping* **15**, 157–64.

(Continued)

**Table 11.2** (continued) Compendium of representative studies involving functional MRI (2000 to mid-2004) that have ethical, legal, and social implications

**Lying and deception**

Spence SA, Farrow TF, Herford AE, Wilkinson ID, Zheng Y, Woodruff PW (2001). Behavioural and functional anatomical correlates of deception in humans. *Neuroreport* **12**, 2849–52.

Stuss DT, Gallup GG Jr, Alexander MP (2001). The frontal lobes are necessary for 'theory of mind'. *Brain* **124**, 279–86.

**Meditating and religious experience**

Lazar SW, Bush G, Gollub RL, Fricchione GL, Khalsa G, Benson H (2000). Functional brain mapping of the relaxation response and meditation. *Neuroreport* **11**, 1581–5.

Wuerfel J, Krishnamoorthy ES, Brown RJ, *et al.* (2004). Religiosity is associated with hippocampal but not amygdala volumes in patients with refractory epilepsy. *Journal of Neurology, Neurosurgery, and Psychiatry* **75**, 640–2.

introduced in legal proceedings as evidence, and experience points to the potential for neuroimaging to bring leniency or justify claims of mitigating circumstances (Lasden 2004; Illes and Racine 2005).

The venture of neuroimaging into the domain of social behaviors—some that are tangible and others not—introduces the possibility of rejuvenating historical insights on human nature and capabilities. The study of emotions and moral reasoning, for example, is bringing new biological perspectives to domains traditionally attributed to philosophy and the social sciences (Greene *et al.* 2001; Greene 2003; Moll *et al.* 2002a, b). Neuroimaging studies of intelligence (Fletcher *et al.* 1995; Gray and Thompson 2004), economics (Glimcher and Rustichini 2004), education (OECD 2002; Goswani 2004), and emotion and personality (Canli *et al.* 2001; Partiot *et al.* 1995; Phan *et al.* 2002) also bring neuroscience to new horizons, while sparking healthy debates, discussion, and cross-fertilization of ideas on the nature of human life (Johnson 2004), art (Kandel and Mack 2003), religious beliefs (Newberg *et al.* 2002), law (Loftus 2003; Lasden 2004), and philosophy (Churchland 1998; Haidt 2001; Damasio 2002; Casebeer 2003; Racine 2005). However, such innovations bring to the foreground the need for an appraisal of the limit of the technology in revealing brain structure and, more critically, the relationship between mind and brain. Hence, what do neuroimages really reveal? Is the lament of some concerned scholars and citizens that we ought to leave some human phenomena unexplored legitimate? Is a picture of the brain worth a 1000 words? If it is, which 1000?

# Imaging human thought still an emerging endeavor

Functional neuroimaging conveys critical information about mental processing in the brain. Unlike the early phrenologists, who believed that complex personality traits were associated with discrete cerebral regions, modern neuroscientists recognize that the brain is composed of interdependent neural networks, such that a given brain region contributes to several mental functions and each function relies on numerous brain regions. Although fMRI has already greatly enhanced our knowledge of the functional brain, or neuro-knowledge as we may call it, the technology has boundaries. From small changes in cerebral blood oxygenation, researchers make inferences about the underlying neuronal activity and how this activity relates to behavioral phenomena. However, the diversity of interpretations to which fMRI data can give rise poses many challenges to investigators involved in the production of this data. Through the exploration of the basic principles of fMRI, the experimental paradigms, and data processing steps that yield colorful brain activation maps, we will show here why both neuroimagers and citizens of science might be cautious of the *bold* conclusions often drawn from fMRI data.

## Deriving meaning from signals

For functional imaging to be possible, there must be measurable physiological markers of neural activity. Techniques like fMRI rely on metabolic correlates of neural activity, not the activity itself. Images are constructed based on blood-oxygenation-level dependent (BOLD) contrast.

BOLD contrast is an indirect measure of a series of processes. It begins with a human subject performing a behavioral task, for example a repetitive finger-tapping task. Neuronal networks in several brain regions are activated to initiate, coordinate, and sustain this finger tapping. These ensembles of neurons require large amount of energy in the form of adenosine triphosphate (ATP) to sustain their metabolic activity. Since the brain does not store its own energy, it must make ATP from the oxidation of glucose. Increased blood flow is required to deliver the necessary glucose and oxygen (bound to hemoglobin) to maintain this metabolic demand.

Since the magnetic properties of oxyhemoglobin and deoxyhemoglobin are different, they show different signal intensities on an MRI scan. When a brain region is more metabolically active, more oxygenated hemoglobin is recruited to that area, which displaces a certain percentage of deoxyhemoglobin. This displacement results in a local increase in MR signal or BOLD contrast. Although direct neuronal response to a stimulus can occur on the order of milliseconds, increases in blood flow, or the hemodynamic response to this increased neural activity, lag by 1–2 s. This hemodynamic response function (HRF) is important in determining the temporal resolution of fMRI.

Blood flow, as with many other physiological processes in the human body, is influenced by many factors including the properties of the red blood cells, the integrity of the blood vessels, and the strength of the heart muscle, in addition to the age, health, and fitness level of the individual. Fluctuations in any of these variables could affect the signal measured and the interpretation of that signal. For example, the velocity of cerebral blood flow decreases with aging (Desmond and Chen 2002; Rosen *et al.* 2002) and similar differences may be induced in pathological conditions (Mazziotta 2000). In comparison, women using hormone replacement therapy may have enhanced cerebrovascular flow. Some medications, such as antihypertensives, can also modify blood flow (Rosen and Gur 2002). Since complete medical examinations are not routinely given to subjects recruited to fMRI studies as healthy controls, it is important to take this potential variability into account when interpreting and comparing fMRI data. Variability in blood flow is especially relevant when evaluating fMRI data taken from a single subject, as might be the case for diagnosing or monitoring psychiatric disease or if fMRI is eventually used by the legal system as a lie detector. We will explore other difficulties in interpreting single-subject fMRI data later in this chapter.

## Spatial and temporal resolution of fMRI

High spatial and temporal resolution are necessary for making accurate interpretations of fMRI data. Advances in MRI hardware over the past decade have greatly increased both, but the ultimate limitation is the concordance of the BOLD signal with underlying neuronal activity.

The units of spatial resolution for an MRI scan of the brain are voxels, or three-dimensional pixels. While modern MR scanners can acquire images at a resolution of less than 1 mm$^3$, the task-dependent changes in the BOLD signal might not be large enough to detect in such a small volume of brain tissue. The measured signal from a voxel is directly proportional to its size—the smaller the voxel, the weaker the signal. In regions like the primary visual or motor cortex, where a visual stimulus or a finger-tap will produce a robust BOLD response, small voxels will be adequate to detect such changes. On the other hand, more complex cognitive functions (i.e. moral reasoning or decision-making) use neural networks in several brain regions and there-fore the changes in BOLD signal in any specific region (i.e. the frontal lobes) might not be detectable with small voxels. Thus larger voxel sizes are needed to capture these small changes in neuronal activity, which results in decreased spatial resolution. fMRI is typically used to image brain regions on the order of a few millimeters to centimeters.

As the voxel size increases, the probability of introducing heterogeneity of brain tissue into the voxel also increases (these are referred to as partial volume effects). Instead of a voxel containing only neuronal cell bodies, it might also contain white matter tracts, blood vessels, or cerebrospinal fluid that artificially reduce the signal intensity from a given voxel. Several other processing steps in the analysis of fMRI data can also have implications for spatial resolution. fMRI data are typically smoothed using a Gaussian filter, which improves the reliability of statistical comparisons but in turn decreases its spatial resolution. Spatial reso-lution is also sacrificed when fMRI data are transformed into a common stereotactic space (also referred to as normalization) for the purposes of averaging or comparing across subjects. Lastly, smaller voxel sizes require increased scanning time, which is often a limiting factor when dealing with certain behavioral paradigms or special subject populations (e.g. children or elderly subjects).

The temporal resolution of fMRI is dependent on the hemodynamic response of the brain and how frequently the response is sampled. The measured hemodynamic response in the brain rises and falls over a period of about 10 s. The more frequently this response is sampled, the better the estimate we can make as to the underlying neural activity. fMRI has on average a resolution on the order of seconds; however, latency differences as small as a few hundred milliseconds can be measured. These differences do not reflect the absolute timing of the neural activity, but rather a relative difference between different types of stimuli or different brain regions. It should also be noted that the BOLD response is non-linear for multiple stimuli activating the same brain region. If the same brain region is activated in rapid succession, the BOLD response to the later stimuli is reduced compared with the initial stimulus.

There is ample evidence to support the relationship between increased neuronal activity and increased BOLD contrast, especially for primary motor and sensory processing. However, it is reasonable to question the indirectness of this methodology for the study of complex mental processes like abstract human thought. As we will see in the next section, there are additional variables inherent in the design of fMRI experiments that can also introduce variability into the data.

## Equating structure and function

As functional neuroimaging relies on task-dependent activations under highly constrained conditions (Desmond and Chen 2002; Kosik 2003), equating structure and function is some-what analogous to equating genes and function. This is fraught with challenges, especially where variability can affect the BOLD signal changes (Kosik 2003). On the most basic level, there are intrinsic properties of the MR scanner that increase variability in the recorded signal from the brain. Technical issues stem from differences between individual MRI sites and scanner drifts. Manufacturer upgrades that may also introduce changes in image quality and other features of a study, however welcome, also require ongoing consideration.

Muscles contracting with swallowing, pulsating large blood vessels, or limbs moving to improve comfort all result in motion artifacts and physiological noise, thus introducing intrasubject variability into the data. Keeping subjects motionless in the scanner is particularly challenging when subjects representing vulnerable populations are needed; patients suffering from executive function dysfunctions or severe memory impairments may find the long period of immobilization taxing. Although algorithms that have been proposed to correct for head movement provide a partial solution, task-related movements can interfere in comparisons between control and experimental groups (Desmond and Chen 2002).

Intersubject variability is also a consideration, especially when understanding of single-subject data is the goal. Aguirre *et al.* (1998) showed that the shape of the hemodynamic response across subjects is highly variable. Thus, if two subjects performed the same task, the levels of BOLD signal may change, and consequently the activation maps might be different. Desmond and Glover (2002) have shown that if one assumes that intersubject variability is about 0.5 percent, the number of subjects needed for 80 percent power at $P <$ 0.05 depends on the percentage signal change. If the assumption is a percentage signal change of about 0.5 percent, then 80 percent power at $P <$ 0.05 will depend on the intersubject variability.

It is also possible that two independent subjects will show different patterns of activation although their behavioral performances are comparable. Although subjects perform the same behavioral task, they might employ different strategies, thereby recruiting different neural networks resulting in different patterns of activation.

When interpreting fMRI activation maps it is important to remember that since changes in the BOLD signal are indirect inferences of neuronal activity, all areas of significant activation may not be task-specific. For example, eye-blink paradigms have been shown to activate the hippocampal formation and the cingulate gyrus; however, lesions of the hippocampal formation do not eradicate the eye-blink conditioning. There are two alternative interpretations for this result. Either the hippocampus is involved in some aspect of eye-blink condition, but is not necessary to elicit the behavioral result, or the hippocampal activations are false positives. A false-positive activation may lead to erroneous conclusions that brain areas are associated with a function when in fact they are not. Therefore fMRI results do not definitively demonstrate that a brain region is involved in a task, but rather that the region is activated during the task (Rosen and Gur 2002).

## Designing an fMRI experiment

Part of the art of fMRI imaging is designing an experimental task that is simple and specific so that behavioral responses can be attributed to an isolated mental process and not confounded by other functions (a concept known as functional decomposition). For this reason, fMRI relies on a subtraction technique where the differences in BOLD signal between a control task and an experimental task lead to conclusions about the neuronal activity underlying the areas of increased activation (Figure 11.1). Therefore, it is essential to design the control and experimental tasks such that the variable of interest is the only thing different between the two tasks. The control condition alone is crucial as it can impact the downstream interpretation of

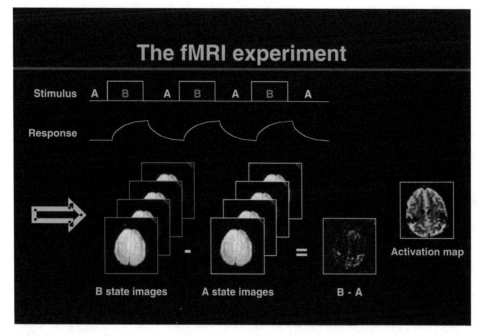

**Fig. 11.1** Experimental (B state) images are subtracted from control (A state) images to achieve regional activation maps with fMRI. Courtesy of G.H. Glover, Lucas MRS/MRI Center, Stanford University Medical Center. Reproduced with permission from *The American Journal of Bioethics* (See also the colour plate section).

images. For example, a researcher is interested in studying the regions of the brain responsible for processing human memory. The experimental task is remembering a list of five words and then subsequently indicating whether a probe item matches one of the words studied. If the control task is a rest condition, then subtracting rest from the memory task would yield a plethora of activated brain regions including visual processing centers, memory and language centers, and motor regions elicited by pushing the response button. In contrast, if the control task is identical to the experimental task in terms of timing and stimulus presentation, but only two words are presented instead of five, then the difference between the experimental and control tasks would be limited to those regions involved with memory.

The design of the psychophysical task itself is crucial for research reliability and validity. Even minor differences in task design, such as word frequency, word familiarity, and visual frequency, have been reported to have a significant impact on activation patterns (Van Orden and Paap 1997; Roskies and Peterson 2001). Some investigators, such as Van Orden, have argued further that task decomposition introduces a *circulus viti sus*—that, in order to isolate the task, we need to know something about its neuronal basis in order to dissect it in relevant and meaningful terms.

Given this paradigm for fMRI experiments, care must be taken when comparing results from different fMRI studies and when extending results outside the scope of the research environment. Just because two studies both used tasks probing the regions of the brain responsive to fear, the activation maps are not necessarily directly comparable. Along the same lines, an image generated from a single subject cannot necessarily be compared with an image representing the average of a group of normal subjects who performed a similar behavioral task.

## Statistical analyses of fMRI data

Among the most challenging issues in neuroimaging is the selection of the statistical treatment of the data. There are several stages of processing that are performed on fMRI data. First, preprocessing prepares the data for statistical analysis. This often includes correcting for motion artifacts, normalizing or transforming the images of each subject's brain into a common stereotactic coordinate system, and smoothing with a Gaussian filter. Secondly, a general linear model (GLM) regression determines for each subject the degree to which changes in signal intensity for each voxel can be predicted by a reference waveform that represents the timing of the behavioral task. The final stage is population inference. This step involves using the GLM results for each subject in a random effects model for making inferences to the population, or inferences regarding differences in the population. With this method, activation differences between experimental conditions or groups can be assessed over all brain regions and results can be reported in a standardized coordinate system. Commercial and freely available software packages for data analysis are widely used, but differences exist in the specific implementation of the statistics.

When the results from the GLM and the random effects model are combined, the result is a statistical parameter map of brain activity. This activation map is typically color coded according to the probability value for each voxel. In most fMRI research conducted using young normal healthy adults, it is desirable to threshold these probability values to minimize the number of false-positive voxels. In this way, researchers can be confident that an activated voxel is indeed correlated with the behavioral task. Since many tens of thousands of statistical comparisons are computed in the GLM, this threshold is usually set at a very conservative level (i.e. on the order of $P = 0.001$). This thresholding procedure can have significant implications for the interpretation of the brain activation maps.

> What constitutes a 'significantly greater' activation than another, is in a way, in the eye of the beholder. . . . lowering the threshold will create more regions that are statistically significant, whereas raising the threshold will reduce the number of significant regions. The choice of the threshold is largely determined by convention among researchers, rather than absolute standards. Reporting brain activation patterns is therefore primarily a statistical interpretation of a very complex dataset, and may be interpreted differently by different researchers. (Canli and Amin 2002)

While group averages are vital for achieving acceptable signal-to-noise ratios, individual differences, from both anatomical and functional variability may become diluted and overshadowed (Beaulieu 2001; President's Council on Bioethics 2004). When dealing with single-subject data, as is the case for presurgical planning, it is often desirable to minimize false-negative voxels in order to avoid erroneously excising potentially healthy tissue (M. P. Kirschen et al., under review). Outside the clinical setting, we can easily extend these considerations to any analytic objective set to pinpoint activation areas for function in individuals:

> . . . the image of an activation pattern from a poorly designed study is visually indistinguishable from one based on an exemplary study. It takes a skilled practitioner to appreciate the difference. Therefore, one great danger lies in the abuse of neuroimaging data for presentations to untrained audiences such as courtroom juries. What can be easily forgotten when looking at these images is that they represent statistical inferences, rather than absolute truths. (Canli and Amin 2002)

Lastly, the interpretability of fMRI activation maps is dependent on how the data are displayed. The color-coded statistical maps are usually overlaid on high-resolution anatomical MR images to highlight the brain anatomy. There are several media for displaying these composite images. The most rigorous is to overlay the functional data onto single anatomical slices in any imaging plane. While this is the most comprehensive means of examining the data, it is often difficult to localize the activations to a particular region, given a particular scan plane, and researchers are limited in the number of slices they can include in a publication or lecture. Alternatively, the activation maps can be presented on a three-dimentional rendered brain. While this technique gives good visualization of the prominent external brain structures, internal regions like the hippocampus or basal ganglia are not well characterized on these models. Researchers often use both of these techniques to examine data, but ultimately choose the one that best highlights the main results of the study for presentation.

Since basic research is usually done to infer characteristics bearing on populations, the extension to individual applications is challenged by a scarcity of normative data that can support, for example, conclusions of abnormal activation (Rosen and Gur 2002). There are risks that measures will vary between individuals or that the meaning of data compared with normal individuals will be difficult to establish. Abnormality and predictive validity could even be more problematic in the context of real-world behaviors, especially those that are potentially value laden or culturally determined (Illes *et al.* 2003).

## Neuroimaging and neuroethics

As we have seen, the methodological complexity of neuroimaging justifies substantial qualifications about the conditions under which knowledge is produced and interpreted. Great competence and skills are needed to perform neuroimaging research, but comparable skills are also needed in scientific communication to transfer the subtleties and the uncertainties of neuroimaging results.

One of the underlying issues within the scope of epistemological awareness relates to why neuroimages are so convincing. To draw a parallel with genomics, the idea that the genome is the secular equivalent of the soul has been legitimately criticized (Mauron 2001) as genomic metaphysics (Mauron 2002). In this sense, the brain may represent a culturally invested organ and, like, or even more than the genome, a specific symbol in our self-identity. One overarching element of evidence for this claim is how smoothly (all things considered) neuroscience informs policy-making and popular culture in comparison to genetics (Racine *et al.* 2005). We propose that the evolution of functional neuroimaging and its possible wide application in the social domain emphasize the need for rethinking researcher responsibility beyond issues of scientific integrity or traditional research ethics. New dimensions of responsibility, such as accountability and reproducibility, public involvement, and outlook on consequences of the technology as identified in ethical discussion of genomics and beyond (Racine 2002), are becoming part of the ethical landscape of neuroimaging (Table 11.3).

## Accountability

Researchers hold integrity as a key value that carries with it accountability for results, whether or not results have yet been reproduced independently. This is translated in major research ethics guidelines such as the World Medical Association's Helsinki Declaration and the Belmont Report that emphasize requirements for the highest degree of integrity from those

**Table 11.3** Four new dimensions of researcher and clinician responsibility

| | |
|---|---|
| Accountability and reproducibility | Accountability for scientific evidence and new approaches to reproducibility |
| Responsiveness | Care within the research setting and extended roles outside |
| Democratic and civic involvement | Partnership in promoting public understanding of the brain and democratic debate |
| Prospective responsibility | Management of real and imagined future uses of neuroimaging |

who perform research. This familiar responsibility may seem straightforward, but the context of neuroimaging brings additional requirements. Today, creativity and innovation characterize the state of the art in neuroimaging and few, if any, studies are formally replicated. The result is studies with small sample sizes that build on each other, but do not necessarily validate initial findings. How can we circumvent this in the future? Should we do so?

We think we should, if we can. Reproducibility is key to hypothesis-driven science that culminates in dissemination of results through the peer-reviewed literature. But reproducibility will require an investment in infrastructure and ethical muscle, and data that are robust enough to withstand cross-platform differences. Cross-institutional collaborations, common analytic methodologies, and database sharing represent potentially economical approaches to achieving this goal, but are accompanied by a host of interesting ethical challenges. For example, in the domain of data sharing, attributions of credit for authorship and other forms of academic currency become complicated when large numbers of investigators are involved in studies and, even more so, when the collaborations cross traditional academic boundaries where different expectations and values may collide. Whether we use a utilitarian framework, where the maximization of beneficial outcomes prevails, or a deontological framework emphasizing inalienable individual rights and freedoms, we must give careful thought to the ground rules needed to facilitate and empower a database-sharing approach. While there is great momentum in encouraging and in some cases requiring the sharing of databases (e.g. GenBank, PhysioNet, *Journal of Cognitive Neuroscience*), the spadework in ensuring equitable access for neuroscience data is not at all complete. Consider, for example, unanswered questions such as: Who should establish, monitor and update rules and ensure an evenness of requirements and fairness among investigators? What processes are needed for handling violations? What range of data should be shared? In what format? How should data be organized by investigators so that they can be shared and used efficiently? What impact will standardizing data acquisition to maximize efficiency have on innovation and scientific creativity? How will data obtained from vulnerable populations be protected, and how will unexpected anomalies detected in secondary analysis be managed? What safeguards are needed in this new era of imaging genomics in which physiological links between functional genetic polymorphisms and information processing have been demonstrated (see also Chapter 12)? These are a few, but nonetheless key questions that will require our continued thought and attention.

## Responsiveness

To discuss our concept of responsiveness, we draw on two examples: unexpected clinical anomalies in research, and direct-to-consumer marketing of neuroimaging services.

Traditional ethics guidelines include the principle of beneficence, a term which translates into the need for careful evaluation of the ratio of risks and benefits involved in a protocol, especially for clinical trials. However, this principle is also particularly relevant in the case where non-clinical neuroimaging reveals an unexpected medical finding such as a tumor or vascular formation in a research subject recruited as a healthy control, or in a patient where the finding is unrelated to the primary purpose of the study. Typically, basic neuroimaging studies in cognitive neuroscience are performed by non-clinicians, many by research fellows and some even by undergraduate students. Unanticipated findings may go unrecognized and thereby leave subjects without appropriate health care. While studies have shown that most of these findings are clinically insignificant, the clinically significant ones vary in frequency and severity varies with age and gender (Illes *et al.* 2002, 2004; Kim *et al.* 2002).

The presence of significant clinical findings in an otherwise non-clinical research setting is a matter of both medical and bioethical concern. Many participants in medical research expect that a physician will review their studies, even though they have acknowledged through the informed consent process that the study does not bear any benefit, clinical or otherwise (M.P. Kirschen *et al.* 2006). This phenomenon, known as the therapeutic misconception, is of particular significance when it is juxtaposed with the discovery of a medical anomaly in the context of research (Hinton 2002). Findings may create anxiety and financial cost if follow-up is needed, and even a benign lesion detected in an asymptomatic subject (Illes *et al.* 2002) has the potential to affect medical insurability (Kulynych 2002). Therefore, while neuroimagers may have an ethical obligation to anticipate detection and disclosure issues in their research, is it reasonable to expect that all procedures for non-clinical neuroimaging include clinician follow-up? On the one hand, scan volume and professional costs would be staggering. On the other hand, the cost of a missed or unreported finding in a research subject who succumbs to a fatal condition within months of a research study could be greater. Responsibility to inform research subjects of incidental findings cannot be easily waived. We believe that some new element of responsibility will require neuroimagers to consider a clinical attitude of beneficence (see also Chapter 14).

Our second example of responsibility bears on the growing dissemination of neuroimaging devices and services in the non-clinical for-profit sector. If we imagine psychometric uses of neuroimaging in matters of personality or employment, like pencil-and-paper tests of the past, what would be the appropriate role of neuroimagers? Today, without physician referral, consumers across the USA and Canada may purchase for themselves CT or MRI head scans whether or not they are symptomatic or functional scans with SPECT to obtain an assessment of attention and memory for themselves or their loved ones.

What obligations do neuroimagers have regarding legitimate or nefarious goals to which neuroimaging might contribute? In the absence of clear deontological obligations to consumers, how would market forces and profit imperatives challenge traditional researcher roles? Is there a special commitment toward the consumer in terms of follow-up? What are the principles to which entrepreneurial neuroimagers must adhere in order to inform consumers properly? Respecting autonomy in the context of the open market may be insufficient. New levels of responsiveness to these new challenges to responsibility are vital.

## Public involvement

Up to this point in our discussion, the necessity for democratic and civic responsibility has been an implicit theme. To be more explicit here, we have observed that neuroscientists, like physicists and geneticists, are becoming increasingly aware of their social and civic responsibilities in fostering public education and dialogue on brain understanding (Racine 2002). We believe that this is, in part, one of the contributions that neuroethics has already made. However, making the public more aware of both the excitement surrounding neuroimaging research and, at the same time, its limits is challenging for even the most committed and eloquent interlocutor. Analysis of the media shows that, in the case of fMRI, proper interpretation of data and the validity and limitations of research are prime concerns and outweigh (in sheer numbers) ethical issues (Racine *et al.* 2005). In this context, what can we expect in terms of epistemological awareness?

In the area of education policy, Georgia's state legislature issued a mandate in 1998 for the distribution of a recording of classical music to all newborn infants with the goal of stimulating intellectual development on the basis of a study published by Rauscher and Shaw in 1995 called 'Listening to Mozart enhances spatial-temporal reasoning: toward a neuropsychological basis' (DiPietro 2000). Early reports promised that discoveries in neuroscience would revolutionize how people think about parenting or early education based on critical periods for development and the role of enriched environments (Bruer 1998; DiPietro 2000). Some also believe that cognitive neuroscience will provide through neuroimaging the possibility of early detection of learning difficulties and enable assessment of education for special needs (Goswani 2004; Illes and Raffin 2005).

However, despite public and political interest in this area of research, there remain many significant challenges. For example, the so-called Mozart-effect of short-term increase in spatial reasoning in adults that justified the Georgia initiative was documented in adults (not in infants) and apparently has no significant lasting effect on IQ (DiPietro 2000). Many concluded that neuroscience-inspired childhood policies are also not the right public health orientation, given the documented detrimental effects of poverty on child development (Bruer 1998; DiPietro 2000; Hinton 2002; see also Chapter 19). The Organization for Economic Cooperation and Development (OECD) qualified interpretation of the data as neuromythology. Nonetheless, these obstacles are not preventing a Minnesota-based private school for underachievers from offering services of brain-based education today, and even suggesting before-and-after PET scans (http://www.calvinacademy.com/brain_based_education_htm).

Examination of some recent examples of research reporting and new social practices also emphasizes the relevance of increasing responsibility. For example, studies of neuromarketing consumer preferences using fMRI to inform marketing strategies have sparked a fierce debate within the neuroscience community and the wider public (Anonymous 2002, 2004). Such debate is precisely why neuroimagers must lead the effort toward multidirectional communication with the public, the media, and other stakeholders:

> Scientific training in the past included the lesson: that it was somehow 'unethical' to speak with the press. 'Good scientists' just didn't engage in dialogue in the public arena, assuming that their statements would be twisted and misconstrued by the uninformed lay public. This elitist attitude, to the good of the public that pays for the research, has come to an end. ( ... ) Neuroscientists as a group are beginning to accept their responsibility for conveying their new data to the public. (Chugani 1998).

This move away from the traditional and unidirectional expert knowledge pathway will enable significant strides to be made in assuring the kind of responsible understanding about neuroimages that must be promoted both within and outside the scientific community.

## Prospective responsibility

With an increasing number of studies that provide tempting ground on which to link 'neuro-types' to phenotypes, the dimension of prospective responsibility defines how we can tackle real and imagined future uses of neuroimaging. To begin to address but a few of the emerging questions, we ask: How will the association between neurotypes and phenotypes be conveyed and managed? What are requirements for protection of privacy (Farah and Wolpe 2004)? Would mind reading give rise to stigmatization of individuals who are considered abnormal, or will it help to destigmatize people by providing better understanding of human differences? Are new forms of prejudicial discrimination to be expected from neurotype testing or neuroprofiling? How will the underlying epistemological issues bridging structure and function be addressed if neurotypes are used to assess intangible human qualities? How will the issues change if a non-invasive, portable, and affordable fMRI device becomes available to study or monitor real-world behaviors in natural contexts (Izzetoglu *et al.* 2004)? History would predict that these are not questions of pure fiction. They deserve our attention without delay.

## Conclusion

The power of the image of the human brain—its structure and function combined—and the hunger of the public for innovations in science and technology fuel perceptions about what an image reveals and, moreover, hopes for what it may mean. However, bridging mind and molecules is anything but a simple task, and its inherent complexity increases as the envelope of frontier neurotechnology is pushed to new extremes. However, if a technology is not ready for a specific application, be it clinical or other, the utilization of neuroimaging may be misin-formed and knowledge may be over-interpreted. What once resided safely in the domain of the academic and medical elite now dangles in the public eye, albeit still on a thin thread, by virtue of the interest of the media, the sheer drive of human curiosity, and the potential social relevance of the research image—to love, hate, trust, deceive. One can read that neuroimaging allows one 'to see past the rhetoric, and directly into the brain to find out exactly what someone believes', and that 'the brain always reveals the truth, no matter what tales we tell' (Persaud 2001). Such deep and previously intangible qualities and abilities of humans have now begun to assume visual-izable concrete features. How those features are reconstructed to have a single face—the face of meaning—underlies a new set of responsibilities for professionals and amateurs alike, respon-sibilities that build on the fundamental dedication to truth in knowledge.

## Acknowledgments

The invaluable help of Marisa Gallo is gratefully acknowledged. This work was supported by the Greenwall Foundation (JI), NIH/NINDS RO1 NS 045831 (JI), The Henry J. Kaiser Family Foundation (JI), the SSHRC and FQRSC (ER) and the Stanford Medical Scientist Training Program (MPK).

## References

Aguirre G, Zarahn E, D'Esposito M (1998). The variability of human, BOLD hemodynamic responses. *NeuroImage* 8, 360–9.

Anonymous (2002). Open your mind (Editorial) *Economist*, 25 May.

Anonymous (2004). Brain scam? (Editorial) *Nature Neuroscience* 7, 683.

Beaulieu A (2001). Voxels in the brain. *Social Studies of Science* 31, 1–45.

Borck C (2001). Electricity as a medium of psychic life: electrotechnological adventures into psychodiagnosis in Weimar Germany. *Science in Context* 14, 565–90.

Bruer JT (1998). The brain and child development: time for some critical thinking. *Public Health Reports* 113, 388–98.

Canli T, Amin Z (2002). Neuroimaging of emotion and personality: scientific evidence and ethical considerations. *Brain and Cognition* 50, 414–31.

Canli T, Zhao Z, Desmond JE, Kang E, Gross J, Gabrieli JDE (2001). An fMRI study of personality influences on brain reactivity to emotional stimuli. *Behavioral Neuroscience* 114, 33–42.

Casebeer WD (2003). Moral cognition and its neural constituents. *Nature Neuroscience* 4, 841–6.

Chugani HT (1998). Neuroscience and public policy. *Public Health Reports* 113, 480.

Churchland PS (1998). Feeling reasons. In Churchland PM, Churchland PS (eds) *On The Contrary*. Cambridge, MA: MIT Press, 231–54.

Cohen D (1972). Magnetoencephalography: detection of the brain's electrical activity with a superconducting magnetometer. *Science* 175, 664–6.

Coyle S, Ward T, Markham C, McDarby G (2004). On the suitability of near-infrared (NIR) systems for next-generation brain–computer interfaces. *Physiological Measurement* 25, 815–22.

Damasio AR (2002). The neural basis of social behavior: ethical implications. In Marcus SL (ed) *Neuroethics: Mapping the Field*. San Francisco, CA: Dana Press, 14–19.

Desmond JE, Chen ASH (2002). Ethical issues in the clinical application of fMRI: factors affecting the validity and interpretation of activations. *Brain and Cognition* 50, 482–97.

Desmond JE, Glover GH (2002). Estimating sample size in functional MRI (fMRI) neuroimaging studies: statistical power analyses. *Journal of Neuroscience Methods.* 2002 118(2): 115–28.

DiPietro JA (2000). Baby and the brain: advances in child development. *Annual Review of Public Health* 21, 455–71.

Farah MJ and Wolpe PR (2004). Monitoring and manipulating brain function: new neuroscience technologies and their ethical implications. *Hastings Center Report* 34, 35–45.

Fletcher PC, Happé F, Frith U, *et al.* (1995). Other minds in the brain: a functional imaging study of 'theory of mind' in story comprehension. *Cognition* 57, 109–28.

Glimcher PW, Rustichini A (2004). Neuroeconomics: the consilience of brain and decision. *Science* 306, 447–52.

Goswani U (2004). Neuroscience and education. *British Journal of Educational Psychology* 74, 1–14.

Gray JR, Thompson PM (2004). Neurobiology of intelligence: science and ethics. *Nature Reviews Neuroscience* 5, 471–82.

Greene JD (2003). From neural 'is' to moral 'ought': what are the moral implications of neuroscientific moral psychology? *Nature Reviews Neuroscience* 4, 846–850.

Greene JD, Sommerville RB, Nystrom LE, Darley JM, Cohen JD (2001). An fMRI investigation of emotional engagement in moral judgment. *Science* 293, 2105–8.

Haidt J (2001). The emotional dog and its rational tail: a social intuitionist approach to moral judgment. *Psychological Review* 108, 814–34.

Hinton VJ (2002). Ethics of neuroimaging in pediatric development. *Brain and Cognition* 50, 455–68.

Horovitz S, Gore JC (2004). Simultaneous event-related potential and near-infrared spectroscopic studies of semantic processing. *Human Brain Mapping* 22, 110–15.

Illes J, Racine E (2005). Imaging or imagining? A neuroethics challenge informed by genetics. *American Journal of Bioethics* 5(2), 5–18.

Illes J, Raffin TA (2005). No child left without a brain scan? A model problem for pediatric neuroethics. *Cerebrum.* 7, 33–46.

Illes J, Desmond JE, Huang LF, Raffin TA, Atlas SW (2002). Ethical and practical considerations in managing incidental findings in functional magnetic resonance imaging. *Brain and Cognition* 50, 358–65.

Illes J, Kirschen MP, Gabrieli JD (2003). From neuroimaging to neuroethics. *Nature Neuroscience* 6, 205.

Illes J, Rosen AC, Huang L, *et al.* (2004). Ethical consideration of incidental findings on adult brain MRI in research. *Neurology* 62, 888–90.

Izzetoglu K, Bunce S, Izzetoglu M, Onaral B, Pourrezaei K (2004). Functional near-infrared neuroimaging. In: *Proceedings 26th Annual International Conference of the IEEE Engineering in Medicine and Biology Society*. Piscataway, NJ: Institute of Electrical and Electronics Engineers.

Johnson S (2004). *Mind Wide Open: Your Brain and the Neuroscience of Everyday Life.* New York: Scribner.

Jung CG (1964). *Man and His Symbols.* Garden City, NY: Doubleday.

Kandel ER, Mack S (2003). A parallel between radical reductionism in science and in art. *Annals of the New York Academy of Sciences* **1001**: 272–94.

Kim BS, Illes J, Kaplan RT, Reiss A, Atlas SW (2002). Incidental findings on pediatric MR images of the brain. *American Journal of Neuroradiology* **23**, 1674–7.

Kirschen MP, Jaworska A, Illes J. Subjects expectations in neuroimaging research. *Journal of Magnetic Resonance Imaging* **23**, 205–9.

Klingberg T, Hedehus M, Temple E *et al.* (2000). Microstructure of temporo-parietal white matter as a basis for reading ability: Evidence from diffusion tensor magnetic resonance imaging. *Neuron* **25**(2), 257–259.

Kosik KS (2003). Beyond phrenology, at last. *Nature Neuroscience* **4**, 234–9.

Kulynych J (2002). Legal and ethical issues in neuroimaging research: human subjects protection, medical privacy, and the public communication of research results. *Brain and Cognition* **50**, 345–57.

Lasden M (2004). Mr. Chiesa's brain. *California Lawyer* 27–30, 61–3.

Lefèvre W, Renn J, Schoepfin U (eds) (2003). *The Power of Images in Early Modern Science.* Basel, Switzerland: Birkäuser Verlag.

Loftus E (2003). Our changeable memories: legal and practical implications. *Nature Reviews Neuroscience* **4**, 231–3.

Mallard JR (2003). The evolution of medical imaging. From Geiger counters to MRI—a personal saga. *Perspectives in Biology and Medicine* **46**, 349–70.

Mauron A (2001). Is the genome the secular equivalent of the soul? *Science* **291**, 831–2.

Mauron A (2002). Genomic metaphysics. *Journal of Molecular Biology* **319**, 957–62.

Mazziotta JC (2000). Window on the brain. *Archives of Neurology* **57**, 1413–21.

Moll J, de Oliveira-Souza R, Bramati IE, Grafman J (2002a). Functional networks in emotional and nonmoral social judgments. *NeuroImage* **26**, 696–703.

Moll J, de Oliveira-Souza R, Eslinger PJ, *et al.* (2002b). The neural correlates of moral sensitivity: a functional magnetic resonance imaging investigation of basic and moral emotions. *Journal of Neuroscience* **22**, 2730–6.

Moll J, de Oliveira-Souza R, Eslinger PJ (2003). Morals and the human brain: a working model. *Neuroreport* **14**, 299–305.

Newberg A, D'Aquili E, Rause V (2002). *Why God Won't Go Away: Brain Science and the Biology of Belief.* New York: Ballantine Books.

OECD (2002). *Understanding the Brain: Toward a New Learning Science.* Paris: OECD.

Partiot A, Grafman J, Sadato N, Wachs J, Hallett M (1995). Brain activation during the generation of non-emotional and emotional plans. *Neuroreport* **6**, 1269–72.

Penfield W and Boldray E (1937). Somatic motor and sensory representation in the cerebral cortex of man as studied by electrical stimulation. *Brain* **60**, 389–443.

Persaud R (2001). Who's telling porkies about racism? Refinements in brain-scanning could soon make the thought police a reality. *Daily Telegraph*, 25 April, p. 21.

Phan LK, Wager T, Taylor SF, Liberzon I (2002). Functional neuroanatomy of emotion: a meta-analysis of emotion activation studies in PET and fMRI. *NeuroImage* **16**, 331–48.

President's Council on Bioethics (2004). Session 5: Neuroscience, brain, and behavior IV: Brain imaging. http://www.bioethics.gov/transcripts/june04/session5.html

Racine E (2002). Éthique de la discussion et génomique des populations. *Éthique Publique* **4**, 77–90.

Racine E (2005). Pourquoi et comment doit-on tenir compte des neurosciences en éthique? Esquisse d'une approche neurophilosophique émergentiste et interdisciplinaire. *Laval Théologique et Philosophique*, **61**, 77–105.

Racine E, Bar-Ilan O, Illes J (2005). fMRI in the public eye. *Nature Reviews Neuroscience* **6**, 9–14.

Rosen AC, Gur RC (2002). Ethical considerations for neuropsychologists as functional magnetic imagers. *Brain and Cognition* **50**, 469–81.

Rosen AC, Bodke ALW, Pearl A, Yesavage JA (2002). Ethical and practical issues in applying functional imaging to the clinical management of Alzheimer's disease. *Brain and Cognition* 50, 498–519.

Roskies Al, Petersen SE (2001). Visualizing human brain function. In: Bizzi E, Calissano P, Volterra V (eds.) Frontiers of Life, Vol III: The Intelligent Systems, Part one: The Brain of Homo Sapiens. New York: Academic Press, 87–109

Stufflebaum RS, Bechtel W (1997). PET: exploring the myth and the method. *Philosophy of Science* 64, S95–106.

Van Orden GC, Paap KR (1997). Functional neuroimages fail to discover pieces of mind in the parts of the brain. *Philosophy of Science* 64, S85–94.

Chapter 12

# When genes and brains unite: ethical implications of genomic neuroimaging

Turhan Canli

## Introduction

The Burning Man Festival in Black Rock, Nevada, is an annual celebration of individual expression and non-conformity. Its theme for 2005 was 'Psyche: the Conscious, the Subconscious and the Unconscious', and encouraged artistic expression related to the self. An appreciation of the individual may not be limited to those who view themselves as the vanguard of counterculture hipness, but may rather reflect a *Zeitgeist* that has also taken hold of an increasing number of researchers in the biological sciences. Geneticists, neuroscientists, and personality psychologists are now on a quest to understand the biological basis of personality and individual differences. In this chapter, I will highlight recent advances in this field of research. I will illustrate how data obtained from neuroimaging scans can predict narrowly defined forms of behavior better than self-report and other behavioral measures, and make the argument that future integration of genetic and life experience data with neuroimaging data will further enhance this capability. I will then identify likely applications of this technology and conclude that a statistically informed cost–benefit analysis may be the most practical approach towards the ethical use of this technology across a diverse set of real-life applications.

## From noise to signal: a new-found appreciation for individual differences in functional neuroimaging

Functional neuroimaging is concerned with the association of mental processes with brain activation patterns. The two most common methods are positron emission tomography (PET) and functional magnetic resonance imaging (fMRI). Both have traditionally relied on averaged data across groups of subjects to determine loci of activation. Intersubject variability diminishes the statistical reliability of such analyses, which explains why investigators eschewed individual differences. Steinmetz and Seitz (1991) drew attention to the difficulty posed by individual differences in PET studies of language processing. They identified diversity in the localization of language and in brain shape as two contributors to intersubject variability, and suggested that studies of cognitive functions should address individual differences with appropriate analysis strategies. Indeed, new approaches to the analysis of individual differences in imaging studies have led to a growth in publications. A search in Medline of the terms 'individual difference', and 'PET' or 'fMRI', produced a total of five publications between 1990 and 94, 11 from 1995–1999, and 57 from 2000–2004.

In the domain of emotion and personality, my colleagues and I developed a research program that exploits individual differences in emotional responsiveness to understand the neural basis of personality (Canli 2004). It is consistent with everyday experience that individuals differ in emotional reactivity. For example, a film clip intended to manipulate the positive or negative mood of the viewer may be effective in some individuals but not in others. Some individuals seek out social contact, whereas others prefer solitude. Some seem unfazed by anything, whereas others are prone to worry. These individual differences in positive and negative emotionality map onto two dimensions of personality—extraversion and neuroticism, respectively (Costa and McCrae 1980; Meyer and Shack 1989; Larsen and Ketelaar 1991; Watson and Clark 1992). These two traits are not opposite ends of the personality spectrum, but rather represent two independent dimensions of personality. Extraversion is associated with positive affect, gregariousness, and excitement seeking (Costa and McCrae 1980; McCrae and Costa 1999). Accordingly, individuals who score high in measures of extraversion (extraverts) are more responsive to positive mood induction procedures than individuals who score low (introverts) (Larsen and Ketelaar 1991). Neuroticism is associated with negative affect—a tendency to feel anxious, self-conscious, or worried (Costa and McCrae 1980; McCrae and Costa 1999). Accordingly, individuals who score high on measures of neuroticism are more responsive to negative mood induction procedures than individuals who score low (Larsen and Ketelaar 1991). A given individual may score high or low in either trait dimension. For example, a student who scores high in both extraversion and neuroticism would probably enjoy going out with friends on a Thursday night, but would also worry about his academic success and his parents' approval.

If emotional reactivity is related to personality, then individual differences in brain activation to emotional stimuli should be associated with participants' measures of extraversion and neuroticism. We tested this hypothesis explicitly in an fMRI study in which participants passively viewed alternating blocks of positive and negative pictures (Canli *et al.* 2001). The subject matter depicted in these pictures was varied and included positive and negative examples of people (e.g. happy or upset), food (e.g., appetizing images of cakes versus rotting food), and animals (e.g., puppies versus snakes). Participants' extraversion and neuroticism scores on a personality trait questionnaire (Costa and McCrae 1992) were correlated with the brain activation data acquired while they viewed the images passively. Consistent with our hypothesis, higher extraversion scores were associated with greater brain activation to positive, compared with negative, emotional stimuli (Figure 12.1). Similarly, higherer neuroticism scores were associated with greater brain activation to negative, compared with positive, emotional stimuli (Fig. 12.1).

The use of a passive viewing task, together with the lack of a neutral baseline condition, complicated the interpretation of the data in this first imaging study of emotion and personality. Therefore subsequent studies were designed to constrain the task to specific cognitive processes. For example, an emotional face-processing task revealed that activation of the amygdala in response to happy faces varied as a function of extraversion (Canli *et al.* 2002): those participants who scored high in the trait exhibited amygdala activation in response to happy, relative to neutral, faces, whereas those participants who scored low did not (Fig. 12.2).

The finding offered one explanation of why previous imaging studies reported contradictory findings with regard to the role of the amygdala in the processing of happy facial expressions: previous studies had not tested participants for personality traits. It is possible that the proportion of extraverts across different study samples may have varied sufficiently to affect the outcome of group-based analyses.

Other studies employed cognitive paradigms designed to test attention for emotional stimuli (Amin *et al.* 2004; Canli *et al.* 2004). These studies associated regions such as the fusiform gyrus, anterior cingulate cortex, and inferior parietal lobule (these areas have previously been identified to be involved in attentional processes) with individual differences in personality

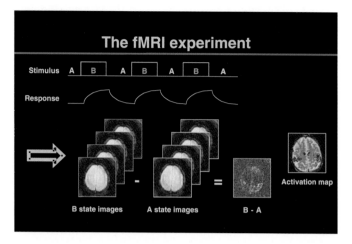

**Fig. 11.1** Experimental (B state) images are subtracted from control (A state) images to achieve regional activation maps with fMRI. Courtesy of G.H. Glover, Lucas MRS/MRI Center, Stanford University Medical Center. Reproduced with permission from *The American Journal of Bioethics*.

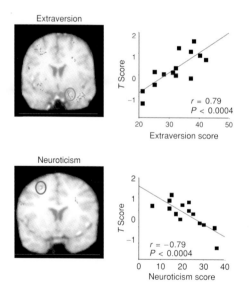

**Fig 12.1** Brain activation to emotional stimuli as a function of personality traits. The top row shows activation associated with extraversion. The top left shows a coronal cut through the region of the amygdala (circled in blue). Colored clusters identify regions where greater activation to positive, relative to negative, pictures (indicated by positive T score values) was associated with higher extraversion scores. The top right scatterplot depicts this association quantitatively for the amygdala. The bottom row shows activation associated with neuroticism. The bottom left shows a coronal cut through the region of the middle temporal gyrus (circled in red). Colored clusters identify regions where greater activation to negative, relative to positive, pictures (indicated by negative T score values) was associated with higher neuroticism scores. The bottom right scatterplot depicts this association quantitatively for the middle temporal gyrus. Data from Canli, *et al.* (2001).

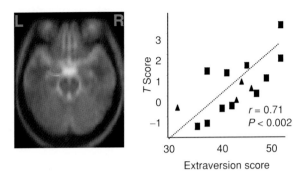

**Fig 12.2** Amygdala activation to happy faces as a function of extraversion. The left panel shows an axial cut through the plane of the amygdala. The red cluster identifies voxels that were significantly activated to happy, relative to neutral, faces as a function of extraversion. L, left; R, right. The right panel shows a scatterplot representing activation (in T scores) from the cluster in the left panel as a function of extraversion. Squares and triangles identify females and males, respectively. Data from Canli, *et al.* (2002).

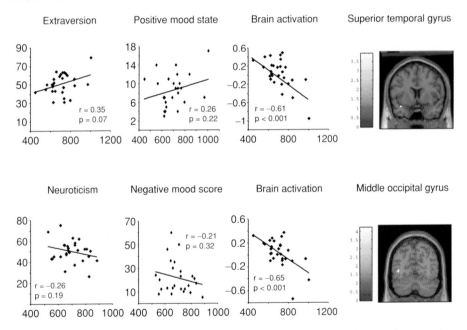

**Fig 12.3** Comparison of three predictors of reaction time (RT). RT to positive (top row) or negative (bottom row) word stimuli was correlated with individual measures of personality traits (first column), mood state (second column), or brain activation (third column) for clusters located in either the superior temporal gyrus (top right) (MNI coordinates: −38, 8, −20; cluster size: 11 voxels; T score: 3.92; Z score: 3.44) or the middle occipital gyrus (bottom right) (MNI coordinates: −40, −68, 2; cluster size: 13 voxels; T score: 4.21; Z score : 3.64). For positive stimuli, extraversion explained 12 percent of the variance in RT, positive mood scores explained 7 percent, and activation in the superior temporal gyrus explained 37 percent. For negative stimuli, neuroticism explained 7 percent of the variance in RT, negative mood scores explained 4 percent, and activation in the middle occipital gyrus explained 42 percent.

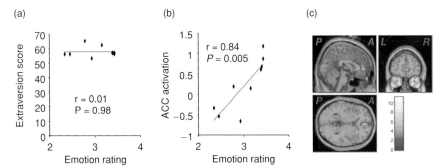

**Fig 12.4** Two predictors of subjective emotional experience. (a) Scatterplot showing association between participants' extraversion scores and mean subjective emotional rating scores in response to positive pictures. (b) Scatterplot showing association between participants' mean ACC activation values in response to positive, relative to neutral, pictures and mean rating scores in response to positive pictures. (c) Cluster in the ACC (1191 voxels; $P = 0.005$, family-wise-error corrected for the region of the entire ACC; most significant voxel located at 2, 50, 2 in MNI coordinates) where activation to positive, relative to neutral, pictures was significantly correlated with subjective emotional arousal ratings of positive pictures. A, anterior; P, posterior; L, left; R, right.

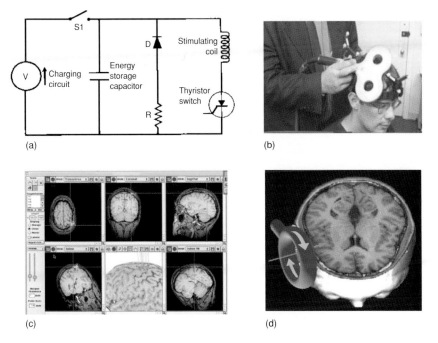

**Fig. 14.1** Illustration of the application of TMS. (a) Schematic diagram of the electric circuit used to induce the TMS pulse. (b) The TMS coil being applied by an experimenter. Both the coil and the subject have a tracking device affixed to them so that the head/coil position can be monitored in real time. (c) Illustration of how the subject's MRI can be used, along with the tracking system which monitors head and coil movement, to display the cortical area being targeted in real-time. (d) Depth of effect of the TMS coil on the human cortex.

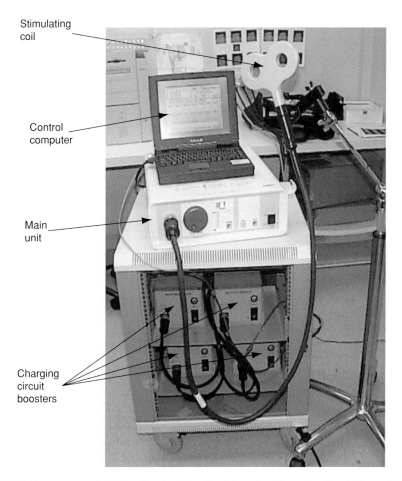

Stimulating coil

Control computer

Main unit

Charging circuit boosters

**Fig. 14.2** TMS equipment including the charging circuit boosters, the main stimulating unit, the control computer, and the stimulating coil.

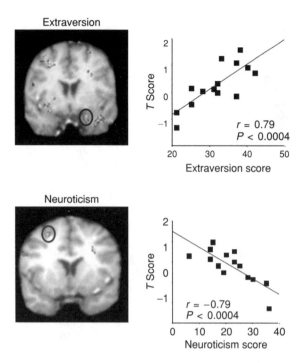

**Fig 12.1** Brain activation to emotional stimuli as a function of personality traits. The top row shows activation associated with extraversion. The top left shows a coronal cut through the region of the amygdala (circled in blue). Colored clusters identify regions where greater activation to positive, relative to negative, pictures (indicated by positive T score values) was associated with higher extraversion scores. The top right scatterplot depicts this association quantitatively for the amygdala. The bottom row shows activation associated with neuroticism. The bottom left shows a coronal cut through the region of the middle temporal gyrus (circled in red). Colored clusters identify regions where greater activation to negative, relative to positive, pictures (indicated by negative T score values) was associated with higher neuroticism scores. The bottom right scatterplot depicts this association quantitatively for the middle temporal gyrus. Data from Canli, *et al.* (2001) (See also the colour plate section)

trait and mood state variables. Considered together, these studies make it clear that there is no single personality spot in the brain. Rather, different tasks engage different neural networks, and individual differences within these networks can be associated with individual differences in personality traits or mood states.

## Does brain activation predict behavior better than personality questionnaires?

Reports of an association between brain activation and personality measures reliably generate the following question: 'Can you predict my personality by simply looking at a brain picture?' My (somewhat tongue-in-cheek) answer is: 'Absolutely (assuming the scan was done using appropriate stimuli, experimental design, analysis methods)—or I could just talk to you for a few minutes'. The point is that we make personality assessments all the time in our social

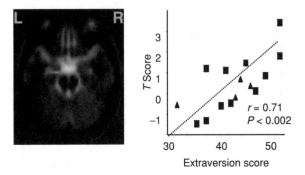

**Fig 12.2** Amygdala activation to happy faces as a function of extraversion. The left panel shows an axial cut through the plane of the amygdala. The red cluster identifies voxels that were significantly activated to happy, relative to neutral, faces as a function of extraversion. L, left; R, right. The right panel shows a scatterplot representing activation (in T scores) from the cluster in the left panel as a function of extraversion. Squares and triangles identify females and males, respectively. Data from Canli, *et al.* (2002) (See also the colour plate section).

interactions. As social beings, we are experts in observing the behavior of others and drawing conclusions about their personality from these observations. Since all behavior is generated by the brain, it should not be too surprising that knowledge about someone's brain state ought to reveal something about that individual's personality.

I believe that the more important question to ask is whether brain imaging data can predict behavior *better* than traditional assessments of personality. Note that this is a different question than was addressed in previous imaging studies (Canli 2004; Canli *et al.* 2004) in which brain activation was correlated directly with self-reported personality scores. Instead, here we are interested in assessing whether some response measure is better predicted by personality scores or by brain activation data. I will consider two cases: in the first case, the response measure is a motor response (reaction time) to emotional word stimuli; in the second case, the response measure is a subjective emotional rating.

For the first case, I present data from a study in our laboratory in which we collected fMRI and reaction time (RT) data from participants during an emotional attention task, the emotional word Stroop Test. This is a simple RT task designed to infer how much a person is distracted by the presence of an emotional stimulus. Emotional and neutral words are printed in different colors, and subjects have to press a button, as quickly as possible, that corresponds to the color of the printed word. Previous studies have shown that individual trait differences can affect task performance: trait anxious subjects respond more slowly to anxiety-related words than to neutral words (Richards *et al.* 1992). The negative meaning of these words distracts the subjects sufficiently to interfere with their task performance. Similarly, subjects who score high in neuroticism may respond more slowly to negative than to neutral words. The empirical question I address is this: Are individual differences in RT better predicted by (i.e. more strongly correlated with) brain activation data, or by mood state or personality trait scores?

Twenty-eight right-handed subjects (16 female) participated in an fMRI study. While they were scanned, they viewed negative, positive, and neutral word stimuli selected from a standardized stimuli set (Bradley and Lang 1999) and matched for arousal and frequency.

Each word was displayed on a computer screen in blue, red, or green, and subjects were instructed to press a button corresponding to the word color as quickly and accurately as possible. Responses were captured by a computer at millisecond resolution for subsequent analysis. Words were shown in four 18-s blocks of negative, neutral, or positive words and fixation crosses (order counterbalanced across subjects) with six word stimuli per block (1.5 s duration, 1.5 s inter-trial interval), and no repetitions of word stimuli.

Whole-brain imaging data were acquired on a 3-T scanner at Yale University's Magnetic Resonance Research Center using standard imaging parameters and fMRI analysis procedures. Correlation analyses were conducted for all behavioral and brain variables of interest. RT in response to positive stimuli was significantly correlated with brain activation to positive (relative to neutral) words, but not with extraversion or positive mood scores (Fig. 12.3, top row). Similarly, RT in response to negative stimuli was significantly correlated with brain activation to negative (relative to neutral) words, but not with neuroticism or negative mood scores (Fig. 12.3, bottom row). Thus, for both positive and negative word stimuli, brain activation in specific loci was much more strongly correlated with RT responses than with

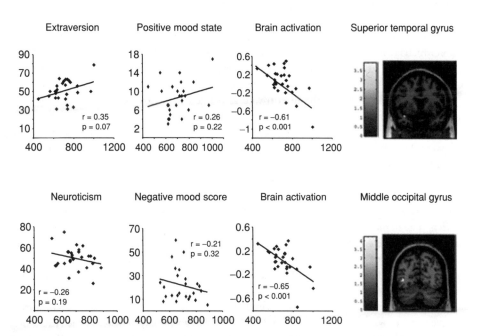

**Fig 12.3** Comparison of three predictors of reaction time (RT). RT to positive (top row) or negative (bottom row) word stimuli was correlated with individual measures of personality traits (first column), mood state (second column), or brain activation (third column) for clusters located in either the superior temporal gyrus (top right) (MNI coordinates: −38, 8, −20; cluster size: 11 voxels; T score: 3.92; Z score: 3.44) or the middle occipital gyrus (bottom right) (MNI coordinates: −40, −68, 2; cluster size: 13 voxels; T score: 4.21; Z score : 3.64). For positive stimuli, extraversion explained 12 percent of the variance in RT, positive mood scores explained 7 percent, and activation in the superior temporal gyrus explained 37 percent. For negative stimuli, neuroticism explained 7 percent of the variance in RT, negative mood scores explained 4 percent, and activation in the middle occipital gyrus explained 42 percent (See also the colour plate section).

subjects' emotional trait and state characteristics. Indeed, variance in RT was better explained by brain activation data than by personality or mood scores by as much as a factor of 10 (see caption to Fig. 12.3).

One can argue that RT is hardly a meaningful measure of personality, or of a behavior worth predicting. I agree to some extent. The above example is intended to provide empirical evidence that data derived from brain scans can be better predictors of behavioral measures than other types of measures. Applications that have real-world relevance have yet to be developed, as I will argue in a later section. However, the association between RT and personality or mood variables was not analyzed arbitrarily, because certain trait or mood states have indeed been shown to correlate with RT responses in this task (Richards *et al.* 1992) and many cognitive paradigms have utilized RT as a measure of individual differences in personality (Matthews and Deary 1998). Perhaps another example, in which the outcome measure is self-reported subjective emotional experience, will seem more relevant.

For the second example, I present data from an imaging study in which participants viewed emotional and neutral pictures and rated their emotional subjective response to these stimuli while being scanned. The question now is: Are self-reported subjective emotional ratings better predicted by (i.e. more strongly correlated with) brain activation data, or by personality trait scores?

In previous work, my colleagues and I identified the anterior cingulate cortex (ACC) as a region which is associated with reactivity to positive stimuli as a function of extraversion (Canli *et al.* 2001, 2004). Therefore the subsequent analysis addresses the question of whether the subjective rating responses of subjects viewing positive words is better predicted by self-reported extraversion or by a brain correlate associated with extraversion (i.e. activation in the ACC in response to positive relative to neutral words).

Nine women completed self-report personality questionnaires (Costa and McCrae 1992) and were scanned as they viewed negative, positive, and neutral pictures presented in random order. Imaging parameters and analysis methods were similar to those in the previous study. Subjects reported on their emotional arousal in response to 32 pictures in each of three affective categories (positive, neutral, or negative), with each picture's membership in a given category determined by available normative ratings (Lang and Greenwald 1993). Subjects made emotional arousal judgments by pressing a four-button box according to the instruction to 'make judgments of how excited or calm you feel when you view each picture. At one extreme of the scale, you are stimulated, excited, frenzied, jittery, wide-awake, aroused. At the other end of the scale, you feel completely relaxed, calm, sluggish, dull, sleepy, unaroused'.

The correlation between self-reported extraversion and self-reported subjective ratings of positive pictures was non-existent. In contrast, there was a very large cluster in the ACC where activation was highly correlated with subjects' ratings. Figure 12.4 illustrates the differences in association between subjective emotional experience ratings as a function of self-reported extraversion (left panel) or as a function of ACC activation (right panel), and shows the cluster from which these activation data were extracted.

Inspection of Figure 12.4 makes it clear why the brain data are superior to the personality data. As can be seen in Figure 12.4(a), the range of the subjects' extraversion data is very narrow, making it very difficult to find significant correlations. In contrast, there is a wide range of brain activation values. Thus, for small samples with restricted range of personality scores, individual differences in brain activation are a far more sensitive tool for detecting significant correlations with behavioral response measures.

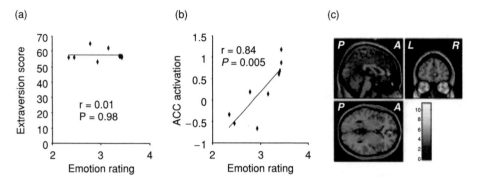

**Fig 12.4** Two predictors of subjective emotional experience. (a) Scatterplot showing association between participants' extraversion scores and mean subjective emotional rating scores in response to positive pictures. (b) Scatterplot showing association between participants' mean ACC activation values in response to positive, relative to neutral, pictures and mean rating scores in response to positive pictures. (c) Cluster in the ACC (1191 voxels; $P = 0.005$, family-wise-error corrected for the region of the entire ACC; most significant voxel located at 2, 50, 2 in MNI coordinates) where activation to positive, relative to neutral, pictures was significantly correlated with subjective emotional arousal ratings of positive pictures. A, anterior; P, posterior; L, left; R, right (See also the colour plate section).

I must conclude this section with a healthy dose of caution. Although I illustrated the potential power of neuroimaging to predict behavior better than RT or self-report measures, these demonstrations are very far from real-life applications. Both the tasks and the behavioral measures used here constitute a very narrow slice of human behavior. They are used in the laboratory to learn about fundamental aspects of brain function, not to predict human behavior in the real world. For any real-life application, one would need to conduct a large-scale scan study to establish the normative range of activation values, against which the data from one individual could later be compared. One would want to include measures of discriminant and convergent validity (Canli and Amin 2002) to assure oneself that the observed association reflects what one thinks it reflects. Dobbs (2005) illustrated the importance of discriminant validity in more concrete terms. He observed '[a]nd while a certain activation pattern may be common to most murderers, for example, too many diseases and characteristics remain unexplored to know that the same pattern couldn't also show up in a Grand Theft Auto fanatic' ('Grand Theft Auto' is a violent computer game).

## Genomic imaging: toward molecular brain mechanisms of personality

Most previous work on the neural basis of personality has relied on self-report questionnaires to reveal neural systems associated with personality. An alternative is to consider measures of genetic variability. Some genes exist in more than one form (polymorphism), and individual differences in genotype have been associated with individual differences in personality.

A specific example is a functional repeat length polymorphism in the transcriptional control region of the serotonin (5-HT) transporter gene (*5-HTT*, *SLC6A4*). The presence or absence of a repetitive sequence in the transcriptional control region of *5-HTT* creates a short (s) and a long (l) variant, with the s variant having a lower 5-HT uptake function. The functional difference in the availability of the 5-HT transporter as a function of genotype is associated with individual differences in personality; individuals who carry one or two copies of the short allele tend to score higher in self-reported anxiety-related traits such as neuroticism or harm avoidance compared with individuals who carry none (Lesch *et al.* 1996).

In a pioneering study, Hariri *et al.* (2002) demonstrated that the *5-HTT* polymorphism is associated with individual differences in brain activation in the amygdala, a region associated with fear and other strong emotions. They asked scan subjects to match pictures of angry and fearful faces, or to match spatial objects. Carriers of the s allele showed greater amygdala activation to the face stimuli than carriers of the l allele. Remarkably, these effects were observed in a small sample (an initial sample of 14 individuals, seven in each genotype group; replicated in a second sample of 14 individuals). Subsequent studies further replicated and extended these results (Furmark *et al.* 2004; Hariri *et al.* 2005; Heinz *et al.* 2005).

The integration of genetic information with neuroimaging data, call it **genomic imaging**, constitutes a powerful tool for learning about the effects that genes have on behavior. Hamer (2002) noted that Hariri *et al.* (2002) reported an effect size that was 10-fold greater than traditional studies in which genotype is associated with self-report measures of behavioral traits. Why should the effect size be so much stronger in a genomic imaging study? Because the brain is the mediator of genetic effects onto behavior (Hamer 2002), because genetic variation is expressed at the neuronal level of analysis, and only from the concert of neuronal activations does behavior emerge. Consequently, the effect of genotype on brain activation is much more direct than its effect on behavior.

However, behavior is not only influenced by genotype. Behavioral genetic studies consistently attribute a substantial proportion of observed variance to environmental factors, and the interaction between genetic and environmental factors has long been acknowledged. A recent set of studies by Caspi and colleagues has identified specific examples of gene–environment interactions in humans (Caspi *et al.* 2002, 2003). For example, individuals who carried one or two copies of the *5-HTT* s allele were significantly more likely to become depressed or show depression-related symptoms in response to stressful life events than individuals who experienced a similar number of stressful life events, but only carried the *5-HTT* l allele (Caspi *et al.* 2003). Similar observations have also been reported for rhesus macaques, for whom allelic variation of *5-HTT* function and early life adversity interact in the modulation central 5-HT system homeostasis and emotionality in later life (Lesch *et al.* 1997; Bennett *et al.* 2002; Barr *et al.* 2004).

For the purpose of predicting behavior, the combination of life history information, genotype, and brain imaging data may yield very precise predictors of future behavior or psychopathology. Although this prediction is untested to date, several possible applications are visible on the not too distant horizon.

## Real-world applications and implications for neuroethics

Real-life imaging applications are motivated by the desire to predict behavior more accurately than is possible with more traditional methods. Several domains can be identified where the motivation to do so is substantial. In matters of homeland security and criminal investigations, one would like to extract truthful testimony from accused defendants or be able to predict confidently whether a convicted felon is going to behave lawfully upon release in the future. This may only apply to relatively few individuals, but other applications may affect a larger percentage of the population. For example, a proportion of working adults may eventually face the prospect of some form of neural screening, and perhaps all consumers will at some point buy products that were test-marketed using neuroimaging techniques. What is the likelihood of these scenarios and is there reason for concern?

## Homeland security and criminal investigations

There is great interest in obtaining information from accused defendants who may not be willing to cooperate in an interrogation or who are suspected of providing false information. A sophisticated form of electroencephalography is being applied commercially by Brain Fingerprinting Laboratories (www.brainwavescience.com). A potential suspect views stimuli that are familiar to him, unfamiliar but irrelevant to the crime, or unfamiliar to any person except the perpetrator of the crime. According to Brain Fingerprinting Laboratories, this method has been used in field tests and actual criminal cases, and has been used by the Federal Bureau of Investigation, an unidentified US intelligence agency, police departments, and other organizations. The scientific concerns with the application of this technology are similar to those identified by Canli and Amin (2002). For example, the choice of stimuli that constitute the appropriate baseline condition is critical to detect a signal. The broader concerns are with regard to access to this technology. For example, could this technology not be used by repressive regimes to extract information from political opponents? Is it acceptable to retrieve information from a defendant's mind without his consent?

Another application may be the assessment of violent offenders during parole board hearings. Its development would be motivated by the desire to use a combination of genetic, life history, and neuroimaging data to predict the likelihood of recidivism. The ground-breaking work of Caspi et al. (2002) has already shown that genotype can moderate the effects of life experience on subsequent antisocial behavior. These authors studied a birth cohort of 1037 children who were repeatedly assessed over a period of 23 years to evaluate the interaction between life experience and genetic variation on subsequent psychosocial behaviors. They reported that a functional polymorphism of the monoamine oxidase A enzyme producing gene (MAOA) moderated the effects of childhood maltreatment on four different measures of antisocial behavior: conduct disorder, conviction of a violent crime by age 26, disposition toward violence, and symptoms of antisocial personality disorder. For all of these measures, the effects of childhood experience of maltreatment on subsequent antisocial behavior were significantly stronger for those individuals who carried the low-activity MAOA variant than for those who carried the high-activity variant. The authors stressed the need for replication and were scrupulous in their discussion of the data in the context of research and clinical applications. Indeed, it would be premature and inappropriate to advocate gene testing as a means of predicting antisocial behavior at the present time. However, there is likely to be much interest in using such data for the development of genomic imaging approaches for just this purpose, by integrating gene × life experience data with forensic neuroimaging methods developed in the study of violent offenders (Canli and Amin 2002).

As these methods will be developed and refined, it is likely that ethical and philosophical concerns will converge on what Dennett (2003) calls the 'specter of creeping exculpation'. If a violent offender can blame his behavior on genetic vulnerability and adverse life experience, together with poorly functioning neural circuits controlling violent impulses, then what moral responsibility is he left to carry? I suspect that the burden of agency—who will be held accountable for bad behavior, to what extent, and under which circumstance—will become one of the dominant themes in future neuroethics debates.

## Recruitment

The recruitment of able employees has traditionally relied on interviews and self-report questionnaires. However, it is evident that applicants are motivated to emphasize those aspects of their personality that they believe will land them the job. Can neuroimaging methods be used to screen applicants? There already exists an imaging literature that has investigated the neural basis of personality traits that may be of interest to future employers, such as extraversion and neuroticism (reviewed by Canli 2004), persistence (Gusnard *et al.* 2003), moral processing (Anderson *et al.* 1999; Greene *et al.* 2001; Modl *et al.* 2002a, 2002b; Singer *et al.* 2004), and cooperation (McCabe *et al.* 2001; Rilling *et al.* 2002, 2004; Decety *et al.* 2004). Therefore it is only a matter of time before employers seek to apply these methods for applicant screening, a prospect that the popular media has already registered (Pepper 2005).

Along with neuroimaging, genetic screening may be used to select the ideal job applicant. For example, military elite commandos may develop a screening process to select for individuals who are not afraid of danger and enjoy the thrill of combat. Gene polymorphisms have already been identified that are associated with harm-avoidance or anxiety-related traits (Lesch *et al.* 1996; Reif and Lesch 2003; Strobel *et al.* 2003a) and with sensation-seeking (Ebstein *et al.* 1996; Benjamin *et al.* 1998, 2000; Strobel *et al.* 2003b). Of course, these associations were obtained in laboratory studies and it is currently unknown whether genetic differences would have any predictive value in the screening of combat troops. This caveat may not dissuade some from developing genomic imaging methods that would seek to maximize predictive information gleaned from these two sources of information.

Dobbs (2005) discussed some of the ethical consequences. He pointed out that the classification of scans as either medical or non-medical information has significantly different legal ramifications. As medical information, federal laws in the United States apply that regulate the use by employers and protect access to such information. On the other hand, there is currently no regulation of non-medical brain imaging.

Additional legal and ethical challenges may come from job applicants who were denied a position on the basis of genomic imaging information. They may challenge the deterministic view that predicts their behavior on the basis of genetic or neuroimaging data when they are otherwise qualified for the position. The debate would center on the question of how to balance a person's history of accomplishments against a forecast of future performance derived from covert measures of mental function or genomic information.

## Neuromarketing

Product marketing is big business, with annual advertising costs of $117 billion (Blakeslee 2004). Similarly, political campaigns are costly, with an estimated $4 billion spent in the American presidential and congressional elections of 2004, a 30 percent increase over federal election costs in 2000 (Weiss 2004). Can neuroimaging be used to improve marketing or campaigning, or to understand better the mental state of consumers or voters? Two imaging studies illustrate this possibility by measuring neural activation associated with consumer responses to products and voter responses to political candidates.

In the first study, brain activation was assessed during a taste test for two very similar sugared soda beverages, Coca Cola® and Pepsi® (McClure *et al.* 2004). When the identity of the beverage was unknown, activation was observed for both drinks and it varied as a function of taste preference in the ventromedial prefrontal cortex (VMPFC), a region associated with reward processing. However, when the brand was identified as Coca Cola®, taste preferences changed and regions such as hippocampus, dorsolateral prefrontal cortex (DLPFC), and midbrain were activated. The authors interpreted the data to suggest that there are two separate systems associated with biasing taste preferences, one based on sensory information and the other based on cultural (i.e. marketing or branding) information. Future work will need to identify which specific cultural elements contribute to these activations and whether these observations extend to other products that have a strong cultural identity.

The second study (Kaplan et al., submitted for publication) was conducted during the 2004 US presidential campaign and collected functional scan data from 10 registered Democrats and 10 registered Republicans as they viewed pictures of the faces of George W. Bush, John Kerry, and Ralph Nader. When participants viewed pictures of the candidate from the opposing party (based on contrasts between brain activation in response to images of George Bush and John Kerry) they showed greater activation in the DLPFC, ACC, insula, and anterior temporal poles than when they viewed pictures of their own party's candidate, and activation was correlated with self-reported emotion ratings. The authors suggested that this activation pattern represents the engagement of both emotional systems (insula and temporal poles) and cognitive control networks (DLPFC and ACC) to manage affect. Importantly, the interpretation of these data is based on prior studies of conflict monitoring, cognitive control, and emotion regulation, which have used very different paradigms. Because this study did not explicitly manipulate levels of cognitive control or emotion regulation, it remains to be shown that the observed activations represent these types of cognitive processes in the context of viewing politically salient stimuli.

Ethical concerns over such studies are raised by critics such as the consumer group Commercial Alert (www.commercialalert.org). Commercial Alert is opposed to this technology because it fears that neuromarketing would further enhance (i) the sale of products that lead to health problems associated with obesity, alcoholism, or type 2 diabetes, (ii) political propaganda, and (iii) degraded values (see Commercial Alert website). The belief is that this technology can identify a 'buy button' in the brain and thus allow the manipulation of individuals' behavior according to the wishes of advertisers.

The three areas of concern for Commercial Alert seem to apply to any methodology that increases marketing effectiveness, and therefore are not uniquely applicable to neuroimaging. With regard to the concern that neuroimaging per se can be used to manipulate behavior, this has no scientific basis: the technology measures, but does not cause changes in brain activation. What about the idea of a 'buy button'? On the one hand, no neuroscientist would seriously claim that a behavior as complex as a buying or voting decision is localized in one brain area. Products or candidates have many attributes (physical, social, economic, emotional) that will be represented across different brain regions. Likewise, the evaluation of these attributes will engage many different cognitive and emotional processes (comparisons against competing products or candidates, conflict monitoring for consistency with one's own beliefs, values, needs, and desires, and cost–benefit analyses) that will be represented across different brain regions. On the other hand, it is conceivable that information gleaned from imaging data may be a better predictor of consumer or voter behavior than more traditional measures such as self-report or focus group polling. There are at least two reasons why this may be so. First, self-report responses and discussion participation in a focus group are subject to social desirability and peer pressures, and therefore may reflect more what a subject thinks is the desired response than his or her true feelings. Secondly, the subject may not be able to articulate affective responses that may influence his consumer or voting behavior, perhaps because these responses are not available to conscious introspection. However, it remains to be shown that neuroimaging can actually produce more accurate predictions of consumer or voting behavior than these other means.

## A heuristic for neuroethical decision-making

Real-world applications of genomic imaging raise a number of questions and concerns. Some are common to all biomedical data, such as privacy and confidentiality. There is the larger question of what constitutes medical versus non-medical uses of neuroimaging, and how to regulate non-medical applications, if at all (Dobbs 2005). There will probably be a legal context, in which conclusions drawn from 'forensic neuroimaging' need to balance the rights of the individual versus the rights of society (Canli and Amin 2002). The overall effort to perfect the predictability of human behavior touches on the question of free will. If we can predict behavior with 100 percent accuracy, which I do not believe we ever will, where does that leave the notion of free will? [For an intriguing answer on how there can be free will in a deterministic world, see Dennett (2003).] The discussion of these and other questions will probably elicit fervent participation by ethicists, scientists, regulators, clergy, philosophers, entrepreneurs, legal and medical societies, insurance companies, and a host of other stakeholders.

I suggest that one useful heuristic for the ethical application of neuroimaging data involves statistical considerations. Biostatisticians and neuroimaging researchers routinely consider factors such as signal-to-noise ratio, confidence range, significance threshold, effect size, and false-positive and false-negative results. These variables quantify the degree of certainty that a particular inference (e.g. there is significant activation in this brain region) is likely to be true and not simply due to chance [the statistical nature of neuroimaging has been discussed in greater depth by Canli and Amin (2002)]. I suggest that this information should be viewed in the context of a cost–benefit analysis. If my statistical inference is wrong, what cost would be incurred? If it is correct, what benefit would be derived? How likely is it that this inference could be incorrect?

The tolerance for an inaccurate prediction may be higher if there is little or no consequence to being wrong. On the other hand, if the stakes are high, then one would want to minimize the risk of an inaccurate prediction. Let us assume that there is significant activation in a brain region that is used to predict behavior, and that the strength of the activation is such that there is only a 1 percent probability that it is due to chance. Is that good enough? I think that the answer depends on the larger context. If the prediction is in regard to hiring an employee, there may not be too much downside in being wrong (in the worst case, the employee will be fired and replaced). If the prediction is in regard to a capital crime, would one be comfortable with the fact that in one out of 100 times an innocent person would be found guilty? Perhaps one in 1000 would be more acceptable odds? Or better, yet, one in 100 000? It turns out that reducing the likelihood of convicting an innocent person wrongly (a statistical false alarm, false positive, or so-called type I error) comes at a cost of increasing the likelihood that someone who is guilty slips through the neuroimaging net (a statistical miss, false negative, or so-called type II error). This is not due to currently imperfect technology that can some day overcome the problem. Rather, it is a fundamental aspect of statistical reality, like the uncertainty principle of statistics.

A similar set of concepts that assesses the association between symptoms and disease is in use in clinical research. The term 'sensitivity' refers to the probability that a screening test is positive when the patient indeed has the disease (a sensitivity of 1.0 indicates that the screening test will turn out positive for every patient who has the disease). The term 'specificity' refers to the probability that a screening test is negative when the patient indeed is disease-free (a specificity of 1.0 indicates that the screening test is always negative for every person who is disease free). Applied to neuroimaging in a high-stakes context, one would want a scan that has supreme sensitivity and specificity.

## Concluding remarks

In this chapter, I have made the point that data from neuroimaging studies may yield better predictors of behavior or truthful testimony than traditional measures such as self-report. These predictors may be further refined by the inclusion of genetic and life experience information. To date, the predictors only apply to narrowly defined behaviors in laboratory, not real-world, settings. However, there is undoubtedly great motivation to move beyond the constraints of behavior studied in academic research institutions. In order to develop a heuristic for the ethical use of neuroimaging across diverse real-life applications, I recommend taking an empirical view and focusing on the statistical aspects of the technology. What is the cost of making an inaccurate prediction, and what is the benefit? This question is most resonant in the domain of criminal justice, where one study found that 7 percent of individuals convicted of a capital crime were found to be innocent on retrial (Liebman *et al.* 2000). On the other hand, 3.3 percent of child molesters who were released in 1994 were rearrested for another sex crime against a child within 3 years, compared with a recidivism rate of less than 0.5 percent over the same period for all non-sex offenders in the United States (Langan *et al.* 2003). Clearly, it would be desirable to develop neuroimaging applications that can reduce the likelihood of tragic errors in sentencing innocents or releasing recidivists. If the downside is that some other applications, such as neuromarketing devoted to boosting sales of sugared beverages, also become part of our culture, then perhaps that is an acceptable price to pay.

## References

Amin Z, Constable RT, Canli T (2004). Attentional bias for valenced stimuli as a function of personality in the dot-probe task. *Journal of Research in Personality* 38, 15–23.

Anderson SW, Bechara A, Damasio H, Tranel D, Damasio AR (1999). Impairment of social and moral behavior related to early damage in human prefrontal cortex. *Nature Neuroscience* 2, 1032–7.

Barr CS, Newman TK, Schwandt M, et al. (2004). Sexual dichotomy of an interaction between early adversity and the serotonin transporter gene promoter variant in rhesus macaques. *Proceedings of the National Academy of Sciencesof the USA* 101, 12358–63.

Benjamin J, Ebstein RP, Lesch KP (1998). Genes for personality traits: implications for psychopathology. *International Journal of Neuropsychopharmcology* 1, 153–68.

Benjamin J, Osher Y, Kotler M, et al. (2000). Association between Tridimensional Personality Questionaire (TPQ) traits and Three functional polymorphisms: dopamine receptor D4 (DRD4), serotonin transporter promoter region 95-HTTLPR) and catechol-O-methyltransferase (COMT). *Molecular Psychiatry* 5, 96–100.

Bennett AJ, Lesch KP, Heils A, et al. (2002). Early experience and serotonin transporter gene variation interact to influence primate CNS function. *Molecular Psychiatry* 7, 118–22.

Blakeslee S (2004). If you have a 'buy button' in your brain, what pushes it? *New York Times*, 19 October.

Bradley MM, Lang PJ (1999). *Affective Norms for English words (ANEW)*. Gainesville, FL: NIMH Center for the Study of Emotion and Attention, University of Florida.

Canli T (2004). Functional brain mapping of extraversion and neuroticism: learning from individual differences in emotion processing. *Journal of Personality* 72, 1105–32.

Canli T, Amin Z (2002). Neuroimaging of emotion and personality: scientific evidence and ethical considerations. *Brain and Cognition* 50, 414–31.

Canli T, Zhao Z, Desmond JE, Kang E, Gross J, Gabrieli JDE (2001). An fMRI study of personality influences on brain reactivity to emotional stimuli. *Behavioral Neuroscience* 115, 33–42.

Canli T, Sivers H, Whitfield SL, Gotlib IH, Gabrieli JD (2002). Amygdala response to happy faces as a function of extraversion. *Science* 296, 2191.

Canli T, Amin Z, Haas B, Omura K, Constable RT (2004). A double dissociation between mood states and personality traits in the anterior cingulate. *Behavioral Neuroscience* 118, 897–904.

Caspi A, McClay J, Moffitt TE, *et al.* (2002). Role of genotype in the cycle of violence in maltreated children. *Science* 297, 851–4.

Caspi A, Sugden K, Moffitt TE, *et al.* (2003). Influence of life stress on depression: moderation by a polymorphism in the 5-HTT gene. *Science* 301, 386–9.

Costa PT Jr, McCrae RR (1980). Influence of extraversion and neuroticism on subjective well-being: happy and unhappy people. *Journal of Personality and Social Psychology* 38, 668–78.

Costa PT, McCrae RR (1992). *Professional Manual of the Revised NEO Personality Inventory and NEO Five-Factor Inventory.* Odessa, FL: Psychological Assessment Resources.

Decety J, Jackson PL, Sommerville JA, Chaminade T, Meltzoff AN (2004). The neural bases of cooperation and competition: an fMRI investigation. *NeuroImage* 23, 744–51.

Dennett DC (2003). *Freedom Evolves.* New York: Viking Penguin

Dobbs D (2005). Brain scans for sale: as brain imaging spreads to nonmedical uses, will commerce overtake ethics? Available online at: http://www.slate.com/id/2112653 (accessed 3 May 2005).

Ebstein RP, Novick O, Umansky R, *et al.* (1996). Dopamine D4 receptor (D4DR) exon III polymorphism associated with the human personality trait of novelty seeking. *Nature Genetics* 12, 78–80.

Furmark T, Tillfors M, Garpenstrand H, *et al.* (2004). Serotonin transporter polymorphism related to amygdala excitability and symptom severity in patients with social phobia. *Neuroscience Letters* 362, 189–92.

Greene JD, Sommerville RB, Nystrom LE, Darley JM, Cohen JD (2001). An fMRI investigation of emotional engagement in moral judgment. *Science* 293, 2105–8.

Gusnard DA, Ollinger JM, Shulman GL, *et al.* (2003). Persistence and brain circuitry. *Proceedings of the National Academy of Sciences of the USA* 100, 3479–84.

Hamer D (2002). Genetics. Rethinking behavior genetics. *Science* 298, 71–2.

Hariri AR, Mattay VS, Tessitore A, *et al.* (2002). Serotonin transporter genetic variation and the response of the human amygdala. *Science* 297, 400–3.

Hariri AR, Drabant EM, Munoz KE, *et al.* (2005). A susceptibility gene for affective disorders and the response of the human amygdala. *Archives of General Psychiatry* 62, 146–52.

Heinz A, Braus DF, Smolka MN, *et al.* (2005). Amygdala-prefrontal coupling depends on a genetic variation of the serotonin transporter. *Nature Neuroscience* 8, 20–1.

Kaplan JT, Freedman J and Iacoboni M. Us vs. them: political attitudes and party affiliation influence neural response to faces of presidential candidates. Submitted for publication.

Lang PJ, Greenwald MK (1993). *International Affective Picture System Standardization Procedure and Results for Affective Judgments: Technical Reports 1A–1C.* Gainesville, FL: University of Florida Center for Research in Psychophysiology.

Langan PA, Schmitt EL, Durose MR (2003). *Recidivism of Sex Offenders from Prison in 1994.* Washington, DC: US Department of Justice, Office of Justice Programs, Bureau of Justice Statistics.

Larsen RJ, Ketelaar T (1991). Personality and susceptibility to positive and negative emotional states. *Journal of Personality and Social Psychology* 61, 132–40.

Lesch KP, Bengel D, Heils A, *et al.* (1996). Association of anxiety-related traits with a polymorphism in the serotonin transporter gene regulatory region. *Science* 274, 1527–31.

Lesch KP, Meyer J, Glatz K, *et al.* (1997). The 5-HT transporter gene-linked polymorphic region (*5-HTTLPR*) in evolutionary perspective: alternative biallelic variation in rhesus monkeys. *Journal of Neural Transmission* 104, 1259–66.

Liebman JS, Fagan J, West V (2000). *A Broken System: Error Rates in Capital Cases, 1973–1995*. New York: Columbia University School of Law.

McCabe K, Houser D, Ryan L, Smith V, Trouard T (2001). A functional imaging study of cooperation in two-person reciprocal exchange. *Proceedings of the National Academy of Sciencesof the USA* **98**, 11832–5.

McClure SM, Li J, Tomlin D, Cypert KS, Montague LM, Montague PR (2004). Neural correlates of behavioral preference for culturally familiar drinks. *Neuron* **44**, 379–87.

McCrae RR, Costa PT Jr (1999). A five-factor theory of personality. In: Pervin LA, John OP (eds) *Handbook of Personality: Theory and Research* (2nd edn). New York: Guilford Press, 139–53.

Matthews G, Deary IJ (1998). *Personality Traits*. Cambridge, UK: Cambridge University Press.

Meyer GJ, Shack JR (1989). Structural convergence of mood and personality: evidence for old and new directions. *Journal of Personality and Social Psychology* **57**, 691–706.

Moll J, de Oliveira-Souza R, Bramati IE, Grafman J (2002a). Functional networks in emotional moral and nonmoral social judgments. *NeuroImage* **16**, 696–703.

Moll J, de Oliveira-Souza R, Eslinger PJ, *et al.* (2002b). The neural correlates of moral sensitivity: a functional magnetic resonance imaging investigation of basic and moral emotions. *Journal of Neuroscience* **22**, 2730–6.

Pepper T (2005). Inside the head of an applicant. *Newsweek*, 21 February, E 24–6.

Reif A, Lesch KP (2003). Toward a molecular architecture of personality. *Behavioral Brain Research* **139**, 1–20.

Richards A, French CC, Johnson W, Naparstek J, Williams J (1992). Effects of mood manipulation and anxiety on performance of an emotional Stroop task. *British Journal of Psychology* **83**, 479–91.

Rilling J, Gutman D, Zeh T, Pagnoni G, Berns G, Kilts C (2002). A neural basis for social cooperation. *Neuron* **35**, 395–405.

Rilling JK, Sanfey AG, Aronson JA, Nystrom LE, Cohen JD (2004). Opposing BOLD responses to reciprocated and unreciprocated altruism in putative reward pathways. *Neuroreport* **15**, 2539–43.

Singer T, Kiebel SJ, Winston JS, Dolan RJ, Frith CD (2004). Brain responses to the acquired moral status of faces. *Neuron* **41**, 653–62.

Steinmetz H, Seitz RJ (1991). Functional anatomy of language processing: neuroimaging and the problem of individual variability. *Neuropsychologia* **29**, 1149–61.

Strobel A, Gutknecht L, Rothe C, *et al.* (2003a). Allelic variation in 5-HT1A receptor expression is associated with anxiety- and depression-related personality traits. *Journal of Neural Transmission* **110**, 1445–53.

Strobel A, Lesch KP, Jatzke S, Paetzold F, Brocke B (2003b). Further evidence for a modulation of novelty seeking by DRD4 exon III, 5-HTTLPR, and COMT val/met variants. *Molecular Psychiatry* **8**, 371–2.

Watson D, Clark LA (1992). On traits and temperament: general and specific factors of emotional experience and their relation to the five-factor model. *Journal of Personality* **60**, 441–76.

Weiss S (2004). *'04 Elections Expected to Cost Nearly $4 Billion*. Washington, DC: Center for Responsible Politics.

## Chapter 13

# Engineering the brain

### Kenneth R. Foster

## Introduction

In 1965, the Spanish neuroscientist José Delgado conducted a spectacular demonstration. He implanted electrodes in the brain of a bull and outfitted the animal with a radiofrequency receiver. Then Delgado stood in a bullring in front of the animal and provoked it to charge. Moments before impact, his assistant pushed a button. The animal suddenly stopped his charge. After several applications of the stimulus, Delgado reported, there was a lasting inhibition of aggressive behavior (Delgado 1969). Delgado's demonstration was an early example of the ability of neuroscience to control behavior. As any reader who 'googles' Delgado will quickly discover, he also provoked endless and at times overheated rhetoric about mind control by neuroscientific methods.

The neuroscience revolution is resulting in dramatic advances in the understanding of brain function. In parallel, there have been astonishing developments in technologies that allow investigators to monitor and control the brain, and use the brain to control the external world. What, exactly, are the ethical issues raised by these technologies, and how are they distinctive from those raised by other medical technologies, such as genetic testing?

I begin with a brief review of some new technologies that have emerged from neuroscience. These devices are intended to stimulate selected regions of the brain or peripheral nervous system for therapeutic purposes, or, more recently, as brain–computer interfaces to allow the brain to exchange information with the outside world through direct recording of potentials measured by means of electrodes implanted in the motor cortex, or placed on the surface of the head.

## Neural prostheses

The National Institutes of Health has had a neural prosthesis program since 1971. This work has borne fruit; a number of neurological devices have been approved for the market and numerous other devices are in advanced developmental stages. Between 1994 and 2003, the US Food and Drug Administration (FDA) approved 19 neurological devices including seven for use with children (Pena *et al.* 2004).

By far the best established of these devices is the cochlear implant. Initially developed during the early 1960s, several devices have received FDA premarket approval and, as of 2002, some 59 000 people worldwide have received the implants, a large fraction of whom are children. Unlike a traditional hearing aid, which simply amplifies sound that enters the ear canal, cochlear implants use a microphone and speech processor to transduce sounds to electrical signals that are applied to the cochlea via an array of electrodes implanted within it.

Auditory brainstem implants, a newer class of device that was first implanted in a patient in 1979, is designed for patients without functioning auditory nerves (a rare condition that typically results from surgery to remove a tumor). The devices employ a microphone and speech processor, as does the cochlear implant, but the stimulation is applied to the brainstem instead of the cochlea. One such device has been approved by the FDA (Toh and Luxford 2002).

Visual prostheses, by comparison, are in much earlier developmental stages. Several classes of such devices are being developed, which are designed to stimulate the visual system at different levels (Hossain *et al.* 2005). One type, popularly known as the artificial retina, is implanted just beneath the retina. It converts light from visual sources into electrical signals that can stimulate the retina for use in patients suffering from vision loss due to retinal degeneration from various conditions (Chow *et al.* 2004). One commercial device (Optobionics) has been undergoing clinical trials since 2000. This silicon-based device consists of approximately 5000 tiny micro-electrode-tipped photodiodes powered by light incident on the retina. The voltages generated by the photodiodes are able to induce visual signals in the remaining functional retinal cells. Other devices, which are designed to stimulate the visual cortex of the brain or optic nerve, are in much earlier stages of development (Schmidt *et al.* 1996; Chowdhury *et al.* 2004). Despite promising results from such studies, at present no patient has had an acceptable level of vision restored, and no large clinical trials have compared the current approaches to this technology (Hossain *et al.* 2005).

At face value, the sheer volume of information that is contained in visual or auditory sensations would be a daunting problem to encode and present to a subject through implanted electrodes. However, people are remarkably adaptable in learning to process stimuli, and a visual or auditory prosthesis can improve the ability of a patient to extract information from stimuli without recreating the electrical activity that would result in the brain if the subject had normal vision or hearing. A striking example of this is provided by the work of Bach-Y-Rita and colleagues on 'vision and vestibular substitution systems' for neural prostheses. These systems enable subjects to process sensory information (and even recognize faces) presented to them via an array of flexible electrodes placed against the tongue (Bach-Y-Rita 2004).

## Deep-brain stimulation

Quite a different class of neural devices provides therapy for a variety of neurological problems through a process called neuromodulation. The American Neuromodulation Society defines the term as 'the therapeutic alteration of activity in the central, peripheral or autonomic nervous systems, electrically or pharmacologically, by means of implanted devices' (http://www.neuromodulation.org/). Much of this work involves the use of implanted devices (most implanted near the spine) for treatment of chronic pain, but other treatments are also covered by this rubric. (The term 'neuromodulation' is also used by some chiropractors in reference to an unrelated treatment for pain, involving mechanical stimulation of the back using a vibrator.)

Deep-brain stimulation uses electrodes implanted in the thalamus for treatment of move-ment disorders, including Parkinson's disease and other conditions, and is well accepted by the medical community (Lozano *et al.* 2002). The treatment is believed to work by disrupting electrical activity in this region of the brain, thereby blocking signals that cause the disabling motor symptoms of Parkinson's disease. One company (Medtronic) has received FDA approval for a deep-brain stimulator for treatment of Parkinson's disease, essential tremor, and dystonia (a rare movement disorder) and, according to the company's website, the device has been used by more than 14 000 people worldwide since 1997.

Deep-brain stimulation has been proposed for treatment of a variety of psychiatric and neurological disorders, including obsessive–compulsive disorder and severe depression

(Aouizerate *et al.* 2004) and epilepsy (Theodore and Fisher 2004). However, despite a number of reports of the therapeutic effectiveness of such treatments in the medical literature, there is a dearth of well-controlled trials demonstrated their effectiveness, and many questions remain. Theodore and Fisher (2004), in a review of the use of deep-brain stimulation for treatment of epilepsy, concluded:

> Although stimulation for uncontrolled epilepsy with electrodes implanted in the brain itself has been done for many years, the initial claims for therapeutic success have not been confirmed by the very few controlled studies that have been done so far. The best structures to stimulate and the most effective stimuli to use are unknown...The risks and expense of stimulation demand careful consideration of its value on an individual basis. Some initial data for both deep brain stimulation and TMS are exciting and encouraging, but it is important to remember that many early reports of therapeutic success are not confirmed by controlled clinical trials. Given the potential for uncon-strained application of medical technology, it is vital that patients who wish to explore these approaches be enrolled in formal studies.

## Pacemaker for mood

One of the more intriguing forms of brain stimulation does not use a brain implant at all, but rather a pacemaker-like device that stimulates the left vagus nerve in the neck (Stimpson *et al.* 2002). The vagus nerve, in addition to serving as a conduit for brain signals to modulate heart rate or secretion of gastric acid, has afferent sensory fibers that convey information to the brain about perceptions of hunger, satiety, and pain. Stimulation of the vagus nerve is believed to modulate the activity of cortical and limbic structures in the brain that are considered relevant to depression (Matthews and Eljamel 2003).

One commercial device, manufactured by Cyberonics Inc. (Houston, TX, USA), is available for vagus nerve stimulation. The device has been under investigation for several years, and by now it has been implanted in several thousand patients for treatment-resistant depression. In June 2004, the FDA Neurological Devices Panel evaluated the premarket approval application for the device. While noting severe weaknesses in the clinical studies used to support the company's claims (lack of placebo controls and blinding in the clinical studies), the panel nevertheless voted to recommend approval of the application, in part because the device offered a last-resort treatment for patients who were otherwise at high risk for suicide. At present (June 2005) no final ruling has been issued by the FDA. The device has been challenged by public citizen, a consumer advocate group, citing concerns about safety and lack of evidence for efficacy.

## Stimulation of the brain with externally applied fields

The brain can also be stimulated by electrical currents that are passed through he skull by means of electrodes placed on the head [transcutaneous electrical stimulation (TES)] or induced in the brain by strong time-dependent magnetic fields from a coil placed near the head [transcutaneous magnetic stimulation (TMS)]. TMS is far more widely used because it avoids the painful shocks produced by TES. Both techniques are unable to target specific cells, but introduce currents in broad regions of the brain.

TMS was originally developed to allow physicians to stimulate the motor cortex for neuro-logical evaluation of patients with movement disorders. More recently, it has been used as therapy for a variety of problems, notably depression (Grunhaus *et al.* 2003), as an alternative to electric shock therapy where it has the advantages of not producing convulsions and avoiding cognitive effects such as the memory loss that often follows electroconvulsive therapy. Despite an at times enthusiastic medical literature on the subject and demands by patients for TMS as an alternative to electric shock therapy, the clinical effectiveness of the treatment remains unclear. Lisanby *et al.* (2002) concluded that 'It is still unresolved whether the magnitude of the effect will turn out to be clinically important'. Other psychiatric applications of TMS under investigation include treatment of mania, schizophrenia, and anxiety disorders. There is likewise a dearth of well-controlled studies that demonstrate the effectiveness of such treatments (Lisanby *et al.* 2002; see also Chapter 14).

## The artificial hippocampus—a brain prostheses?

Whereas the artificial retina, cochlear implant, and the deep-brain stimulator stimulate or inhibit nervous system activity by means of electrical currents passed into the body, other devices in very early stages of development are intended to mimic brain function directly. The difference is roughly similar to that between applying a voltage from a test source to affect the operation of a computer and designing a computer chip to work within the computer itself.

In 2003 a spate of media coverage appeared about the so-called artificial hippocampus developed by Theodore Berger at UCLA. The device, fabricated from a silicon chip, was designed to mimic the electrophysiological responses of the hippocampus in rats, as measured in an extensive series of electrophysiological experiments in the animals. This device was frequently described in media reports as a 'brain prosthesis'. The hippocampus is involved in the encoding of experience to form long-term memories, and a prosthetic hippocampus might help patients with memory impairment due to damage to this brain structure. However, the device is in very preliminary stages of development and Berger's tests, which were widely described in the lay media but not so far in a conventional scientific journal, involved rat brain slices and not living animals.

## Brain–computer interfaces

The applications discussed above basically involve one-way communication of signals to the brain. There are also rapid advances in developing technologies to communicate in the opposite direction, recording signals from the brain and decoding them into a form that can be processed by a computer–the brain–computer interface (Donoghue 2002; Wolpaw *et al.* 2002; Musallam *et al.* 2004).

Developing such interfaces is a new and highly active research field. A recent international meeting on brain–computer interfaces held in 2002 included 92 investigators from 38 different research groups in the United States, Canada, China, and Europe (Vaughan *et al.* 2003). A recent search of the Medline database for 'brain–computer interface' produced 126 papers, most published since 2000.

Some of this work has been motivated by the desire to interface neurons to electrical circuits for engineering applications. Indeed, a press release dated October 2004 from the University of Florida describes the work of bioengineering professor Thomas DeMarse who used an aggregation of 25 000 cultured rat neurons in a Petri dish with an array of electrodes to control a jet flight simulator. (At the time of writing, this work had not been published in a peer-reviewed journal.)

Of more immediate practical use, and the motivation for most of the work currently underway, is the desire to develop systems that allow severely disabled people to communicate or manipulate their surroundings, using signals recorded from their brains. Such a device might, for example, allow a 'locked-in' patient (who has normal cognitive function but is completely paralyzed) to type information into a computer, send e-mail, or control the movement of an artificial limb. The signals are recorded from the motor cortex using implanted electrodes; or from the surface of the head.

Progress toward developing usable brain–computer interfaces has been spectacular. In 2002, a group led by John Donoghue (Brown University) described an experiment in which monkeys with implants in the motor cortex manipulated a joystick with their paws to control the cursor on a computer display (Serruya *et al.* 2002). The cortical signals were simultaneously processed by computer and also used to control the cursor. Eventually, the investigators disabled the joystick and the monkeys continued to control the cursor by thought alone. Recently, Donoghue formed a company (Cyberkinetics Inc., Foxboro, MA) that is developing a system called Braingate. The system, presently being tested under an FDA investigational device exemption, uses electrodes implanted in the heads of paralyzed patients, with the aim of allowing them to control a computer. In October 2004, it was reported that a paralyzed man was able to send e-mail using the device (Khamsi 2004).

A different company (Neural Signals Inc., Atlanta GA) is developing a system, reported to be in phase II trials, called the Brain Communicator that uses either an electrode implanted 5 mm under the surface of the brain or an electrically conductive screw that penetrates the skull but does not enter the brain. In 2004 investigators affiliated with the company reported the successful use of human cortical signals to control two assistive technology tools, a virtual keyboard speller and a computer-simulated digit (Kennedy *et al.* 2004).

In December 2004, Wolpaw and McFarland (2004) described a brain–computer interface employing a cap with 64 electrodes that enabled subjects (including two partially paralyzed individuals in wheelchairs) to control a computer cursor using EEG signals recorded from the surface of the head. It is clearly not a large step to using such signals to control prosthetic devices, wheelchairs, and other devices, which would be of great benefit to disabled people. In March 2004, it was reported that a group at Massachusetts Institute of Technology Media Lab Europe, Dublin, Ireland had developed a video game controlled by EEG signals, which are relayed to the computer using wireless communications (http://medialabeurope.org/mindgames).

Despite the rapid advances in the state of art in brain–computer interfaces, a number of technical problems limit the range of applications that can be developed (Mussa-Ivaldi and Miller 2003). Brain signals can be recorded either intracortically, from electrodes implanted in the brain, or from EEG signals recorded from electrodes on the scalp or inserted into the skull against the dura. The former approach requires the patient to submit to brain surgery. Recording signals non-invasively from the scalp (or minimally invasively from electrodes screwed into the skull) avoids this necessity. However, the bandwidth of an EEG signal (the rate at which information can be transmitted) is far smaller than that of signals from implanted microelectrodes. EEG-based methods are limited to a very slow rate of information transfer from the subject, currently about 20–30 bits/min.

Recording signals from cortical neurons allows much faster rates of information transfer. However, positioning the electrode is critical. Moreover, the present state of the art allows investigators to record from a relative handful of neurons in the motor cortex (7–30 in the system used by Donoghue's group), whereas thousands of motor neurons are involved in the simplest body movement.

One might think that decoding the signals, to determine the intent of the subject, would be an immense problem. However, this difficulty is avoided by employing training routines that use feedback. Animals and human subjects can learn to control the computer by regulating their EEGs or the rates of firing of the cortical neurons that are being recorded. In the words of Helms Tillery *et al.* (2003), 'an animal's ability to regulate the motion of a cortically controlled device is not crucially dependent on the experimenter's ability to estimate intention from neuronal activity'.

Signals from the brain can even provide a new medium for communication. 'Couple's nervous system linked by implants in limbs' read the headline of a news story in the *New Zealand Herald* (Collins 2004): 'When Kevin Warwick lifted his finger, his wife Irena felt as if a bolt of lightning ran down her palm and into her own finger'. The couple had had electrodes surgically implanted in their arms and linked by radio signals to a computer, forming a link between their nervous systems. 'It was like my wife communicating with me,' the man said.

## Controlling behavior electrically

The use of electric stimulation to control the mind or behavior has been discussed for many years, and there is a body of serious scholarship as well as popular books by scientists on the subject. In his book addressed at the public, *Physical Control of the Mind*, Delgado (1969) described experiments that applied electrical stimulation via implanted electrodes to the brains of cats, monkeys, and other animals. Delgado could change the diameter of the animals' pupils, cause the animal to flex a limb, open its mouth, yawn, walk upright (in monkeys), or inhibit or stimulate aggressive behavior. Stimulating the brain in one female monkey 'evoked a rage response expressed by self-biting and abandoning her baby... ignoring the appealing calls of [the baby]' (Delgado 1969). Delgado invented a device, called the Stimoceiver, which could be activated by remote control to stimulate the brain via implanted electrodes, and demonstrated its use in the bull as described at the beginning of this chapter.

Robo-Rat, described by Talwar and coworkers at the State University of New York, is a far more sophisticated example of the use of electrical stimulation to control the behavior of an animal. In one experiment (Talwar *et al.* 2002) the investigators implanted several electrodes in the brains of rats that were connected to radio frequency receivers attached to the animals' backs. One set of electrodes elicited sensations of whisker movement (which rats use to sense the presence of nearby surfaces as they move about in the dark); a third electrode was implanted in the pleasure center of the brain. The investigators taught the rats to respond to their commands, transmitted from as far as 500 m away.

## Nanotechnology and more

The technological advances discussed above resulted in part from advances in the scientific understanding of the function of the brain, and in part from advances in techniques to measure and control the electrical behavior of cells. While both are enabling, they are also limiting factors in developing technologies for monitoring and controlling the brain and therapeutic applications.

Nanotechnology (a loose catch-all term for technologies whose only common feature is small scale) will certainly result in great improvements in instrumentation. For example, a number of groups are experimenting with silicon chips that interface to neurons, and the size of the arrays (i.e. number of cells that can be recorded from and controlled) will continue to expand. We can assume that, as time goes on, implants will become smaller, smarter, more effective, and less expensive, and their implantation in the brain will be less destructive of brain tissue.

There is considerable speculation in official circles about 'convergent' science and technologies, including nanotechnology, biotechnology, information technology, and cognitive science (NBIC) and their possible applications. Certainly the military and security services are aware of potential applications of this convergence. The Defense Advanced Research Projects Agency (DARPA) which, according to its website, seeks 'to identify and pursue the most promising technologies...and to develop those technologies into important, radically new military capabilities', has a program in brain–computer interfaces.

Recently, there have been major conferences in the United States and Europe to evaluate the potential of NBIC. The report of one National Science Foundation (NSF) sponsored conference is instructive (Roco and Bainbridge 2002). The NSF report describes a host of potential benefits of NBIC technologies. These include:

> enhancing individual sensory and cognitive capabilities,...highly effective communication techniques including brain-to-brain interaction, perfecting human–machine interfaces including neuromorphic engineering, sustainable and 'intelligent' environments including neuro-ergonomics, enhancing human capabilities for defense purposes, reaching sustainable development using NBIC tools, and ameliorating the physical and cognitive decline that is common to the aging mind.

The European conference, which was supported by the European Commission with a report issued in summer of 2004 (Nordmann 2004), included a panel of 25 high-level scientists, officials from government and industry, philosophers, and a few self-described futurologists. Its discussion ranged over potential technological developments, together with the ethical, legal, and societal aspects of converging technologies. The panel envisioned several potential military applications of convergent technologies. Some applications would use insects or small mammals controlled by electrodes in the brain. Others would utilize implants in the brain to monitor the stress levels in war-fighters, releasing therapeutic drugs or hormones as necessary. The report predicted the use of implants connected to sensory organs or to brain-cortex areas to allow pilots to respond more quickly to sudden threats. However, the report noted, 'communicating complex sensory impressions or thoughts...requires fundamental progress in brain research and a reduced barrier against human experiments'.

The European panel predicted that these convergent technologies would take 10–20 years to mature. With the present state of the art of the brain–computer interface being limited to recording from a few dozen neurons, and using these recordings to control the motion of a cursor on a computer screen, such developments may take even longer, or they may never occur. Also a long way off is the invention, colorfully suggested by Google co-founder Larry Page, of a Google chip for the brain (Orlowski 2004).

## Fantasies

Any discussion of the ethical implications of neuroscience must pay careful attention to what can and cannot be done with presently foreseeable technology. For several reasons, this is more difficult than might appear. One problem is the considerable amount of hype, or at least wildly optimistic discussion, in the news media (and even more so on Internet discussion groups) concerning what brain implants (and more generally NBIC technologies) will be able to accomplish.

The problem of maintaining perspective is exacerbated by the endless speculation about mind control by hostile government agents by means of electromagnetic fields, electromagnetic weapons, and so on that can be found on the Internet. Even the scientific literature on the biological effects of electromagnetic fields is unreliable in many places, with reports of effects of fields that cannot be independently confirmed and speculation about possible weak-field effects (Foster 2003). Judging from numerous websites and occasional calls to this author, a great many individuals are convinced that the government has found some way to read the thoughts of a person by recording electromagnetic fields emitted by the brain or from implanted circuits in the brain or other body parts.

The problem of maintaining balance is also exacerbated by the history of American security agencies in pursuing bizarre research programs, including the notorious research on mind control using LSD and other drugs conducted by the US Central Intelligence Agency (CIA) in the 1950s (Moreno 2000). While these scandals are now history, there is still great interest in some government circles about the possibility of monitoring or affecting the mind using electromagnetic fields. In the summer of 2003, this author participated in a workshop run by a consulting company on behalf of security agencies at which experts were asked about the current state of art of the subject. Individuals who are inclined to believe in Orwellian tendencies of the government can find enough items of evidence to keep their fantasies alive, however far from reality they might be.

The use of electrical stimulation to control the brain is an especially fertile area for fantasy. For example, Delgado's stunt with the bull and the more recent Robo-Rat experiments have provoked endless Internet discussion about their implications. One website describes the Robo-Rat as a 'remote-control automaton, a living machine' and speaks of a secretive company that is developing this technology to produce 'Remote Control Human Drones' (http://www.uncoveror.com/roborat.htm). There were also complaints about the 'insult to their [the animals'] dignity involved in turning them into involuntary cyborgs' (Meek 2002).

In reality, the Robo-Rat experiments used a clever electrophysiological technique to stimulate sensory organs and to reward the rats—an effective way to train and control the animal. This approach is undoubtedly far more effective than using a mechanical apparatus to stimulate the animals' whiskers and provide food pellets, but it is hardly equivalent to turning them into 'involuntary cyborgs'. Investigators might trigger profound behavioral or emotional changes by electrical stimulation of the brain but, thankfully, turning animals or humans into automatons or 'involuntary cyborgs' remains in the realm of science fiction.

Finally, fantasies about mind control and tampering with the content of people's minds are part of American culture, for example movies such as the *Manchurian Candidate* (1962) and *Eternal Sunshine of the Spotless Mind* (2004). Numerous websites speculate about uploading and downloading memories to people's brains, and erasing memories. Such capabilities would raise important ethical issues, if they existed, but they remain far in the future—perhaps forever in the future if current ethical standards remain in place and institutional review boards continue to monitor human studies.

Fantasies about mind control with electric or magnetic fields fail the test of plausibility on several levels. At the simplest level, there is the problem of how to get sufficient levels of electrical currents to the tissues that are to be excited. Medical treatments involving stimulation of the brain require use of implanted electrodes (which involves brain surgery) or powerful magnetic coils placed close to the head (which requires specialized and very obvious equipment). The electric currents that are induced within the head by electric or magnetic fields in the environment at any ordinary level are far below those needed to excite neural tissue, and are far smaller than currents that are naturally present in the brain due to normal physiological processes.

A much more fundamental problem is the sheer complexity of any project that would read or revise memories, emotions, thoughts, or other functions of the mind. The brain comprises about a hundred billion neurons, each synapsing with thousands of other neurons. Scientists can record from a few dozen neurons at a time with implanted electrodes, or else record the aggregate activity of billions of neurons through measurements of electrical potential on the surface of the head. Using functional magnetic resonance imaging scientists can detect changes in the electrical activity of the brain associated with emotions or cognition, representing the combined effects of perhaps billions of neurons.

By passing electrical currents into the brain, scientists can induce profound physiological, cognitive, and behavioral changes, as Delgado and many other investigators have shown. Stimulation of the brain using implanted electrodes has 'blocked the thinking process, inhibited speech and movement ... evoked pleasure, laughter, friendliness, verbal output, hostility, fear, hallucinations, and memories' (Delgado 1969, p. 71).

It is one thing to induce broad changes in behavior or emotion, for example by indiscriminately stimulating billions of brain cells. It is quite another to attempt to control the brain in any precise way, to explore or change the contents of thoughts and memories, or to affect behavior in any controllable way: 'If we developed sufficiently sensitive measures at the neuronal level we might be able to record feelings, but we would never be able to play them back. Creating an emotion requires synaptic changes in so many areas of the brain that it would be impossible to recreate' (LeDoux 2000). Since the precise way that the brain encodes memory is largely unknown, the ability to upload or download memories will only be realized in the very distant future, if ever.

More generally, fantasies about mind control reflect a mechanistic view—that the mind can be manipulated by pushing the levers of the brain. (Even the operation of the visual and auditory implants and brain–computer interfaces discussed above cannot be understood in such simplistic terms.) The brain may be a deterministic system, comprised of billions of neurons that operate according to strictly determined rules. How the mind is related to all this neural activity is, of course, an unsolved and age-old problem. Despite the rapid advances in neuroscience, one can still make a powerful case that people remain free to make their own decisions (Gazzaniga and Steven 2004).

## Ethical implications of implanted neurotechnologies

In one of the few ethical analyses of brain implants by bioethicists, McGee and Maguire (2001) envisioned three stages in the use of brain implants. The first, which accounts for most present applications, is the use of neural implants to develop prostheses for severely disabled individuals. These include cochlear and visual implants, brain–computer interfaces for communication by paralyzed individuals, and so on. The second stage will include the use of implanted devices to enhance the function of otherwise fully enabled persons. The third stage, McGee and Maguire predict, will be the use of brain implants by 'those involved in very information intensive businesses, who will use these devices to develop an expanded information transfer capability'. Google chips for the brain, for example.

Each of these stages of use will raise distinctive ethical issues, they believe, with steadily increasing urgency for ethical analysis. 'Inasmuch as this technology is fraught with perilous implications for radically changing human nature, for invasions of privacy and for governmental control of individuals,' they conclude, 'public discussion of its benefits and burdens should be initiated, and policy decisions should be made as to whether its development should be proscribed or regulated, rather than left to happenstance, experts and the vagaries of the commercial market.'

While the three-stages of the development of brain implants that McGee and Maguire envision is reasonable enough, the factual basis of the technologies, which must be considered in any ethical analysis, becomes more and more obscure at each level. It is difficult to conduct an insightful ethical analysis of a scenario that is, at present, merely science fiction.

The second stage of the use of brain implants, as described by McGee and Maguire, is to enhance the function of otherwise fully enabled persons. It is difficult to imagine exactly what applications might develop. One could certainly construct analogues of cochlear or visual implants to allow people to 'hear' ultrasound or 'see' infrared energy. But why bother? In a person with normal vision, for example, it would be far simpler just to provide night vision goggles. And who would submit to brain surgery to receive such implants?

One could, conceivably, devise brain–computer interfaces to speed up the reactions of military pilots, as mentioned in the 2004 European Commission report (Nordmann 2004). However, the gap between the requirements for such applications to succeed and the present state of the art is very great. Present technology allows people to control cursors on a computer display or send e-mail using a device that records the EEG. Neither application demands high-speed or high-reliability communication. The demonstration of these technologies proves nothing about the feasibility of high-speed high-reliability control of the sort that would be required to maneuver an aircraft or operate a weapons system in combat. We can expect, in a holiday shopping season in the very near future, to be able to buy flight-simulator games for computers that are controlled by the player's EEG. If those succeed (and young people become amazingly adept at playing computer games) we might be in a better position to discuss using brain signals to control the real thing.

Developing such technologies will also be limited by current ethical standards for human research, and (at least in the United States) military research is conducted under ethical guidelines that are consistent with those in the civilian world (Moreno 2000). What institutional review board, operating under current bioethical guidelines, would approve experimental protocols involving brain surgery for such purposes? The same could be said for other foreseeable applications of neuroscience. An implant to inhibit sexual desire might be attractive to a pedophile faced with the alternative choice of indefinite incarceration in a mental hospital after release from prison. The military would certainly be interested in implants that might reduce soldiers' anxiety or allow faster and more secure communication among war-fighters. But what present-day institutional review board would approve the research needed to accomplish this?

However, some ethical issues are clearly apparent, even though they might not be specific to neural implants. One is the need to protect human subjects from adverse effects of experimentation. Nobody can truthfully say that he understands all potential effects of surgery on the brain or the electrical stimulation of brain tissue. Brain–computer interfaces, by their very novelty, will be unpredictable in their effects on patients. 'The technology [of brain–computer interfaces] is a little premature to commercialize,' Duke University neuroscientist Miguel Nicolelis was quoted in a recent article in *Forbes*. 'We have to be very careful. It's like gene therapy. If we make one mistake, the whole field is dead' (Moukheiber 2004).

Indeed, there have been unexpected side effects of neural implants, which have raised unforeseen ethical problems. Deep-brain stimulation has been reported to have serious psychiatric effects in some patients (Piasecki and Jefferson 2004). Recently, physicians described the plight of a 62-year-old man who had been treated with a deep-brain stimulator for

Parkinson's disease (Leentjens *et al.* 2004). He had developed a manic state as a result of the treatment, with unpredictable chaotic behavior and mental incompetence. Adjusting the stimulation parameters of the device reduced these problems, but at the cost of recurrence of his motor symptoms that left him debilitated.

> Ultimately, there seemed to be only two alternatives: to admit the patient to a nursing home because of serious invalidity, but mentally in good condition, or to admit the patient to a chronic psychiatric ward because of a manic state, but with acceptable motor capacity and ADL functions. Thorough ethical evaluation followed. When not being stimulated, the patient was considered competent to decide about his own treatment; in this condition the patient chose for the second option. In accordance with his own wishes he was therefore legally committed to a chronic ward in the regional psychiatric hospital. (Leentjens *et al.* 2004)

Such devastating side effects are apparently uncommon; however, few deep-brain stimulators are in use and the likelihood of such mishaps is difficult to judge.

The use of brain implants in severely disabled, and therefore vulnerable, patients raises difficult ethical issues. As Fins (2000, 2003) has pointed out, deep-brain stimulation has an element of disrepute because of its perceived resemblance to discredited psychosurgery of the past, despite the vast difference that exists between modern techniques for neuromodulation and the psychosurgery that was practiced a half century ago. Fins noted the need for 'balancing access to novel therapies versus protection of vulnerable study populations, rational evaluation of study design and research strategies, informed consent, and the importance of achieving societal consensus for this line of scientific inquiry' (Fins 2000). Given the rush to develop applications of deep-brain stimulators, functional magnetic stimulation, and other therapies for a host of neurological and psychiatric problems, the cautions note by Fins are entirely sensible.

The cochlear implant is a good example of a new medical technology that has negative consequences unanticipated by its developers. Intended as a device to help profoundly deaf individuals, the cochlear implant raised great concerns, and considerable hostility, among large parts of the deaf community. The deaf community is held together by sign language, and children who receive the implants at a prelingual stage (the preferred time for implantation) are not inclined to learn sign language—a threat to the community. Parents of deaf children have had to choose whether to allow their children to receive the devices, often under pressure from members of the deaf community to withhold the implants. The case in favor of providing cochlear implants to prelingually deaf children has been made by bioethicists such as Levy (2002). In recent years the intensity of the debate appears to have subsided. In part, this may be a result of the steady improvement of cochlear implants, which has made the decision by parents to have them implanted in their children much easier. Whether similar controversies will arise with other types of brain implant remains to be seen.

More generally, other critics have complained that the focus on developing high-technology prostheses, while valuable, detracts attention from the social needs of the patient by medicalizing a situation that the patient perceives in social terms:

> Many bio/gene/nano technology applications (predictive testing, cures, adaptation) focus on the individual and his or her perceived shortcomings. They follow a medical, not a social evaluation of a characteristic (biological reality) and therefore offer only medical solutions (prevention or cure/adaptation) and no social solutions (acceptance, societal cures of equal rights and respect). Furthermore the use and development focus of bio/gene/nanotechnology as it is perpetuates the medical, intrinsic, individualistic, defect view of disability. Not often discussed by clinicians,

academics in general, or the general public is the view, commonly expressed by disabled people, that the demand for the technology is based too much on the medical model of disability and hardly acknowledges the social model of disability. (Wolbring *et al.* 2002)

These issues are perhaps more acute with the technologies discussed in this chapter than they are with heart pacemakers, for example, because they are intimately and fundamentally related to a person's communication with the outside world. But similar points could be made about medical care in general, and care of people with disabilities in particular. It is not sufficient to view the patient's problems in strictly medical terms; one should also consider the social definition of disability and the needs of the patient. That said, it is hard to raise ethical objections to attempts for example, to provide a locked-in patient with a means to communicate with the outside world.

While not directly related to neuroscience, the use of implanted microchips to track humans is already here, and their ethical implications (mostly privacy concerns) can be severe. An implantable identification chip called the VeriChip is presently being marketed under an FDA premarket approval granted in 2002. Another company, Applied Digital Solutions, will soon begin marketing its own implantable tracking chip called Digital Angel. In early 2005, the United States government had reportedly issued contracts to four companies to develop radiofrequency identification chips for passports, which would beam information about the passport owner to a reader nearby (http://www.rfidgazette.org/2005/01/us_government_a. html). Some applications have undisputed benefits of ethical significance; a major medical school is reportedly considering the implantation of identification chips in cadavers to stop the sale of body parts by medical school staff.

There is a long history of use of animals in wartime, including efforts to train or modify animals for military purposes. In one bizarre experiment carried out by the CIA in the 1960s (but only reported in 2001 after the release of newly declassified documents) investigators embedded a microphone and radio transmitter in a cat, threading the antenna up the animal's tail—a walking listening station: 'The idea of Project "Acoustic Kitty" was for the hapless animal to sidle up to Soviet bloc spies, perch on nearby park benches or window sills, and allow its CIA masters to listen in' (Watson 2001). The cat, being a cat, wandered away from the investigators during the first experiment. It was 'run over by a taxi as it made its way towards its first assignment and the project was abandoned'.

With modern technology, it would be easy to improve on this experiment. The investigator who carried out the Robo-Rat experiment has proposed mounting small television cameras on a rat and sending it into a dangerous or otherwise inaccessible area, guided by a human with a radiofrequency transmitter. Using implanted electrodes to deliver stimuli and rewards is clearly a highly effective way to train an animal, or a human for that matter. The training and control can be done from a distance thanks to communications technologies, and perhaps even from across the globe via the Internet. A number of practical applications may exist (although how much attention a rat will pay to a pleasurable sensation induced by an electrode when faced with serious external threats to its existence remains an open question). The ethical implications of using this approach to train and control an animal are not necessarily different from those raised by other less effective methods. However, it raises the possibility of increased use of higher animals for military applications, which raise ethical issues of a different sort. For example, for years the US Navy has had a program to train dolphins to locate enemy divers and mines in harbors, which has been limited by the independence of these animals. No doubt the security services and military are experimenting with this promising new technology right now.

Bioethics, or its new subspecialty neuroethics, can play an important positive role in shaping the evolution of ethical standards to respond to new scientific and technical developments in brain science. However, a larger problem may be challenges to ethical standards resulting from political developments, and not just the continuing evolution of science and technology. The 2001 terrorist attacks have led to a noticeable decrease in civil liberties in the United States and elsewhere, and to practices by the military and security agencies that, at the very least, might be questioned on ethical grounds. What would be the consequences for Western democracies of another major terrorist attack? Will there will be a 'reduced barrier against human experiments' (Nordmann 2004) for developing new neuroscience technologies for military or security uses? If so, the neuroethics community has an obligation to be part of the discussion.

So we end with some essential questions about engineering the brain. What will the boundaries be for human implants and for the experimentation needed to make them work? Will they be decided by animal experimentation or tested immediately in people in real time? Who will decide? Most importantly, will future developments lead to reduced barriers to human experimentation, and what role should the bioethics and neuroethics communities play in such a process of revision of ethical standards? Whose values will prevail? Although only time will tell, this is truly a very interesting and most important time to be paying attention.

# References

Aouizerate B, Cuny E, Martin-Guehl C, *et al.* (2004). Deep brain stimulation of the ventral caudate nucleus in the treatment of obsessive–compulsive disorder and major depression. Case report. *Journal of Neurosurgery* 101, 682–6.

Bach-Y-Rita P (2004). Tactile sensory substitution studies. *Annals of the New York Academy of Science* 1013, 83–91.

Chow AY, Chow VY, Packo KH, Pollack JS, Peyman GA, Schuchard R (2004). The artificial silicon retina microchip for the treatment of vision loss from retinitis pigmentosa. *Archives of Ophthalmology* 122, 460–9.

Chowdhury V, Morley JW, Coroneo MT (2004). Surface stimulation of the brain with a prototype array for a visual cortex prosthesis. *Journal of Clinical Neuroscience* 11, 750–5.

Collins S (2004). Couples' nervous system linked by implants in limbs. *New Zealand Herald*, 6 July.

Delgado JMR (1969). *Physical Control of the Mind.* (New York: Harper and Row).

Donoghue JP (2002). Connecting cortex to machines: recent advances in brain interfaces. *Nature Neuroscience* 5 (Suppl), 1085–8.

Fins JJ (2000). A proposed ethical framework for interventional cognitive neuroscience: a consideration of deep brain stimulation in impaired consciousness. *Neurological Research* 22, 273–8.

Fins JJ (2003). From psychosurgery to neuromodulation and palliation: history's lessons for the ethical conduct and regulation of neuropsychiatric research. *Neurosurgery Clinics of North America*, 14, 303–19.

Foster KR (2003). Limiting technology: issues in setting exposure guidelines for radiofrequency energy. In: Ma J.-G. (ed) *Third Generation Mobile Communication Systems: Future Developments and Advanced Topics.* New York: Springer-Verlag, 57–77.

Gazzaniga MS, Steven MS (2004). Free will in the twenty-first century. In: Garland B (ed) *Neuroscience and the Law.* New York: Dana Press, 51–70.

Grunhaus L, Schreiber S, Dolberg OT, Polak D, Dannon PN (2003). A randomized controlled comparison of electroconvulsive therapy and repetitive transcranial magnetic stimulation in severe and resistant nonpsychotic major depression. *Biological Psychiatry* 53, 324–31.

Helms Tillery SI, Taylor DM, Schwartz AB (2003). Training in cortical control of neuroprosthetic devices improves signal extraction from small neuronal ensembles. *Reviews in the Neurosciences* 14, 107–19.

Hossain P, Seetho IW, Browning AC, Amoaku WM (2005). Artificial means for restoring vision. *British Medical Journal* 330, 30–3.

Kennedy PR, Kirby MT, Moore MM, King B, Mallory AM (2004). Computer control using human intracortical local field potentials. *IEEE Transactions on Neural Systems and Rehabilitation Engineering* 12, 339–44.

Khamsi R (2004). Paralysed man sends e-mail by thought. News@nature, 11 October.

Leentjens AF, Visser-Vandewalle V, Temel Y, Verhey FR (2004). Manipulation of mental competence: an ethical problem in case of electrical stimulation of the subthalamic nucleus for severe Parkinson's disease. *Nederlands Tijdschrift voor Geneeskunde* 148, 1394–8 (in Dutch).

LeDoux J (2000). *Daily Express*, 31 December.

Levy N (2002). Reconsidering cochlear implants: the lessons of Martha's Vineyard. *Bioethics* 16, 134–53.

Lisanby SH, Kinnunen LH, Crupain MJ (2002). Applications of TMS to therapy in psychiatry. *Clinical Neurophysiology* 19, 344–60.

Lozano AM, Dostrovsky J, Chen R, Ashby P (2002). Deep brain stimulation for Parkinson's disease: disrupting the disruption.*Lancet Neurology* 1, 225–31.

McGee EM, Maguire GQ (2001) Implantable brain chips: ethical and policy issues. *Medical Ethics (Burlington, Mass)* 1–2, 8. Available online at: http://www.bu.edu/wcp/Papers/Bioe/BioeMcGe.htm

Matthews K, Eljamel MS (2003). Vagus nerve stimulation and refractory depression: please can you switch me on doctor? *British Journal of Psychiatry*, 183, 181–3.

Meek J (2002). *The Guardian*, 2 May.

Moreno JD (2000). *Undue Risk*. New York: W.H. Freeman, 189–200.

Moukheiber Z (2004). Mind over matter, *Forbes Magazine*, 15 March 15.

Musallam S, Corneil BD, Greger B, Scherberger H, Andersen RA (2004). Cognitive control signals for neural prosthetics. *Science* 305, 258–62.

Mussa-Ivaldi FA, Miller LE (2003). Brain–machine interfaces: computational demands and clinical needs meet basic neuroscience. *Trends in Neurosciences* 26, 329–34.

Nordmann A (2004). *Foresighting the New Technology Wave—Expert Group State of the Art Reviews and Related Papers*, 14 June 2004. Available online at http://europa.eu.int/comm/research/conferences/2004/ntw/pdf/final_report_en.pdf

Orlowski A (2004). Google founder dreams of Google implant in your brain. *The Register (UK)*, 3 March.

Pena C, Bowsher K, Samuels-Reid JM (2004). FDA-approved neurologic devices intended for use in infants, children, and adolescents. *Neurology* 63, 1163–7.

Piasecki SD, Jefferson JW (2004). Psychiatric complications of deep brain stimulation for Parkinson's disease. *Journal of ClinicalPsychiatry* 65, 845–9.

Roco MC, Bainbridge WS (eds) (2002). *Nanotechnology, Biotechnology, Information Technology and Cognitive Science*. Washington, DC: National Science Foundation. Available online at http://www.technology. gov/reports/2002/NBIC/Content.pdf

Schmidt EM, Bak MJ, Hambrecht FT, Kufta CV, O'Rourke DK, Vallabhanath P (1996). Feasibility of a visual prosthesis for the blind based on intracortical microstimulation of the visual cortex. *Brain* 119, 507–22.

Serruya MD, Hatsopoulos NG, Paninski L, Fellows MR, Donoghue JP (2002). Instant neural control of a movement signal. *Nature,* 416141–2.

Stimpson N, Agrawal, N, Lewis G (2002). Randomised controlled trials investigating pharmacological and psychological interventions for treatment-refractory depression. Systematic review. *British Journal of Psychiatry* 181, 284–94.

Talwar SK, Xu S, Hawley ES, Weiss SA, Moxon KA, Chapin JK (2002). Rat navigation guided by remote control. *Nature* 417, 37–8.

Theodore WH, Fisher RS (2004). Brain stimulation for epilepsy. *Lancet Neurology* 3, 111–18.

Toh EH, Luxford WM (2002). Cochlear and brainstem implantation. *Otolaryngologic Clinics of North America* 35, 325–42.

Vaughan TM, Heetderks WJ, Trejo LJ, et al. (2003). Brain–computer interface technology: a review of the Second International Meeting. *IEEE Transactions on Neural Systems and Rehabilitation Engineering* 11, 94–109.

Watson CR (2001) CIA's pet project for a purrfect spy fails. *The Times*, 5 November.

Wolbring G (2002). Science and technology and the triple D (disease, disability, defect). In Roco MC, Bainbridge WS (eds) *Nanotechnology, Biotechnology, Information Technology and Cognitive Science*. Washington, DC: National Science Foundation, 208.

Wolpaw JR, McFarland DJ (2004). Control of a two-dimensional movement signal by a noninvasive brain–computer interface in humans. *Proceedings of the National Academy of Sciences of the USA* 101, 17849–54.

Wolpaw JR, Birbaumer N, McFarland DJ, Pfurtscheller G, Vaughan TM (2002). Brain–computer interfaces for communication and control. *Clinical Neurophysiology* 113, 767–91.

Chapter 14

# Transcranial magnetic stimulation and the human brain: an ethical evaluation

Megan S. Steven and Alvaro Pascual-Leone

## Introduction

Transcranial magnetic stimulation (TMS) is a neuroscientific technique that induces an electric current in the brain via application of a localized magnetic field pulse. The pulse penetrates the scalp and skull non-invasively and, depending on the parameters of stimulation, facilitates or depresses the local neuronal response with effects that can be transient or long lasting. While the mechanisms by which TMS acts remain largely unknown, the behavioral effects of the stimulation are reproducible and, in some cases, are highly beneficial. As the applications of and access to this technique become increasingly pervasive, scientific engagement is needed to define the ethical framework in which research with TMS should be translated to application. In this chapter we review the technique in detail and discuss safety as the paramount ethics issue for TMS. We further examine the ethical arguments for and against neuroenhancement with TMS and how the framework for acceptable practice must differ for patient and non-patient populations.

## A TMS primer

TMS is a relatively new neurophysiologic technique that allows the safe, non-invasive, and relatively painless stimulation of the human brain (Pascual-Leone *et al.* 2002; Walsh and Pascual-Leone 2003). TMS can be used to complement other neuroscience methods to study the pathways between the brain and the spinal cord and between different neuronal structures. It can be used further to validate the functional significance of neuroimaging studies in determining the causal relationship between focal brain activity and behavior. Most relevant for the present chapter is the way in which modulation of brain activity by repetitive TMS (rTMS) can transiently change brain function and be utilized as a therapeutic tool for treatment of a variety of neurological and psychiatric illnesses.

The principles that underlie TMS were discovered by Faraday in 1831. A pulse of electric current flowing through a coil of wire generates a magnetic field [Fig. 14.1(a)]. The rate of change of this magnetic field determines the induction of a secondary current in a nearby conductor. In TMS, the stimulating coil is held over a subject's head [Fig. 14.1(b)] and, as a brief pulse of current is passed through it, a magnetic field is generated that passes through the subject's scalp and skull without attenuation (only decaying by the square of the distance) [Fig. 14.1(d)]. This time-varying magnetic field induces a current in the subject's brain that depolarizes neurons and generates effects depending on the brain area targeted. Therefore, in TMS, neural elements are not primarily affected by the exposure to a magnetic field, but rather by the current induced in the brain by electrodeless non-invasive electric stimulation.

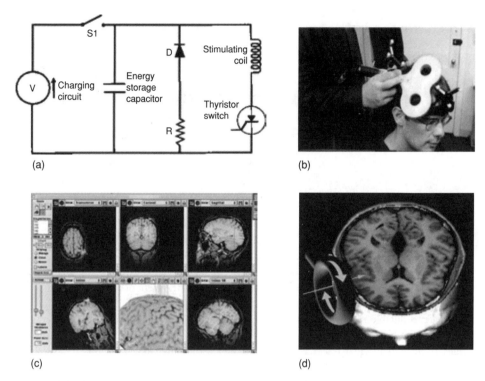

(a)

(b)

(c)

(d)

**Fig. 14.1** Illustration of the application of TMS. (a) Schematic diagram of the electric circuit used to induce the TMS pulse. (b) The TMS coil being applied by an experimenter. Both the coil and the subject have a tracking device affixed to them so that the head/coil position can be monitored in real time. (c) Illustration of how the subject's MRI can be used, along with the tracking system which monitors head and coil movement, to display the cortical area being targeted in real-time. (d) Depth of effect of the TMS coil on the human cortex (See also the colour plate section).

In the early 1980s, Barker and colleagues developed the first compact magnetic coil stimulator at the University of Sheffield. Soon after, TMS devices became commercially available. The design of magnetic stimulators is relatively simple. Stimulators consist of a main unit and a stimulating coil. The main unit is composed of a charging system, one or more energy storage capacitors, a discharge switch, and circuits for pulse shaping, energy recovery, and control functions (Fig. 14.2). Different charging systems are possible; the simplest design uses step-up transformers operating at line frequency of 50–60 Hz. Energy storage capacitors can also be of different types. The essential factors in the effectiveness of a magnetic stimulator are the speed of the magnetic field rise time and the maximization of the peak coil energy. Therefore large energy storage capacitors and very efficient energy transfer from the capacitor to the coil are important. Typically, energy storage capacity is around 2000 J and 500 J are transferred from the capacitors into the stimulating coil in less than 100 $\mu$s via a thyristor, an electronic device that is capable of switching large currents in a few microseconds. The peak discharge current needs to be several thousand amperes in order to induce currents in the brain of sufficient magnitude to depolarize neural elements (about 10 mA/cm$^2$).

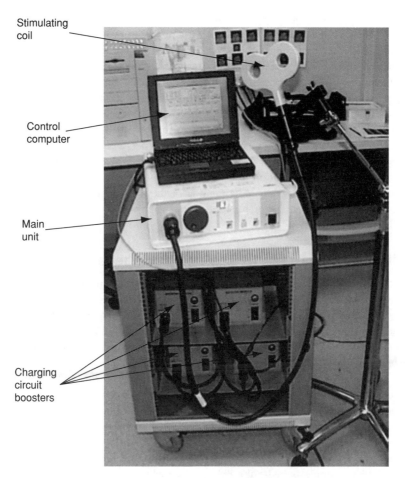

Stimulating coil

Control computer

Main unit

Charging circuit boosters

**Fig. 14.2** TMS equipment including the charging circuit boosters, the main stimulating unit, the control computer, and the stimulating coil (See also the colour plate section).

During transcranial magnetic brain stimulation only the stimulating coil needs to come into close contact with the subject [Fig. 14.1(b)]. Stimulating coils consist of one or more well-insulated coils of copper wire, frequently housed in a molded plastic cover, and are available in a variety of shapes and sizes. The geometry of the coil determines the focality of brain stimulation. Figure-of-eight coils, also called butterfly or double coils (Fig. 14.2), are constructed with two windings placed side by side and provide the most focal means of brain stimulation with TMS available to date. Current knowledge, largely based on mathematical modeling, suggests that the most focal forms of TMS available today affect an area of $0.5 \times 0.5$ cm at the level of the brain cortex (Wagner *et al.* 2004). Stimulation is restricted to rather superficial layers in the convexity of the brain (cortex or gray–white matter junction) and direct effect onto deep brain structures is not yet possible. Digitization of the subject's head and registration of the TMS stimulation sites onto the magnetic resonance image (MRI) of the subject's brain addresses the issue of anatomical specificity of the TMS effects by identifying the actual brain target in each experimental subject [Fig. 14.1(c)]. The use of optical digitization and frameless stereotactic systems represents a further improvement by providing online information about the brain area targeted by a given coil position on the scalp.

The precise mechanisms underlying the brain effects of TMS remain largely unknown (Pascual-Leone *et al.* 2002; Robertson *et al.* 2003). Currents induced in the brain by TMS primarily flow parallel to the plane of the stimulation coil (approximately parallel to the brain's cortical surface when the stimulation coil is held tangentially to the scalp). Therefore, in contrast with electrical cortical stimulation, TMS preferentially activates neural elements oriented horizontally to the brain surface. Exactly which neural elements are activated by TMS remains unclear and, in fact, might be variable across different brain areas and different subjects. The combination of TMS with other neuroimaging and neurophysiologic techniques provides an enhanced understanding of the mechanisms of action of TMS and a novel approach to the study of functional connectivity between different areas in the human brain.

## TMS in clinical neurophysiology and neurobehaviorial studies

In clinical neurophysiology, TMS is primarily used to study the integrity of the motor fibers that connect the brain with the spinal cord ('central motor pathways') (Kobayashi and Pascual-Leone 2003). TMS is applied to the motor cortex and motor-evoked potentials are recorded using electromyography and surface electrodes tapped over the belly and tendon of the target muscle(s). Frequently, in order to interpret the results fully, motor cortex TMS has to be combined with peripheral nerve, nerve plexus, or spinal root stimulation. Such studies can provide important diagnostic and prognostic insights in patients with motor neuron disease (e.g. Lou Gehrig's disease), multiple sclerosis, stroke, or spinal cord lesion. The specific sites of stimulation, the recorded muscles, maneuvers used for facilitation of the motor-evoked potentials, and the evaluation of the different response parameters have to be tailored to the specific questions asked.

The development of generalized techniques offers the opportunity of widening the clinical uses of TMS. For example, paired-pulse TMS can be used to study intracortical excitability and to provide insight into the pathophysiology of movement disorders such as Parkinson's disease or the mechanisms of action of different medications. rTMS can be used in the study of higher cortical functions, for example the non-invasive determination of the language-dominant hemisphere. Finally, the integration of TMS with image-guided frameless stereotactic techniques can be used for non-invasive cortical mapping and thus can aid in the presurgical evaluation of neurosurgical patients [see Fig. 14.1(c)]. In addition to such clinical applications, TMS provides a unique tool for the study of causal relationships between brain activity and behavior. TMS delivered appropriately in time and space can transiently block the function of neuronal networks, allowing the creation of a time-dependent 'virtual lesion' in an otherwise healthy brain.

When rTMS trains of stimuli are applied to a given brain area at different stimulation frequencies, modulating the level of excitability of a given cortical area beyond the duration of the stimulation itself is possible (Pascual-Leone *et al.* 1998). Remarkably, depending on the stimulation frequency and intensity, potentiation or depression of cortical excitability can occur (Maeda *et al.* 2000). The possibility of enhancing behavior by applying rTMS at parameters that potentiate cortical excitability is intriguing and could have a profoundly positive impact on neurorehabilitation and skill acquisition. Since a variety of neuropsychiatric conditions are associated with disturbed cortical activity, as documented by neuroimaging and neurophysiological studies, 'forced normalization' of such disturbed cortical excitability might lead to symptom improvement. However, this potential also raises a number of ethical concerns that warrant attention.

## TMS: ethics, clinical research, and therapeutic potential

Guidelines for human subjects research in the United States are articulated in the *Belmont Report* (United States National Commission 1979). This report defines three governing principles that remain the gold standard for human subject research ethics: respect for persons, beneficence, and justice (see also Chapter 9).

The first principle of respect and the third principle of justice are well addressed in the TMS literature, especially with discussion of the basic ethical treatment of subjects (e.g. consent, exclusion and inclusion criteria) (Green 2002; Illes *et al.*, in press). The first clause of the second principle is considered at length in the literature on the guidelines for the safe use of single-pulse TMS as well as rTMS on the normal human brain (Wassermann 1998; Hallett *et al.* 1999). Taking this into account, we focus specifically on the issues of beneficence, and on finding the appropriate balance between benefit and risk of TMS.

The potential benefits of TMS for furthering the understanding of the workings of the human brain and for encouraging neurological enhancement and recovery are significant. By monitoring the effects of TMS on a specific neural node and the time course of those effects, TMS can give us new knowledge about the usage of that particular node (reviewed by Pascual-Leone *et al.* 2000). In the clinical population, TMS has shown promise for treatment of depression (reviewed by Gershon *et al.* 2003; Paus and Barret 2004), Parkinson's disease, writer's cramp (Siebner *et al.* 1999), and chronic pain (Pridmore and Oberoi 2000), as well as rehabilitation for motor neglect, motor stroke (Mansur *et al.*, 2005), and aphasia (Martin *et al.* 2004; Naeser *et al.* 2005a,b), among others (Table 14.1).

When conducting new treatment trials with TMS, it is appropriate to recruit patients who have exhausted other less risky forms of treatment, and who have a severe form of a neurological disorder; however, one must also be aware of the potential for diminished individual autonomy in such 'desperate' patients (Miller and Brody 2003; Minogue *et al.* 1995). While

**Table 14.1** Clinical applications of TMS research currently being pursued in research laboratories worldwide

| | |
|---|---|
| Acute mania | Obsessive–compulsive disorder |
| Aphasia<br>Auditory hallucinoses<br>Bipolar disorder<br>Depression | Pain<br>  Visceral pain<br>  Atypical facial pain<br>  Phantom pain |
| Epilepsy<br>  Myoclonic epilepsy<br>  Focal status epilepticus | Parkinson's disease<br>Post-traumatic stress disorder<br>Schizophrenia |
| Focal dystonia | Stuttering |
| Neglect | Tics |

such patients might be more likely to participate in clinical trials even when risks are not minimized because the trials represent a last resort, careful oversight by an institutional review board can provide necessary safeguards and advocacy. This idea is utilized in the US Food and Drug Administration (FDA) clinical trials and it would appear reasonable to adapt this to the TMS field.

TMS, especially rTMS, remains an experimental technique. Side effects are possible and strict safety guidelines need to be followed to avoid adverse events. There are relative and absolute contraindications to TMS (Wassermann 1998; Hallet *et al.* 1999). Examples of these contraindications include metal anywhere in the head (excluding the mouth), cardiac pacemakers and implanted medication pumps, intracranial or intracardiac electrodes, raised intracranial pressure, pregnancy, a history of seizures, a family history of epilepsy, and patients taking medications that might increase the risk of seizures. The main safety concern when using TMS is its potential to induce a seizure, even in subjects without any predisposing illness. This risk is low (in the order of $\leq 1$ in 1000 studies) and is essentially limited to the application of rTMS. Approximately 10–20 percent of subjects studied with TMS develop a muscle tension headache or a neck ache. These are generally mild discomforts that respond promptly to aspirin, acetaminophen (Tylenol®), or other common analgesics. rTMS can also cause ringing in the ears (tinnitus) or even transient hearing loss if the subjects do not wear earplugs during the studies. Furthermore, TMS can cause mild and very transient memory problems and other cognitive deficits, and mood and hormone changes (these rare adverse effects are usually resolved within hours of cessation of TMS).

The major risk of TMS is the risk of producing a seizure. The likelihood of inducing a seizure is small (only nine seizures induced by rTMS have been reported worldwide) but is increased with increasing frequency and intensity of stimulation and with family history of seizure and/or ingestion of pro-epileptic drugs. The parameters of TMS that have produced seizures during experimentation are well known and documented (Wassermann 1998; Hallett *et al.* 1999), and it is important to note that there are no reports of seizure in subjects who were treated with TMS parameters administered within the safety guidelines (Wassermann 1998). Nonetheless, TMS has only been studied for approximately 20 years and the data on potential long-term effects in humans remain insufficient. Although animal studies using TMS have not indicated any risks of brain damage or long-term injury, caution remains imperative.

Since safety guidelines (Wassermann 1998) were generated from information on TMS of the healthy adult human brain, little is known about the appropriate safety guidelines for patient populations and for the developing brain. Great care must be taken when conducting studies involving such populations, and the fact that there are unknown risks because of incomplete safety data should be appropriately described to patients. For example, patients with infarcts or neurological disorders that cause cortical atrophy should be stimulated with great care as the presence of excess cerebrospinal fluid (CSF) can alter the electromagnetic field properties, and stimulation near CSF could cause adverse effects (Wagner *et al.* 2004).

Only seven pediatric patients are reported in the rTMS literature (reviewed by Walter *et al.* 2001). These patients all had psychiatric disorders and one reported an adverse effect (tension headache). Even though rTMS offers the potential for treating developmental disorders like autism, childhood depression, and obsessive–compulsive disorder among others, it is still not appropriate to carry out research on children until safety parameters are known for the developing brain. Clinical trials on children who have medication-refractory focal epilepsy represent a reasonable entry point given the current state of the art.

# Ethical considerations of TMS in basic neuroscience research

Previously, scientists relied on naturally occurring lesions in the human brain (from stroke or other brain damage) to draw conclusions about the functioning of specific neural regions. However, such data are imprecise, irreversible, and do not always occur in isolation from other neurological disorders. Since TMS (at least single-pulse TMS) has only a transient effect, it can be utilized to investigate the importance of a given brain area in the normal functioning human brain by creating a temporary 'virtual lesion' (Pascual-Leone *et al.* 2000; Walsh and Pascual-Leone 2003). For this reason, TMS is used to investigate a myriad of neuroscientific questions about the functioning of the normal human brain.

Some studies have aimed at understanding the early sensory processing system (Amassian *et al.* 1989; Corthout *et al.* 1999) using single-pulse TMS at different time-points after visual stimulation, while others have investigated higher visual processing (Ashbridge *et al.* 1997) with the same relatively safe parameters. Motor processing is also studied extensively with single-pulse TMS on normal subjects (Robertson *et al.* 2003; De Gennaro *et al.* 2004; Theoret *et al.* 2004).

rTMS studies at rates of repetition well below safety limits are also conducted on normal subjects to investigate phenomena varying from self-recognition (reviewed by Keenan *et al.* 2000) to sequence learning (Robertson and Pascual-Leone 2001). However, some studies utilize rTMS at parameters nearing the limit of safety guidelines. Further ethical consideration is needed here.

For example, researchers have recently begun to investigate the induction of long-term depression (LTD) and long-term potentiation (LTP) (the mechanisms of neuroplasticity) using rTMS protocols in the normal human brain (Iyer *et al.* 2003; Huang *et al.* 2004). These studies, while scientifically worthwhile, challenge the risk–benefit ratio. The benefit of such research is that learning how to induce LTD and LTP could have implications for treatment of diseases like depression, epilepsy, Parkinson's disease, and other neurological disorders. However, the risks are also quite high. As described above, increasing the length and rate of stimulation both contribute to the higher risk of seizure. LTP induction requires only 20–190 s, but must be applied at 50 Hz (in the theta range). The parameters necessary to induce LTD are not of as much concern because they involve stimulation at a relatively low repetitive rate (6 Hz followed by 1 Hz), although it must be applied for a long period of time (20 min). However, the greatest risk is that both forms of stimulation attempt to produce a long-term effect without a priori knowledge of know how long this effect will last and what the outcome will be for the subject.

Is the increased risk of seizure and the unknown transience of the effect an ethically responsible risk to undertake given the lack of benefit for the subjects involved? Would not the same studies on animal models yield appropriate conclusions and a lesser ethical concern? Here, it seems, that the principle of beneficence might well be revisited.

# TMS and neuroenhancement

Is neuroenhancement in the non-patient population, i.e. non-therapeutic uses of TMS for enhancing cognitive or affective function, ethical? Does the benefit of increasing mental facility above and beyond natural levels justify an increased risk, as neurorehabilitation benefits might justify increased risk in the patient population?

The idea that targeted brain stimulation (excitatory or inhibitory) can enhance or beneficially alter cognitive function has not been lost on the Hollywood film industry [see *Total Recall*

(1990) or *Eternal Sunshine of the Spotless Mind* (2004)], let alone the scientific community. However, this is not a futuristic issue, as recent studies using TMS and other forms of non-invasive stimulation, such as direct current stimulation, are exploring neuroenhancing applications in the normal population (Antal *et al.* 2004; Kobayashi *et al.* 2004). For instance, Kobayashi *et al.* (2004) discovered that by inhibiting cortical activity in the right motor cortex (which controls the left hand), the reaction time to a sequential finger movement task can be increased in the right hand without affecting the performance in the left hand Similarly, Hilgetag *et al.* (2001) found enhanced attention to the ipsilateral field of a person's spatial environment in normal subjects following suppression of the parietal cortex by rTMS. Others have reported facilitatory behavioral effects of rTMS on working memory, naming, abstract thinking, color perception, motor learning, and perceptual learning (reviewed by Theoret *et al.* 2003).

Snyder *et al.* (2003) reported that latent savant-like qualities could be revealed in normal control subjects following low-frequency rTMS to the left frontotemporal cortex. Subjects (11 right-handed males) performed a battery of tests before, immediately after, and 45 min after rTMS treatment. These tests included drawing animals from memory, drawing novel faces from images provided by the researcher, and proofreading. Of 11 subjects, four showed dramatic stylistic changes in drawing immediately after rTMS compared with the drawings produced before and 45 min after stimulation. This TMS-induced unmasking of increased artistic and language abilities was surprising to the subjects. One subject, who wrote an article about his experiences, commented that he 'could hardly recognize' the drawings as his own even though he had watched himself render each image. He added: 'Somehow over the course of a very few minutes, and with no additional instruction, I had gone from an incompetent draftsman to a very impressive artist of the feline form' (Osborne 2003).

Whether or not savant-like capabilities can be revealed in all persons is a matter of debate. Snyder *et al.* (2003) conducted a study with only minimal success, suggesting that factors like sex, age, genes, and environment might play a role in determining whether or not TMS can induce savant-like responses in the normal population (just as these factors probably play a role in whether or not neurological damage leads to savant symptoms in the patient population). However, it remains a distinct possibility that TMS could soon induce reliable neuroenhancement of motor, attentional, artistic, or language abilities in the normal human brain as more recent studies by Young *et al.* (2004) have shown.

## Weighing the dynamic capabilities of the brain and our moral values

In the not too distant future, we could have students using their at-home TMS machines to 'zap' their parietal lobes before taking SATs, or their prefrontal cortices before going to art class. Some believe that enhancement by neurostimulation is no different than enhancement by education, as both are presumably a result of altering neuronal firing and modulating brain plasticity (Pascual-Leone *et al.* 1998). There exist ethicists who argue both for (Caplan 2003) and against (Sandel 2002; Kass 2003) enhancement. Michael Sandel, a member of the President's Council on Bioethics, raises the concern that enhancement poses a threat to human dignity. Sandel believes that '... what is troubling about enhancement is that it represents the triumph in our time of wilfulness over giftedness, of dominion over reverence, of molding over beholding' (Sandel 2002). However, the capacity of being molded (plasticity) is an intrinsic property of the human brain and represents evolution's invention to enable the nervous system to escape the restrictions of its own genome and thus to adapt to environmental pressures, physiological changes, and experiences. Dynamic shifts in the strength of pre-existing connections across distributed neural networks, changes in task-related cortico-cortical and cortico-subcortical coherence, and modifications of the mapping between behavior and neural activity take place continuously in response to any and all changes in afferent input or efferent demand. Such rapid ongoing changes might be followed by the establishment of new connections through dendritic growth and arborization. Plasticity is not an occasional state of the nervous system; instead, it is the normal ongoing state of the nervous system throughout the lifespan. Therefore we should not conceive of the brain as a stationary object capable of activating a cascade of changes that we shall call plasticity, nor as an orderly stream of events driven by plasticity. We might be served better by thinking of the nervous system as a continuously changing structure of which plasticity is an integral property and the obligatory consequence of each sensory input, each motor act, association, reward signal, action plan, or awareness. In this framework, notions of psychological processes as distinct from organic-based functions or dysfunctions cease to be informative. Behavior will lead to changes in brain circuitry, just as changes in brain circuitry will lead to behavioral changes. Therefore all environmental interactions, and certainly educational approaches, represent interventions that mold the brain of the actor. Given this perspective, it is conceivable that neuromodulation with properly controlled and carefully applied neurophysiological methods could be potentially a safer, more effective, and more efficient means of guiding plasticity and thus shaping behavior. Plasticity is a double-edged sword, to be sure, and harbors dangers of evolving patterns of neural activation that might in and of themselves lead to abnormal behavior. Plasticity is the mechanism for development and learning, as much as it can be the cause of pathology.

Therefore the challenge we face as scientists is to learn enough about the mechanisms of plasticity to be able to determine the parameters of TMS that will *optimally* modulate neuronal firing for patients, and perhaps for the non-patient population. Defining 'optimal' is the accompanying immediate ethical challenge. Overcoming inequities of access to the underserved and coercion will follow (Farah *et al.* 2004).

TMS scientists and neuroethicists would do well jointly to take the lead in pursuing these issues further and in ensuring that utilization parameters of TMS for neurorehabilitation and enhancement become clearly defined.

## Acknowledgments

The work on this article was supported by K24 RR018875, RO1-EY12091, RO1-DC05672, RO1-NS 47754, RO1-NS 20068, and R01-EB 005047. The authors would like to thank Mark Thivierge for the invaluable administrative support.

## References

Amassian VE, Cracco RQ, Maccabee PJ, Cracco JB, Rudell A, Eberle L (1989). Supression of visual perception by magnetic coil stimulation of human occipital cortex. *Electroencephalogry and Clinical Neurophysiology* 74, 458–62.

Antal A, Nitsche MA, Kruse W, Kincses TZ, Hoffman KP, Paulus W (2004). Direct current stimulation over V5 enhances visuomotor coordination by improving motion perception in humans. *Journal of Cognitive Neuroscience* 16, 521–7.

Ashbridge E, Walsh V, Cowey A (1997). Temporal aspects of visual search studied by transcranial magnetic stimulation. *Neuropsychologia* 35, 1121–31.

Caplan AL (2003). Is better best? A noted ethicist argues in favor of brain enhancement. *Scientific American* **289**, 104–5.

Corthout E, Uttl B, Walsh V, Hallett M, Cowey A (1999). Timing of activity in early visual cortex as revealed by transcranial magnetic stimulation. *Neuroreport* **10**, 2631–4.

De Gennaro L, Cristiani R, Bertini M, *et al.* (2004). Handedness is mainly associated with an asymmetry of corticospinal excitability and not of transcallosal inhibition. *Clinical Neurophysiology* **115**, 1305–12.

Farah MJ, Illes J, Cook-Deegan R, *et al.* (2004). Neurocognitive enhancement: what can we do and what should we do? *Nature Reviews Neuroscience* **5**, 421–425.

Gershon AA, Dannon PN, Grunhaus L (2003). Transcranial magnetic stimulation in the treatment of depression. *American Journal of Psychiatry* **160**, 835–45.

Green R (2002). Ethical issues. In: Pascual-Leone A, Davey N, Wassermann EM, Rothwell J, Puri B (eds) *Handbook of Transcranial Magnetic Stimulation*. London: Edward Arnold.

Hallett M, Wassermann EM, Pascual-Leone A (1999). Repetitive transcranial magnetic stimulation. In: Deuschl G, Eisen A (eds) *Recommendations for the Practice of Clinical Neurophysiology: Guidelines of the International Federation of Clinical Neurophysiology*. Amsterdam: Elsevier Science.

Hilgetag CC, Theoret H, Pascual-Leone A (2001). Enhanced visual spatial attention ipsilateral to rTMS-induced 'virtual lesions' of human parietal cortex. *Nature Neuroscience* **4**, 953–7.

Huang YZ, Edwards M, Rounis E, Bhatia KP, Rothwell JC (2004). Theta burst stimulation of the human motor cortex. *Neuron* **45**, 201–6.

Illes J, Gallo M, Kirshen MP (2005). An ethics perspective on the use of transcranial magnetic sitmulation (TMS) for human neuromodulation. *Behavioral Neurology*, in press.

Iyer MB, Schleper N, Wassermann EM (2003). Priming stimulation enhances the depressent effect of low-frequency repetitive transcranial magnetic stimulation. *Journal of Neuroscience* **23**, 10867–72.

Kass LR (2003). Ageless bodies, happy souls: biotechnology and the pursuit of perfection. *New Atlantis* **1**, 9–29.

Keenan JP, Wheeler MA, Callup GG, Pascual-Leone A (2000). Self-recognition and the right prefrontal cortex. *Trends in Cognitive Science* **4**, 338–44.

Kobayashi M, Pascual-Leone A (2003). Transcranial magnetic stimulation in neurology. *Lancet Neurology* **2**, 145–56.

Kobayashi M, Hutchinson S, Theoret H, Schlaug G, Pascual-Leone A (2004). Repetitive TMS of the motor cortex improves ipsilateral sequential simple finger movements. *Neurology* **62**, 91–8.

Maeda F, Keenan JP, Tormos JM, Topka, H, Pascual-Leone A (2000). Modulation of cortico-spinal excitability by repetitive transcranial magnetic stimulation. *Clinical Neurophysiology* **111**, 800–5.

Mansur C, Fregni F, Boggio PS, *et al.* (2005). A sham-stimulation controlled trial of rTMS of the unaffected hemisphere in stroke patients. *Neurology*, **64**, 1802–4.

Martin PI, Naeser MA, Theoret H, *et al.* (2004). Transcranial magnetic stimulation as a complementary treatment for aphasia. *Seminars in Speech and Language* **25**, 181–91

Miller FG, Brody H (2003). A critique of clinical equipoise. Therapeutic misconception in the ethics of clinical trials. *Hastings Center Report* **33**, 19–28.

Minogue BP, Palmer-Fernandez G, Udell L, Waller BN (1995). Individual autonomy and the double blind controlled experiment: the case of desperate volunteers. *Journal of Medicine and Philosophy* **20** 43–55.

Naeser MS, Martin PI, Nicholas M, *et al.* (2005a). Improved naming after TMS treatments in a chronic, global aphasia patient—case report. *Neurocase*, **11**, 182–93.

Naeser MS, Martin PI, Nicholas M, *et al.* (2005b). Improved picture naming in chronic aphasia after TMS to part of right Broca's area, an open-protocol study. *Brain and Language* **93**, 95–105.

Osborne L (2003). Savant for a day. *New York Times*, 22 June, sect 6, p 38, col 1.

Pascual-Leone A, Tormos JM, Keenan J, Catala MD (1998). Study and modulation of cortical excitability with transcranial magnetic stimulation. *Journal of Clinical Neurophysiology* **15**, 333–43.

Pascual-Leone A, Walsh V, Rothwell J (2000). Transcranial magnetic stimulation in cognitive neuroscience—virtual lesion, chronometry and functional connectivity. *Current Opinion in Neurobiology* 10, 232–7.

Pascual-Leone A, Davey N, Wassermann EM, Rothwell J, Puri B (eds) (2002). *Handbook of Transcranial Magnetic Stimulation.* London: Edward Arnold.

Paus T, Barrett J (2004). Transcranial magnetic stimulation (TMS) of the human frontal cortex: implications for repetitive TMS treatment of depression. *Journal of Psychiatry and Neuroscience* 29, 268–79.

Pridmore S, Oberoi G (2000). Transcranial magnetic stimulation applications and potential use in chronic pain: studies in waiting. *Journal of Neurological Science* 182, 1–4.

Robertson EM and Pascual-Leone A (2001). Aspects of sensory guidance in sequence learning. *Experimental Brain Research,* 137, 336–45.

Robertson EM, Theoret H, Pascual-Leone A (2003). Studies in cognition: the problems solved and created by transcranial magnetic stimulation. *Journal of Cognitive Neuroscience* 15, 948–60.

Sandel MJ (2002). What's wrong with enhancement. http://www.bioethics.gov/background/sandelpaper.html

Siebner HR, Tormos JM, Ceballos-Baumann AO, *et al.* (1999). Low-frequency repetitive transcranial magnetic stimulation of the motor cortex in writer's cramp. *Neurology* 52, 529–37.

Snyder AW, Mulcahy E, Taylor JL, Mitchell DJ, Sachdev P, Gandevia SC (2003). Savant-like skills exposed in normal people by suppressing the left fronto-temporal lobe. *Journal of Integrative Neuroscience* 2, 149–58.

Theoret H, Kobayashi M, Valero-Cabre A, and Pascual-Leone A (2003). Exploring paradoxical functional facilitation with TMS *Supplements to Clinical Neurophysiology* 56, 211–19.

Theoret H, Halligan E, Kobayashi M, Merabet L, Pascual-Leone A (2004). Unconscious modulation of motor cortex excitability revealed with transcranial magnetic stimulation. *Experimental Brain Research* 155, 261–4.

United States National Commission for the Protection of Human Subjects of Biomedical and Behavioral Research (1979). *Belmont Report: Ethical Principles and Guidelines for the Protection of Human Subjects Research.* Washington, DC: US Government Printing Office.

Wagner TA, Zahn M, Grodzinsky AJ, Pascual-Leone A (2004). Three-dimensional head model simulation of transcranial magnetic stimulation. *IEEE Transactions on Biomedical Engineering* 51, 1586–98.

Walsh V, Pascual-Leone A (2003). *Neurochronometrics of Mind: Transcranial Magnetic Stimulation in Cognitive Science.* Cambridge, MA: MIT Press.

Walter G, Tormos JM, Israel JA, Pascual-Leone A (2001). Transcranial magnetic stimulation in young persons: a review of known cases. *Journal of Child and Adolescent Psychopharmacology* 11, 69–75.

Wassermann EM (1998). Risk and safety in repetitive transcranial magnetic stimulation. *Electroencephalography and Clinical Neurophysiology* 108, 1–16.

Young RL, Ridding MC, Morrel TL (2004). 'Switching skills on by turning off parts of the brain' *Neurocase.* 2004 Jun; 10(3): 215–22.

Chapter 15

# Functional neurosurgical intervention: neuroethics in the operating room

Paul J. Ford and Jaimie M. Henderson

## Introduction

Evaluating ethics in neurosurgical practice requires a re-evaluation and recalibration of the analysis found in other areas of neuroethics. Neurosurgical practice adds complexities to the neuroethics discussion because of the structure of surgical teams, popular perceptions of surgery and surgeons, and the relatively transitory nature of patient–surgeon relationships. Although neurosurgical ethics does not constitute an ethic separate from general medical ethics, surgical ethics, or neuroethics, significant unique textures must be taken into account. Neuroethical issues discussed in other chapters of this book have relevance and must be recognized when evaluating ethically appropriate neurosurgical practices. For instance, the ethical implications of emerging neuroimaging cannot be ignored if neurosurgeons rely upon these images for guidance in surgery. Similarly, the issues of cognitive capacity must be understood in order to evaluate informed consent processes (see also Chapter 9). The interesting challenges come in integrating these concerns into the events of neurosurgery.

In order to focus the discussion even further, this chapter covers ethical challenges faced by surgeons practicing functional neurosurgery. The exploration of issues surrounding this set of surgeries presents especially interesting problems given the effects, potential or actual, on patient's quality of life in the attempt to restore or normalize a function. In order to elucidate these issues, we set the context by briefly discussing the special challenges of surgical ethics in general, define 'functional neurosurgery', and review the past, present, and expected future of functional neurosurgery. After setting this context, we address a variety of prominent ethical issues. We pay special attention to the context in which issues arise and reflect on ethical challenges to functional neurosurgery as a discipline.

## General surgical ethics

Until recently, particular ethical issues of surgery were largely ignored. Professional journals describe the need both to develop ethics curricula tailored specifically for surgical residents and to include more ethics discussions in journal publications (Hanlon 2004; Polk 2004) Regulations mandating ethics content in resident education have prompted further attention to the ethical issues of subspecialties such as surgery. In the small literature that exists, the established issues of surgical ethics include such things as:

> informed consent, confidentiality, advance directives, and the determination of death—through the range of surgical patients, from elective and high-risk patients to poor-risk and dying patients, to

intra-professional and inter-professional issues, surgical innovation and research, and financial aspects of surgery... (McCullough *et al.* 1998)

These elements play significant roles in the treatment of surgical patients. Given the complexities of patients and health care systems, there are no formulaic ways of addressing ethics problems for all cases. The surgeon and other relevant providers must first be able to identify when ethical challenges arise. The problems quoted above provide a valuable list of classes of potential problems. Subsequently, participants must reflect on and balance salient ethical features of each particular case in order to resolve identified dilemmas well.

The complex processes of surgery provide one type of ethical texture that should be considered. Surgical ethics begins at the time of a patient's referral and continues through postoperative follow-up. Ethical practice relates not only to activities in the operating room, but also to activities of accepting a patient for surgery, preoperative preparation, and post-operative care. Clearly, ethical considerations are fundamentally rooted in what will, is, or has happened in the operating room under the direction of the surgeon(s). However, those activities fall within the context of a temporally related group of activities. Many ethical dilemmas can be avoided by having appropriate preparation or good processes in place. Considering 'ethics in the operating room' means considering the ethics of practice for the entire time surrounding the actual operating room event.

Given the complexity of contemporary health care, surgeons navigate intricate webs of professional and patient relationships. The surgeon relies on the patient both as a patient and as a paying client (or at least as a billing unit). The surgeon relies on other physicians for referrals of potential surgical candidates and for collaboration in research. Conflicts of interest may take the form of financial incentives as well as professional obligations that may be contrary to patient interests. These matters must be transparent when considering surgical options, both in deciding the type of surgery as well as whether to offer any surgery.

Surgeons can be challenged in leading teams and in negotiating interprofessional roles. These complex roles include professional reputation as well as economic incentives. Ethical land mines litter the pathway of these interactions. Much of the surgeon's information relies on subspeciality advice and interpretation. In neurosurgery this can be the neurologist, neuroradiologist, neurophysiologist, or neuropsychologist. Surgeons need to acknowledge the influences, positive and negative, that these subspecialties may have on decision-making.

Further, in considering a patient's best interests and desires, surgeons must recognize the competing interests of patients and their social supports. Patients and their social supports interact with surgeons only during a relatively well-defined window of time. The swing of Western bioethics has been toward viewing patients as needing to make autonomous decisions that are uninfluenced by the interests of others. However, humans seldom make decisions isolated from a social structure and continue to have obligations to others throughout their lives. This translates into health care choices. Recognizing the important role of those who are relationally close (usually families/caregivers) in decision-making is important. (Seaburn *et al.* 2004) These relations can elucidate patient values and best interests given a particular social milieu (Neil-Dwyer *et al.* 2001). Although good ethical practice dictates that patients are not unduly influenced, i.e. coerced, this does not mean that patients should have their regular influences removed while giving consent for surgery. Generally, the small window of interface prior to surgery does not give the surgeon ample time to make a full evaluation of complex relations and how they interface with a patient's decision-making or health. Although surgical teams rely a great deal on referring physicians to identify these conflicts, it is important to watch for warning signs that ethical problems may be present. This is particularly true when dealing with 'functional' surgeries that have a potential to alleviate the caregiver's burden at the expense of other aspects of a patient's health.

The complex surgical dynamic also includes interface with pharmaceutical and device manufacturers. Conflicts of interest in commercial enterprises continue to concern many in the health care community (Trojanowski 1999; Morreim 2004). Balancing patient benefits, societal needs for collaborative work with industry to improve surgery, and commercial interests of companies and surgeons requires great care. Again, transparency and disclosure of conflicts of interest provide necessary, but not always sufficient, conditions for good ethical surgical practice.

Since the anatomy of individual patients and the surgical techniques of individual surgeons vary considerably, standards of practice can be difficult to characterize. Often a surgeon must improvise during surgery. Deciding whether the alterations are simply an exercise of professional judgment or part of a research innovation can be difficult. Those improvisations/innovations do not necessarily lend themselves well to standard research methods developed to govern drug development. These elements of surgical practice have given rise to discussions about appropriate process and regulation of innovative practices in surgery (Gillett 2000). A surgeon's professional prerogative to employ his skill and judgment in unique cases must be balanced against a need to generalize knowledge and provide best care for groups of patients.

Surgical education and training present challenges to informed consent, patient trust, and good individual care. In medical practice, treatment by a resident physician can usually easily be reviewed and reversed if necessary. However, in surgical procedures (as well as in some diagnostic medical procedures) errors are generally more difficult to reverse. This raises the challenge of training new surgeons while retaining patient safety and trust. Training provides a societal benefit that may have some cost to individuals. Although most training programs occur in high-volume centers, and recent correlations have been made between better outcomes and higher volumes of surgeries (Birkmeyer et al. 2002), significant issues remain about the level of disclosure to patients about who actually makes the incision that is ethically necessary.

Gaining informed consent for surgical procedures contains a number of generic challenges. First, a patient needs to have confidence in his surgeon while still understanding that complications may actually occur. This necessitates a balance of optimism with reality. Secondly, a surgeon should have confidence in his practice. Thirdly, the procedure itself may not have clear boundaries in duration or scope. The consent process should cover not only the actual time in the operating room, but also the preoperative evaluations and postoperative recovery. Finally, informed consent involves the patient's understanding and agreeing to go forward with the therapeutic modality and not simply signing a complex legal form. These elements apply to therapy as well as research in differing degrees. We will discuss this at greater length in the later section on neurosurgical ethics.

As addressed in the next section, functional brain surgery has an interesting and somewhat checkered past. When the brain is involved in surgery, there are special overlays of issues both technically and perceptively. Brain function remains somewhat mysterious, with small variations in individual brains making significant functional differences. Recognizing that the brain has a central importance in the organization of patients as persons makes performing brain surgery perceptively different from other types of surgeries. Given that cognition and independence are privileged traits in our cultural understandings, a sense of desperation can deeply influence patients in their desire to go forward with risky neurosurgical procedures or to decline relatively benign neurosurgical procedures. As we discuss in later sections, it can be difficult for patients to weigh the potential of a decrease in cognition, change in personality, or loss of memory as complications of surgeries. The public perceptions of neurological surgeries are deeply influenced by such stories as that of Phineas Gage, people waking after being 'brain dead', and the proliferation of frontal lobotomies (as described below). These elements add interesting textures to the ethics issues in functional neurosurgery, since they cultivate both fascination and distrust.

## Functional neurosurgery: past, present, and future

Functional neurosurgery aims to improve the function of the nervous system by altering the underlying physiology by either destruction or augmentation of the various pathways involved in normal nervous system function. This contrasts with anatomical procedures, in which anatomical lesions are removed regardless of the potential effect on the underlying function of the nervous system. As defined by Iskandar and Nashold (1995), there are six broad categories of functional disorder: abnormal involuntary movements, spasticity, pain, psychiatric disorders, epilepsy, and neuroendocrine disorders. The first five of these are most relevant to our discussion.

### Movement disorders

Surgeons began manipulation of the nervous system for the treatment of movement disorders around the turn of the twentieth century. In 1909, Sir Victor Horsley excised portions of the motor cortex in a patient with continuous uncontrolled involuntary movements (Horsley 1909). The patient's condition improved, ushering in the age of surgical treatment for movement disorders. Other surgeons, encouraged by Horsley's success, performed destructive procedures in other parts of the motor system with mixed success. Browder described sectioning the internal capsule via a transventricular approach. Unfortunately, this procedure universally created motor weakness and spasticity, and in the majority of cases the abnormal movements recurred with time. In 1939, Meyers resected the head of the caudate nucleus in a patient with tremor, with subsequent dramatic improvement in symptoms and no hemiparesis. He then embarked on a series of experiments in the destruction of various deep nuclei, achieving relatively good results but with a surgical mortality of 15 percent (Meyers 1958).

In 1952, Irving Cooper was performing a pedunculotomy in a patient with parkinsonian tremor when he accidentally severed the anterior choroidal artery, which supplies portions of the basal ganglia. He aborted the procedure and the patient subsequently awoke from surgery with marked reduction in tremor. This led Cooper to embark on a series of anterior choroidal artery ligations, with good relief of tremor in 65–75 percent of patients, but with a mortality rate 10 percent (Cooper 1954). Although these results strongly suggested that the basal ganglia could be an effective target for the treatment of movement disorders, it was clear that less invasive methods were necessary.

The use of precise mathematical methods for targeting deep-brain structures had previously been described by Horsley and Clarke (1908). Their apparatus for recording from the deep cerebellar nuclei in monkeys was based on skull landmarks and the relationship of these landmarks to an atlas of brain structures. The technique was called stereotactic surgery, a compound word derived from the Greek *stereos* (solid or three-dimensional) and the Latin *tactus* (to touch). Unfortunately, the variability of the human brain and skull prevented the use of such an apparatus for human neurosurgery until a method could be devised for relating the structure of the brain to the coordinate system of the stereotactic device. In the late 1940s, Spiegel and Wycis linked skull radiography with a stereotactic instrument to produce the first practical system for human stereotactic surgery (Spiegel *et al.* 1947). Other investigators soon followed suit, with rapid application of stereotactic techniques to the treatment of movement disorders.

Stereotactic interventions such as pallidotomy and thalamotomy soon became standard treatment for Parkinson's disease and tremor. Although their efficacy for the treatment of movement disorders was modest, the morbidity was relatively low compared with the highly invasive procedures that had preceded them. The landscape of Parkinson's disease treatment changed dramatically in the late 1960s with the introduction of L-dopa. Stereotactic surgery declined dramatically with the realization that L-dopa was both safer and more effective. However, the limitations of medication became apparent after years of treatment. Patients began to develop abnormal involuntary movements (dyskinesia) and wide fluctuations in motor symptoms. In the late 1980s, Laitinen re-introduced pallidotomy as an effective treatment for patients who had developed motor complications from medication (Laitinen *et al.* 1992). Stereotactic surgery for movement disorders again became viable.

Stimulation of the brain was first attempted in patients with chronic pain and psychiatric disorders (Heath and Mickle 1960). Several investigators reported on targets for pain, and patients had electrodes implanted which were intermittently stimulated. It had long been known that stimulation of a structure before lesioning could help predict the eventual effect of a particular lesion placement. It was this observation that led Benabid and colleagues to chronically implant electrodes into the thalamus of a patient who had a prior contralateral thalamotomy in order to avoid the known risks of bilateral lesioning (Benabid *et al.* 1987). By this time, technology had advanced to the point that a fully implantable stimulation system, based on cardiac pacemaker technology, was feasible. Chronic deep-brain stimulation has subsequently proved to be an effective treatment for medically refractory Parkinson's disease (Krack *et al.* 2003).

## Epilepsy

Surgery for epilepsy has been practiced since the early part of the nineteenth century, when trephination was used for post-traumatic epilepsy. However, epilepsy surgery truly began when the electrical nature of the brain was demonstrated convincingly in animal studies. Fritsch and Hitzig (1870) showed that stimulation of the motor cortex of the dog could cause movements of the contralateral body (Fritsch and Hitzig 1870), leading the way to Penfield's detailed studies of human motor and sensory function in the early twentieth century. The discovery of electroencephalography by Berger in 1929 was eventually validated in 1935 by Adrian and Matthews, with the result that epileptic foci could be reliably localized in the brain. Localization of function with recording and stimulation became commonplace (see also Chapter 11), and mapping procedures are now routinely carried out to characterize electrically responsive sites in patients undergoing brain surgery. In patients with pathology close to critical brain areas, these operations are often carried out with the patient awake, allowing test stimulation of such vital functions as speech, vision, and cognition. Resective surgeries for epilepsy have a significant range of invasiveness that includes corpus callosotomy (a disconnection of communication between hemispheres), lesionectomy, lobectomy, and hemispherectomy.

## Pain

Pain is an integral part of human experience. Thus it is not surprising that attempts to treat pain date back to the beginning of recorded history. For instance, electric fish were used by the ancient Egyptians after it was discovered that electric shocks could relieve pain. Several societies, including the Assyrians, Babylonians, and Egyptians, practiced trephination and other physical procedures.

Pain treatment advanced very little during the Middle Ages, although electrotherapy, massage, and exercise were still practiced. The roots of contemporary surgical treatment of pain can be traced back to a report by Ambroise Paré (1598):

> In the course of bleeding King Charles IX for the smallpox, Antoine Portail's lancet had injured a superficial nerve with the production of intense pain and contraction of the arm. After more than three months of suffering the king happily recovered, but Paré stated in his commentary that, had other remedies not been successful, he was prepared to use boiling oil in the wound or to have severed the nerve completely...Maréchal, surgeon to Louis XIV, inaugurated neurotomies for tic douloureux toward the end of the seventeenth century. (White and Sweet 1955)

The beginning of a modern understanding of pain has been attributed to Descartes, who produced the first depiction of the pain pathway as a string connecting the skin to the brain. As knowledge of neuroanatomy and neurophysiology grew, the existence of a separate pathway dedicated to pain became more clearly defined. Many different types of destructive procedure were designed to interrupt these pathways, with greater or lesser efficacy depending on the painful disorder being treated. These ablative procedures sometimes produce lasting cures, but more frequently merely add a sensory deficit without relieving pain.

In 1965, Melzack and Wall published their influential gate control theory which revolutionized the understanding and treatment of pain (Melzack and Wall 1965). Simply stated, the theory describes a gating mechanism in the spinal cord by which painful stimuli can be overridden by innocuous stimuli. By electrically stimulating sensory nerves, this gate can be 'closed', leading to pain relief. This theory formed the basis for peripheral nerve and spinal cord stimulation, which have been successfully used to treat a wide variety of neuropathic pain syndromes.

Even before these experiments, neurosurgeons had learned that stimulation of the central nervous system could alleviate pain. Heath (1954) reported pain relief in patients who had undergone stimulation of the septal region for treatment of psychiatric disorders. Mazars et al. (1960) used anatomical knowledge of nociceptive pathways to devise a procedure to stimulate the termination of the spinothalamic tract in the thalamus. This technique was later used by several investigators to treat many types of neuropathic pain. For a time, deep-brain stimulation was used for a variety of pain syndromes. Despite reasonably good successes in some conditions, there was insufficient evidence to support its widespread use for the treatment of pain, and the FDA re-classified deep-brain stimulation for pain as an experimental procedure (Bendok and Levy 1998).

## Psychiatric disorders

The treatment of psychiatric disorders may arguably have been among the first uses of neurosurgery. Stone age skulls have been found with well-healed trephinations, and written records of trephining to release demons or evil humors date back to 1500bc (Feldman and Goodrich 2001). However, intentional lesioning of the brain to treat psychiatric disorders was based on observations in patients who had sustained brain injuries with subsequent changes in personality. Perhaps the most famous case of this type is that of Phineas Gage, a 25-year-old railroad worker. On 13 September 1848, an accidental explosion drove a 3 cm steel rod into his left cheek, through both frontal lobes, and out through the skull near the sagittal suture. He was treated by a local physician, John Harlow, who reported the case in a letter to the *New England Journal of Medicine* in 1848 (Harlow 1848). According to Harlow, Gage's personality was now

> ... fitful, irreverent, indulging at times in the grossest profanity (which was not previously his custom), manifesting but little deference for his fellows, impatient of restraint or advice when it conflicts with his desires, at times pertinaciously obstinate, yet capricious and vacillating, devising many plans of future operation, which they are no sooner arranged than they are abandoned in turn for others appearing more feasible.

Observations in patients such as Gage, coupled with experimental work showing specialization of the cerebral cortex in laboratory animals (Fritsch and Hitzig 1870), led to the consideration of surgical interventions for psychiatric disease in humans. Gottlieb Burckhardt was the first investigator to publish the results of cortical excision for psychiatric disease. In his initial report of six patients, three were considered successes, two considered partially successful, and one patient died (Burckhardt 1891). Burckhardt's results were not received enthusiastically, and he performed no further operations. However, the social climate of the early 1900s provided a fertile environment for the further development of surgical procedures for psychiatric disease.

In the early years of the twentieth century, there were few available treatments for patients with psychiatric illness. Asylums became overcrowded, and physicians caring for the hundreds of thousands of intractable patients were desperate for any method which might offer hope of returning them to a useful life. Thus, when Egas Moniz introduced prefrontal leucotomy in 1935 (Moniz 1937), there was widespread enthusiasm for the procedure. Moniz eventually won the Nobel Prize for the development of this surgical technique, and frontal lobe surgery was heralded by the popular press. In 1936, Freeman and Watts performed the first lobotomy in the United States. By 1942 they had performed 200 lobotomies, with a reported 63 percent of patients showing improvement (Freeman and Watts 1942). At about this time, Freeman developed a technique for performing lobotomies using an icepick-like device called an orbitoclast. The instrument was introduced through the orbit with a mallet, and the frontal lobe was severed with a back-and-forth movement. The entire procedure took only 15–20 min, and Freeman visited hundreds of hospitals and asylums performing thousands of lobotomies. Non-surgeons and even personnel without medical training began performing the procedure, with the result that 60 000 psychosurgical procedures were performed between 1936 and 1956. Because of the indiscriminate use of psychosurgical procedures, many neurosurgeons and psychiatrists began expressing grave concerns that presaged the eventual abandonment of psychiatric surgery in all but a few centers. The introduction of chlorpromazine in 1954 provided a medical alternative which was safer, cheaper, and more effective than the available surgical options, and marked the beginning of the end for psychosurgery (Feldman and Goodrich 2001).

## The future of functional neurosurgery

Future advances in functional neurosurgery grow from two major parallel avenues of investigation: understanding of brain function and advances in therapeutic interventions. Although major progress has been made in the understanding of neurodegenerative diseases, our knowledge of the intricacies of brain functions such as movement, speech, cognition, and perception remain woefully inadequate. As basic science research reveals more precisely how these systems function normally and how they fail, targets for therapeutic interventions will become evident. Stem cell transplantation, gene therapy, and targeted delivery of medications will continue to advance in sophistication, with the eventual goal of complete restoration of normal nervous system structure and function. Marked advances in technology for brain–machine interfaces have already led to paralyzed persons controlling devices by brain signals alone, i.e. implantable chips. This technology will advance to the point not only of restoring lost brain function, but also of augmenting the function of the normally functioning brain. Ethical concerns will thus play an ever-increasing role as our power to affect the function of the nervous system continues to grow at a rapid pace.

## Ethics in functional neurosurgery

The review of growth of functional neurosurgery and surgical ethics now allows for a further discussion of particular ethical challenges. The selected topics below give a brief account of challenges faced in functional neurosurgery that add further detail to some of the issues raised in general surgical ethics. Similar to all surgical ethics, informed consent and balancing of risks and benefits are central. Equal to these in importance are societal and research issues as further functional neurosurgical procedures and devices develop.

### Informed consent

Informed consent is a continuous activity formally signified by a document or an initial conversation, i.e. informed consent involves a continuous agreement to go forward with a particular treatment modality. A patient or surrogate must be informed of all relevant information, voluntarily wish to proceed, and have the capacity to understand the implications of the particular decision (Scarrow and Scarrow 2002). The burden of consent varies depending on a number of factors that include potential benefits, risks, degree of understanding, and time sensitivity. The level of consent required in order for a patient to agree to a procedure also varies depending on whether the procedure deals with research, therapy, or some combination thereof. Most functional neurosurgeries are elective procedures for a chronic or degenerative disorder. They are elective in that they are not life saving (although selected epilepsy surgeries have the potential to decrease mortality rates from seizures). Since the problems corrected by functional neurosurgery involve the central nervous system, and the central nervous system influences the way people think, evaluating a patient's capacity to make decisions can be difficult. As discussed below, this becomes even trickier when the potential risks involve psychological impairment or cognitive loss as well as motor or sensory loss. The psychological state of a patient who has functional impairments, especially chronic pain, can make a robust informed consent process challenging.

Neurosurgeons perform some functional neurosurgical procedures while the patient remains awake. This is done for preservation of valued patient function through brain mapping or to evaluate the most effective placement of stimulators and lesions. The most common instances of awake craniotomies involve resections near the eloquent or motor cortices for tumors or focal epilepsy and lesioning or deep-brain stimulation for movement disorders. Revoking consent during awake surgery provides an interesting vehicle to elucidate a number of ethical challenges to informed consent, since the patient may attempt to revoke consent in the midst of the surgical procedure. During most of these awake surgeries, the patient retains a significant level of decision-making capacity. If a patient requests that the surgery be discontinued, the surgeon must make a number of important decisions about whether to halt the procedure and, if so, how quickly and in what way. In reacting to this situation, the surgeon could invoke 'therapeutic privilege' in order to override the need for patient consent to continue. This is a paternalistic principle that allows a medical practitioner to ignore the patient's wishes for some obvious and greater good. Although it is seldom appropriate to invoke therapeutic privilege, in a clearly harmful situation it can be utilized. Since functional neurosurgery usually involves quality of life rather than mortality prevention, this invocation does not generally apply. However, before allowing a patient to halt such a procedure, the surgeon has an ethical obligation to inform the patient of the potential loss of benefit, be certain that the patient is reasonable in his request, and make it clear to the patient that the surgery can only be discontinued in a safe manner. In this way, the surgeon looks for an informed revocation of consent. If the surgeon believes that the surgery has not been the cause of a temporary loss of capacity and that the patient is making an informed revocation, then he must decide whether halting the procedure would egregiously harm the patient. If halting the procedure can be performed safely, there is not a significant increase in mortality risk, and halting would not constitute an unacceptable deviation from standards of practice, then the surgeon is on weak ethical grounds if he continues. It must be understood that a particular expression of a desire to stop does not force the surgeon to discontinue the procedure. Clear procedures should be in place and known by the patient regarding how this type of expression will be handled.

This instance of intraoperative revocation of consent provides an example of the challenges of ethics in the operating room as well as prior to the instance. In the midst of surgery is a poor time to attempt to make an important ethical decision because of time constraints and stress. However, the surgeon still needs to undertake a quick balancing of harms, benefits, respect for persons, and justice to the degree possible. Once this instance arises once in the operating room, it is important to review the processes in place for consent to elucidate whether better ways may be implemented to avoid this dilemma.

The question of how to handle a request to halt surgery becomes slightly more complex when part of the neurosurgery involves a research protocol. Generally consent can be more easily revoked during research procedures than during proven therapeutic endeavors. The researcher/surgeon performing the procedure under a protocol needs to be concerned with what parts of the remaining surgery have known benefit and what parts are experimental. These elements should be clearly outlined in the informed consent process and rediscussed as the surgeon evaluates an informed revocation. As mentioned above in the section on general surgical ethics, good process and preparation can help to avoid these types of problems in both the therapeutic and research areas.

At times, functional neurosurgery involves the implantation of devices that modulate neural functioning. Those neuromodulators may have side effects that have a detrimental impact on a patient's social life without the patient having the ability to recognize the change as a problem. For instance, an induced mania may make a patient feel great, but impair his quality of life because of severely impaired decision-making. An internal device is somewhat different from psychiatric medications that can be discontinued without the consent of the patient. This poses a conflict between medical paternalism and patient autonomy in who controls the settings of the internal device. To avoid these issues, consent should be sought in advance for follow-up and postoperative care. The ethical questions about functional neurosurgical devices continue to evolve alongside the technological advances. The implementation of 'Ulysses contracts', documents that waive the right to change one's mind, may be well intentioned but are not generally enforceable. A competent patient's ability to control his body remains and cannot be waived.

Between control of programming neuromodulators and revocation of intraoperative consent, many neurosurgical programs build safeguards into patient selection criteria to exclude patients at risk of either declining to continue surgery or refusing to have stimulator settings altered. Since there are no definitive tests to predict whether a patient will change his mind or will not be able to handle a surgery, a justice question arises about unfairly excluding patients who would not be a problem balanced against including patients who would have a problem. For instance, excluding all parkinsonian patients with an anxiety disorder from neuromodulation would exclude many patients who only have a very mild anxiety directly related to their frustrations about lack of function. This blanket exclusion would probably not be appropriate since many patients with mild anxiety have had no problems undergoing awake procedures. However, too lax a restriction would cause patients with severe anxiety to undergo only partial operations. Neurosurgical ethics includes the careful and consistent selection of patients who are likely to continue to consent to the entire process of therapy.

Finally, functional neurosurgery often comprises last-chance therapy for patients. These are often experimental or off-label procedures. The desperation of a patient in intractable pain, who can no longer care for himself because of Parkinson's disease, or who cannot leave his house because of obsessive–compulsive disorder should not be underestimated. Although desperation does not necessarily cause a patient to formally fall into the 'vulnerable population', health care providers should be particularly careful that patients have full understanding of the risks and that the health care provider undertakes the procedure with good conscience.

## Risk–benefit: the surgeon's responsibility beyond informed consent

Although informed consent constitutes the bedrock of current ethical practice, informed consent does not make everything permissible or required. Ethical guidelines for health care always include some articulation of a responsibility to benefit patients and to avoid harming them (beneficence/non-malfeasance). In this way, neurosurgeons have obligations to use professional judgments in excluding patients from surgery even if patients or their families demand the procedure. There are limits to patients' choices, just as there are limits to surgeons' paternalism. The above discussion of therapeutic privilege begins to address this point. There are at least two very difficult types of scenarios that demonstrate these limits: suspicion of psychogenic causes and innovation.

Psychogenic causes of diseases provide particularly difficult confounding elements to functional neurosurgery for a number of reasons. First, a psychogenic cause of a functional problem may be wrongly classified as non-organic simply by means of elimination of known organic causes. Secondly, there may be an organic disease present with a psychogenic overlay. For most neurofunctional disorders, there exists no definitive way of deciphering whether a disease is primarily psychogenic or organic. Fortunately, with regard to epilepsy surgery there are clear correlations between EEG patterns and epileptic seizures (Kellinghaus *et al.* 2004; Papavasiliou *et al.* 2004) By careful evaluation, psychogenic seizures can be distinguished from actual seizures. However, diseases such as dystonia, Tourette's syndrome, or trigeminal neuralgia do not have clear physiological indications to discriminate psychogenicity. These present true ethical dilemmas where values come into conflict. The surgeon does not want to keep beneficial therapy from those who could have their suffering alleviated. Also, the surgeon does not want to unnecessarily harm patients for whom no real chance of benefit may be obtained from the surgery. These must be balanced in some way by the surgeon, given informed consent does not dissolve the problem.

The above ethical dilemma could be avoided by developing better ways of differentiating organic from psychogenic causes. Two types of patient deception need ethical mention in this respect. First, a team may consider performing the procedure, or some semblance of it, as a placebo. However, a placebo effect may be very transitory, given the risk of transference of cured symptoms to other manifestations. Given the risks of many functional neurosurgical procedures, this risk–benefit does not generally balance. Secondly, an evaluation using deception may be considered. This may be ethically acceptable, but the patient still needs to be informed to the degree possible while still making the evaluation effective. For example, a patient could be told: 'Sometimes I will be giving you a test of pills that actually do not contain medication'. A great deal of uncertainty may still exist even with the use of the second type of deception. Neurosurgeons must balance elements of risks and benefits in light of significant uncertainty.

Our society's strong belief in 'doing' must be balanced with recognizing the limits of our abilities. This belief invokes the metaphor of galloping in on a white horse with a last-ditch effort to apply an innovative procedure. Relating back to the history of functional neurosurgery, we should question the risk–benefit ratio of Meyer's resections of the head of the caudate nucleus to reduce tremor. His mortality rate of 15 percent appears unjustifiable in comparison with the potential benefits (see above). Likewise, Cooper's anterior choroidal artery ligation with a mortality rate of 10 percent appears to have unbalanced risks. Just because a patient's tremor has been refractory to all known effective treatments does not mean that we should try procedures that have not been shown to be effective or that have significant mortality risks. This is particularly true when the functional neurosurgery is primarily a cosmetic neurosurgery for social purposes. These are considerations of risk–benefit as well as appropriate processes for innovating.

A surgeon may ethically turn down a patient for surgery based on conscience or professional judgment that risks are unbalanced. When a surgeon comes to this conclusion he must then decide whether or not to help the patient to find a surgeon who will perform the surgery. An example would be a pain patient asking for his arm to be amputated when the surgeon is convinced that amputation would not help, would be outside standard surgical practice, and would be harmful to the patient. The ethical values to be balanced in these cases revolve around patient abandonment, professional obligation to facilitate patient transfer, and not being party to unnecessary patient harm.

## Societal consideration: economics and enhancement

Functional neurosurgeries, especially those involving complex devices, can be very expensive. All health care systems have limits to resources with implicit or explicit rationing built into the systems. As a matter of social justice, explicit conversations need to take place concerning which patients should have priority. Much of this depends on selecting a view of justice/fairness. For some, the sickest patients impose greater obligations on us to relieve their suffering than those who are less sick. Others would take the stance that the less sick can be maintained as active workers and members of society and thus will benefit everyone by keeping them more functional. Yet others would consider justice as being served by random selection from all of those who could garner some benefit from the intervention. One example of explicit rationing is the Australian governmental advisory committee report that recommends supplying deep-brain stimulators only for the sickest Parkinson's patients. This is recommended because the system could not afford to have everyone receive the treatment modality (Medical Services Advisory Committee 2001). Explicit recognition and discussion of the underlying views of justice conform to good ethical standards. Societal costs of futile neurosurgical interventions need to be balanced against our respect for patient preferences and goals (Toms 1993).

A particularly interesting subquestion of rationing involves whether a patient with a terminal condition should receive expensive functional neurosurgery if it will provide palliation for only a matter of months. Many deem this to be cost ineffective and thus an unethical use of resources. Yet, many surgeries could conceivably enhance a person's life for that short period through improvement in cognition or physical mobility. Any guiding ethical principle keeping terminal patients from these surgeries needs to be consistent with criteria for non-terminal patients, which would include the length of potential benefit. This is not only an economic concern, but also a concern for the amount of operative harm/suffering persons should be exposed to when they have a limited life expectancy. This question resides at the intersection of societal interests, individual autonomy, and professional judgments of risk and benefit.

The newest and most innovative treatment may not be the most effective or have the most responsible cost–benefit ratio. This can be seen in the aggressive use of spinal instrumentation (plates, screws, and pins) as well as robotic or stereotactic surgery. Often device companies aggressively market products to surgeons and patients (Trojanowski 1999). Patients will often believe that the newest and highest technology solution is the most effective solution. The efficacy of the surgery depends a great deal on the comfort and training of a surgeon, i.e. the tool is only as good as the workman. Although industry provides an important component for improvement in neurosurgical intervention, there are ethical challenges to the degree of influence that companies have on patient and surgeon decision-making.

Enhancing function by means of neurosurgery provides the final social issue of this section. Surgery's goal is to improve patients' lives. In general, functional surgery aims at alleviating suffering and restoring function to a 'normal' state. However, some of the procedures now, or in the future, could be adapted to enhance one's abilities beyond the normal. Like genetic enhancement, concerns involve social injustice, devaluation of traits within boundaries historically considered to be normal, uncertainty about long-term consequences, and use of resources for unnecessary or vain purposes (Parens 1998). These questions of enhancement and justice figure prominently in the development of future neurosurgical innovations.

## Research and innovation

Improvements in functional neurosurgery have depended on experimentation, innovation, and often leaps of faith. As with all research, current functional neurosurgery research is expected to comply with principles articulated in the *Declaration of Helsinki* (World Medical Association 2002) and the *Belmont Report* (United States National Commission 1979). In reviewing the history of functional neurosurgery, it becomes apparent that these principles have not always strongly held sway in practice. The processes that brought about many of the improvements and breakthroughs in neurosurgery would no longer be considered ethically justified. Current regulations are much more stringent on the ways in which innovation can take place. There is an expectation that a surgeon will not explore brain areas unrelated to the immediate purpose of the operation during procedures, and that there will be a clear preoperative explanation of the planned surgery, i.e. informed consent, and good evidence for a positive risk–benefit ratio.

Ethical issues in research on functional neurosurgery differ greatly from many other types of human systems since the brain remains imperfectly understood, there is significant variation in the mapping of functional locations between individuals brains, and the brain is central to a person's identity and cognition. Although functional imaging, such as functional MRI, continues to help surgeons map individual patient's brains better, a great deal remains unknown (see Chapter 11). Because of the complexity of human brains, animal models can be of only limited help. This complexity has kept us from having a robust and accurate theoretical foundation on which to build research. Functional neurosurgical research often occurs through happenstance or clinical observation of what works. Historically, this is exemplified by Cooper's accidental severing of an artery and Benabid's application of continuous electrical stimulation. Finally, because of the high cost of research and the difficulty in standardizing surgical procedures across institutions, the research agenda of functional neurosurgery is plagued with small numbers of enrolled patients which poses challenges to the generalizability of research results. Many surgical devices are approved after relatively small trials and thus fairly weak evidence (Bhandari *et al.* 2004). All these elements make these research endeavors fraught with ethical challenges of providing good generalizable data in an efficient and beneficial way that minimizes harm.

An editorial exchange between Cosgrove and Aouizerate and colleagues provides an example of the types of challenges to expanding functional neurosurgical practice by means of research. In discussing a case report on the effectiveness of deep-brain stimulation for medically refractory obsessive–compulsive disorder with severe depression, Cosgrove (2004) warns of the challenges in appropriately performing further research while urging researchers to grasp this opportunity to learn more: 'These early efforts must go forward only with the highest ethical, moral, and scientific standards to ensure that this historic opportunity is not wasted'. Aouizerate *et al.* (2004) respond with a list of ethically necessary conditions to perform the research. Two conditions of particular interest are 'DBS [deep-brain stimulation] procedures being performed by extensively experienced neurosurgical teams' and 'collaboration of multi-disciplinary investigative teams'. Part of the backdrop of these cautionary comments includes the worry that a technique will be adopted before being fully and rigorously explored. Historical examples of technologies being adopted too hastily include Moniz's leucotomy and Horsley's motor cortex excisions (discussed above). Cosgrove shows an intense curiosity and belief that the potential to explore new therapies should not be lost, while still tempering this with good processes that protect patients. This example is textured even further given the challenges of past psychosurgery. Moving forward in neurosurgical research needs to be cognizant of the accusations of past attempts at social control as well as overzealous application (Pressman 1998; Fins 2003).

Research methods in functional neurosurgery themselves create significant challenges. Double-blind placebo-controlled trials, derived from pharmaceutical research, have become the gold standard for research in general. Recent studies, such as the transplantation of fetal cells for Parkinson's disease, have further supported the usefulness of placebos in neurosurgical research. The use of placebos allows for a very robust type of knowledge. However, there are lesser types of knowledge that can be usefully gained without placebos that minimize harm to human subjects. A great deal of debate surrounding placebo procedures in neurosurgical research continues (Bernat 2002). More appropriate for most types of surgery is either the use of historical controls or the implementation of a cross-over designs where a device is turned on or off.

Even before ethical research methods come into play, a research question must be selected. There are ethical challenges regarding which questions are worth pursing and what priority is given to the various worthy research questions. Restoring function to something like a normal state is a type of enhancement for an individual. If a person can have their function enhanced to a normal state, is it appropriate to research ways of enhancing function to a greater than normal state. The ethical question comes in how many resources should be applied to technologies that will make average people's lives better instead of focusing on improving the lives of those who endure horrible suffering or lack average functions. Again, this question involves a stance on what justice means in this context.

An equivalent issue to the funding of enhancement research lies in the problems of orphan diseases. Functional neurological diseases that are rare may not be lucrative for industry to explore. Hence these diseases may be ignored even if patients suffer horribly. It is important that research agendas maximize the general good, be economically viable, and address those who suffer most. Treatment for orphan neurological diseases should not be ignored in favor of more lucrative diseases. The open ethical question is: Who funds these very expensive neurosurgical trials?

Finally, there is the question of convenience and exploration outside a protocol during a surgery, i.e. exploring brain areas unrelated to the immediate purpose of the operation. These explorations need to conform to best current standards of practice and should be avoided unless they are either under protocol or for the individual patient's best interest. This means respecting the need for review boards to vet research, while recognizing that review boards depend on individual researchers/innovators to consider carefully the burden of risk of each change and evaluation of standard practice.

## Conclusion

Functional neurosurgeons must be cognizant of a multitude of ethical concerns in standard practice, innovation, and research. The privileged status of the brain, the uncertainty involved in outcomes, and the complexity of cases add significant textures to the ethical concerns of functional neurosurgery. The ethical issues cannot be reduced to or solved by impeccable informed consent or some formulaic ethics process. Good standards of practice need to be developed, and surgical teams need to be attentive in identifying special ethics problems. The further development of functional neurosurgery needs to be undertaken with a clear understanding of the costs and ethical implications.

## References

Aouizerate B, Cuny E, Guehl D, Burbaud P (2004). Response to: Deep brain stimulation and psychosurgery. *Journal of Neurosurgery* 101, 575–6.

Benabid AL, Pollak P, Louveau A, Henry S, de Rougemont J (1987). Combined (thalamotomy and stimulation) stereotactic surgery of the VIM thalamic nucleus for bilateral Parkinson disease. *Applied Neurophysiology* 50, 344–6.

Bendok B, Levy RM (1998). Brain stimulation for persistent pain management. In Gildenberg PL, Tasker RR (eds) *Textbook of Stereotactic and Functional Neurosurgery*. New York: McGraw-Hill, 1539–46.

Bernat J (2002). *Ethical Issues in Neurology* (2nd edn). Boston, MA: Butterworth Heinemann, 469–94.

Bhandari M, Busse JW, Jackowski D, *et al.* (2004). Association between industry funding and statistically significant pro-industry findings in medical and surgical randomized trials. *Canadian Medical Association Journal* 170, 477–80.

Birkmeyer JD, Siewers AE, Finlayson EV, *et al.* (2002). Hospital volume and surgical mortality in the United States. *New England Journal of Medicine* 346, 1128–37.

Burckhardt G (1891). Uber Rindenexcisionen, als Beitrag zur operativen Therapie der Psychosen. *Allgemeine Zeitschrift für Psychiatrie psychischgerichtliche Medizin* 47, 463–548.

Cooper IS (1954). Surgical occlusion of the anterior choroidal artery in parkinsonism. *Surgical Gynecology and Obstetrics* 99, 207–19.

Cosgrove GR (2004). Deep brain stimulation and psychosurgery. *Journal of Neurosurgery* 101, 574–5.

Feldman RP, Goodrich JT (2001). Psychosurgery: a historical overview. *Neurosurgery* **48**, 647–59.

Fins JJ (2003). From psychosurgery to neuromodulation and palliation: history's lessons for the ethical conduct and regulation of neuropsychiatric research. *Neurosurgery Clinics of North America* **14**, 303–19.

Freeman W, Watts J (1942). *Psychosurgery: Intelligence, Emotion and Social Behavior Following Prefrontal Lobotomy for Mental Disorders.* Springfield, IL: Charles C. Thomas.

Fritsch G, Hitzig E (1870). Uber die elektrische Erregbarkeit des Grosshirns. *Archives of Anatomical Physiology* **37**, 300–32.

Gillett G (2000). How should we test and improve neurosurgical care? In: Zemam A, Emanuel L (eds) *Ethical Dilemmas in Neurology.* London: Harcourt Brace, 87–100.

Hanlon CR (2004). Surgical ethics. *American Journal Surgery* **187**, 1–2.

Harlow JM (1848). Recovery from the passage of an iron bar through the head. *Boston Medical and Surgical Journal* **39**, 389–92.

Heath RG (1954). *Studies in Schizophrenia.* Cambridge, MA: Harvard University Press.

Heath RG, Mickle WA (1960). Evaluation of 7 years' experience with depth electrode studies in human patients. In: Ramey ER, O'Doherty DS (eds) *Electrical Studies in Anesthetized Brain.* New York: Harper and Row, 214–17.

Horsley V (1909). The function of the so-called motor area of the brain. *British Medical Journal* **2**, 1286–92.

Horsley V, Clarke RH (1908). The structure and functions of the cerebellum examined by a new method. *Brain* **31**, 45–124.

Iskandar BJ, Nashold BS Jr (1995). History of functional neurosurgery. *Neurosurgery Clinics of North America* **6**, 1–25.

Kellinghaus C, Loddenkemper T, Dinner DS, Lachhwani D, Luders HO (2004). Non-epileptic seizures of the elderly. *Journal of Neurology* **251**, 704–9.

Krack P, Batir A, Blercom NV, *et al.* (2003). Five-year follow-up of bilateral stimulation of the subthalamic nucleus in advanced Parkinson's disease. *New England Journal of Medicine* **349**, 1925–34.

Laitinen LV, Bergenheim AT, Hariz MI (1992). Leksell's posteroventral pallidotomy in the treatment of Parkinson's disease. *Journal of Neurosurgery* **76**, 53–61.

McCullough LB, Jones JW, Brody BA (1998). Principles and practice of surgical ethic. In: McCullough LB, Jones JW, Brody BA (eds) *Surgical Ethics.* New York: Oxford University Press, 3–14.

Mazars G, Roge R, Mazars Y (1960). Stimulation of the spinothalamic fasciculus and their bearing on the pathophysiology of pain. *Revue du Practicien* **103**, 136–8.

Melzack R, Wall PD (1965). Pain mechanisms: a new theory. *Science* **150**, 108–9.

Medical Services Advisory Committee (2001). *Deep Brain Stimulation for the Symptoms of Parkinson's Disease.* Canberra, Australia: MSAC.

Meyers R (1958). Historical background and personal experiences in the surgical relief of hyperkinesia and hypertonus. In Fields WS (ed) *Pathogenesis and Treatment of Parkinsonism.* Springfield, IL: Charles C Thomas, 229–70.

Moniz E (1937). Prefrontal leucotomy in the treatment of mental disorders. *American Journal of Psychiatry* **93**, 1379–87.

Morreim HE (2004) High-profile research and the media: the case of the AbioCor artifical heart. *Hastings Center Report* **34**, 11–24.

Neil-Dwyer G, Dorthey L, Garfield J (2001). The realities of postoperative disability and the carer's burden. *Annals of the Royal College of Surgeons of England* **83**, 2145–8.

Papavasiliou A, Vassilaki N, Paraskevoulakos E, Kotsalis C, Bazigou H, Bardani I (2004). Psychogenic status epilepticus in children. *Epilepsy and Behavior* **5**, 539–46.

Parens E (1998). Is better always good? The Enhancement Project. In: Parens E (ed) *Enhancing Human Traits: Ethical and Social Implications.* Washington, DC: Georgetown University Press, 1–28.

Polk HC (2004). Is ATLS a mechanism for teaching core competency in ethics? *American Journal of Surgery* **187**, 6.

Pressman JD (1998). Epilogue: the new synthesis. *Last Resort: Psychosurgery and the Limits of Medicine*. New York: Cambridge University Press, 401–42.

Scarrow AM, Scarrow MR (2002). Informed consent for the neurosurgeon. *Surgical Neurology* **57**, 63–8.

Seaburn DB, McDaniel SH, Kim S, Bassen D (2004). The role of the family in resolving bioethical dilemmas: clinical insights from a family systems perspective. *Journal of Clinical Ethics* **15**, 263–75.

Spiegel EA, Wycis HT, Marks M, Lee AJ (1947). Stereotactic apparatus for operations on the human brain. *Science* **106**, 349–50.

Toms SA (1993). Outcome predictors in the early withdrawal of life support: issues of justice and allocation for the severely brain injured. *Journal of Clinical Ethics* **4**, 206–11.

Trojanowski T (1999). New technologies and methods in neurosurgery—ethical dilemmas. *Acta Neurochirurgica*, **74**, 83–87.

United States National Commission for the Protection of Human Subjects of Biomedical and Behavioral Research (1976). *Psychosurgery*. Washington, DC: US Government Printing Office.

United States National Commission for the Protection of Human Subjects of Biomedical and Behavioral Research (1979). *Belmont Report: Ethical Principles and Guidelines for the Protection of Human Subjects Research*. Washington, DC: US Government Printing Office.

White JC, Sweet WH (1955). *Pain: Its Mechanisms and Surgical Control*. Springfield, IL: Charles C Thomas.

World Medical Association (2002). *Declaration of Helsinki: Ethical Principles for Medical Research Involving Human Subjects. World Medical Association General Assembly, Washington 2002*. New York: World Medical Association.

Chapter 16

# Clinicians, patients, and the brain

Robert Klitzman

## Introduction

Neuroethical issues pose a series of significant challenges for physicians and patients in clinical settings. Physicians play important roles as gatekeepers in the use of neurotechnology, and face dilemmas in ordering and interpreting neurodiagnostic tests, initiating and continuing treatments, prognosticating, making other clinical assessments, and communicating and interacting with patients concerning these and related decisions. Increasingly, these challenges confront neurologists and psychiatrists, primary care doctors, family doctors, internists, nurses, and others. How will health care providers view and approach advances in neurotechnology and the ethical challenges that these developments pose? The growing field of translational medicine has faced challenges and controversy about how bench *versus* patient-oriented research should be emphasized and integrated into clinical practice (Bigio and Bown 2004; Schechter *et al.* 2004). Given the numerous medical and psychosocial factors involved, technological advances need to be incorporated appropriately into clinical care, neither too slowly nor too swiftly, with sensitivity to how patients and providers perceive these advances.

Specific challenges further depend on the nature of different brain diseases, from psychiatric conditions such as depression, schizophrenia, and personality disorders, to neurological disorders such as dementia, and those with genetic or infectious etiologies. However, the ethical issues involved cut across diagnostic categories. In general, ethical issues in psychiatry and neurology have been the subjects of long and distinguished scholarship (Applebaum *et al.* 1987). Neuroethics blends with these two older fields. Yet to discuss all the ethical issues that arise in neurology and psychiatry is beyond the scope of this chapter. In psychiatry alone, clinical ethical challenges have been the subject of textbooks over many decades (Stone 1984) that have examined a range of issues such as assessments of capacity to make informed decisions about starting or terminating treatments, criteria for the insanity defense in legal settings, and criteria for involuntary hospitalization and treatment. Aspects of these issues may be included within neuroethics, depending on how that term is construed, especially as neurotechnologies advance understandings of the biological bases of psychiatric and neurological disorders.

In this chapter, I will focus on where and how several key neuroethical issues converge and diverge in diagnosis and treatment. First, I will examine the broad obstacles that exist to addressing neuroethical problems optimally in clinical settings. Secondly, I will explore ways that these barriers manifest themselves specifically in diagnostic tests that use neuroimaging and neurogenomics, and other clinical scenarios that involve treatment interventions. I will discuss several sets of predicaments that appear likely to emerge, although others will no doubt confront clinicians as neurotechnology continues to advance. Some of the areas examined below may dovetail with those explored elsewhere in this volume. However, it is important to view these neuroethical issues through the prism of doctor–patient interactions in order to understand how the issues are perceived and molded within the complex and nuanced dynamics of physician–patient encounters.

## Neuroethics challenges in the clinical setting

In general, doctors and patients confront a number of institutional and personal obstacles to approaching neuroethical issues optimally. In the current health care system, physicians often have little time to spend with patients to communicate or to discuss patient misunderstandings that arise. Managed care does not cover costs of all tests equally, and this limitation can shape which diagnostic or therapeutic procedures physicians choose. The rise of the Internet, and of direct marketing of diagnostic tests and treatments by private companies, has increased the amount of information and the strength of preferences that many patients have when they enter physicians' offices. Patients now often request or refuse specific tests or treatments based on what they have seen on film, television, or the Internet. At the same time, within the dynamic of the physician–patient relationship, complex webs of meaning, trust, and emotions of hope, fear, guilt, or frustration can also shape how technological advances are perceived and approached.

Historically, the introduction of new technologies into the clinical practice of neurology and psychiatry has been characterized by initial enthusiasm and hope that is later tempered and gives way to more caution. Over the centuries, but particularly in the last 50 years, technological advances have been incorporated into clinical practice in a range of ways, with varying degrees of ultimate success. For example, in the early twentieth century, prefrontal lobotomies were heralded and introduced as a cure for refractory psychiatric disorders, leading to the award of a Nobel Prize in medicine to Egas Moniz in 1949. At first, this new intervention was widely used, only later to be viewed more warily. Similarly, in the mid-twentieth century, electroconvulsive therapy was used commonly and for a wide variety of psychiatric conditions; today it is used considerably less.

Other challenges to clinical encounters derive from the fact that, in general, physicians are poorly trained in communication skills and ethics, for example in obtaining informed consent (McLean and Card 2004). A high proportion of physicians have difficulty communicating with patients, with physicians disagreeing 50 percent of the time with patients about the patient's main initial problem (Starfield *et al.* 1981). Poor communication can lead to poor medical management (Kidd *et al.* 2005) and decreased patient satisfaction (Little et al 2001). Physicians have difficulty discussing with patients sensitive but important topics such as end-of-life care; they raise the topic, but often in ways that are too vague to be useful and without eliciting or exploring patients' values (Tulsky *et al.* 1998). Furthermore, physicians have been found to miss important emotional and cultural cues from patients (Suchman *et al.* 1997, Johnson *et al.* 2004), and to be poorly trained to grapple with issues that they confront in medical ethics (Christakis *et al.* 1994). In addition, medical errors and shortcomings are not always dealt with in ways that can most enhance subsequent care (Bosk 2003).

Daniel Kahneman received the 2002 Nobel Prize in Economics for suggesting that individuals commonly view probabilities subjectively, using biases and heuristics, overvaluing the odds of bad events, and undervaluing the probabilities of good events. For example, in decision-making, rare but traumatic outcomes are over-weighed (Tversky and Kahneman 1981). The interpretation of statistical information is affected by how it is framed, either positively or negatively (Shiloh and Sagi 1989), and numerical estimates have been found to be more effective than verbal ones (Welkenhuysen *et al.* 2000). Thus biases and heuristics may distort patients' perceptions of risks (Redelmeier *et al.* 1993).

Biases in decisions can also stem from other personal characteristics of physicians. For example, gender, religion, and time since training can shape numerous decisions, including physician prescribing patterns (Bodkin *et al.* 1995). These types of obstacles manifest themselves in a variety of ways with regard to different diagnostic tests and treatments. Below I focus on how these barriers appear in neuroimaging and neurogenomics specifically, and in a few representative therapeutic interventions.

# Neuroimaging

## Diagnosis

Over time, neuroimaging studies such as functional MRI (fMRI) will no doubt become increasingly incorporated into clinical care. Such a trend will surely bring many benefits to patients by improving understanding of the biology, diagnosis, and treatment of brain diseases. However, misunderstandings about the diagnostic power of this technology are equally significant. These misunderstandings may arise from unrealistic expectations or hope and media hype. Responses of the insurance industry may further complicate this scenario. On the one hand, physicians may favor the potential efficiency of technological diagnosis rather than lengthy clinical assessments. Yet given the high potential costs involved, insurance companies may make the approval processes for scans highly burdensome, and some patients who might benefit from these procedures may not be able to obtain them. Thus physicians' attempts to save time may be pitted against insurance companies' efforts to reduce costs.

Concomitantly, neurotechnologies are spreading from clinical and scientific arenas to commercial uses. Direct marketing of diagnostic tests will no doubt mount; patients who can afford to pay for scans out of pocket may do so. Already, we see advertisements to 'Test to see if you have Alzheimer's' or 'Scan your brain to maximize your creativity!' (e.g. www.amenclinic.com). These phenomena raise difficult issues of what the roles of clinicians and neuroscientists should be in such situations, and whether and how individual professional decisions should be guided and monitored. Clearly, these tests may not be conducted as part of ongoing physician–patient relationships in which physicians and patients have, hopefully, some element of comfort together based on a history of interactions over time. Ideally, within a stable physician–patient relationship, the physician will know how the results fit within the overall context of a patient's life and other medical concerns—viewing such findings relative to the patient's functioning or fears. The trust between physicians and patients entails beliefs on the part of patients that physician decisions will be appropriate (Mechanic 1998; Mechanic and Meyer 2000). What then should a clinician say if patients are considering getting an outside imaging study, or have decided to do so? Should the clinician encourage or discourage this behavior and, if so, based on what criteria (Illes *et al.* 2003)? A physician may accede to pressure from a patient, even when it is not optimal or appropriate. Yet both individuals will then have to confront the results, which may be complex or of unclear significance, as described below.

## Interpretation of findings

In framing and presenting neuroimaging results to patients, clinicians face several critical challenges. Questions arise with regard to a number of parameters. What if subclinical findings of uncertain significance appear on a neuroimaging study (e.g. below average sizes of certain neurological structures or functioning)? What exactly should patients then be told, and how? How should clinicians explain such apparent, although clinically insignificant, findings? What if early possible signs of dementia or Alzheimer's disease are detected? How should physicians frame these results in order to offer hope?

Neurotechnologies may encourage clinicians and patients to embrace reductionism in pursuit of a biological cause of a psychiatric or neurological disorder. Indeed, neurotechnologies blur the distinctions between the biological and the psychological in ways that can shift understandings of personality. As it is, clinicians differ in their views of whether psychiatric diseases, for instance, are biologically or psychologically caused (Bodkin *et al.* 1995). Related to this phenomenon, in the film *The Eternal Sunshine of the Spotless Mind*, a scientist is able to locate and erase specific memories in the brain. Such possibilities may raise expectations, fears, and disturbing ethical questions for patients that clinicians may have to address concerning abilities to isolate specific memories, erase them, and alter identity or emotional states as a result (see also Chapter 21).

Among patients, neurological and psychiatric conditions themselves will complicate interpretations of results. For example, a paranoid patient may resist undergoing an imaging study, and suspiciously misinterpret the motives of physicians, or the results of the procedure. Depressed patients may feel more distraught, seeing results as indicating that their brain is somehow damaged in a way that they may feel cannot be ameliorated. Obsessive or other highly anxious patients may be overly concerned about subclinical findings, and nervous about small findings that a clinician may feel to be unimportant although nonetheless real. Diagnoses themselves may change due to new neurotechnologies in ways that create questions and pressures for medical educators. Single-disease entities that are now thought to manifest themselves somewhat differently in different individuals may come to be seen as consisting of heterogeneous pathophysiologies. Thus, Alzheimer's disease might eventually be seen as comprised physiologically of several different disorders. Similarly, schizophrenia, major depression, or multiple sclerosis may be found to be terms applied to similar common pathways of heterogeneous abnormalities. New clinical subtypes of diseases may be recognized, and existing symptomatic subtypes may be found to have physiological bases resulting from deficits in wholly different areas of the brain. How then should physicians already in practice be educated concerning new approaches to etiologies, diagnoses, and treatment, especially as these are still evolving? Clinicians may vary widely in the degree to which they have access to or embrace these new technologies. What guidelines and standards of care and education are needed or feasible?

## Neuroimaging and treatment

In the future, treatment for a variety of psychiatric and neurological conditions may become more customized as specificity about the involvement of different portions of the brain is revealed with advanced technology. This scenario may come to resemble that of pharmacogenomics in which, it is anticipated, treatment will be tailored for individuals with particular genotypes. This development in turn may increase pressures on clinicians (to assure the accuracy of interpretation of imaging studies) and on medical physicists (for increasingly detailed and precise methods).

In transferring neuroimaging information to the treatment setting, clinicians will also have to confront the ways in which advances in neuroscience may challenge notions of the patient's responsibility for symptoms. For example, if neurological structures become associated with predispositions for violence, violence may be seen as being less volitional. The stakes here are potentially high. To believe that a disease, or behavior, has a definite cause allows a patient to assign blame for the disorder, and suggests that the disease may have a definite and ready cure. The patient and physician may gain a sense of having potential control over the ailment. To a reductionist, if a disease such as depression or schizophrenia is caused by brain chemistry, it is therefore not caused by the individual, i.e. it is not voluntary or the fault of the individual. Thus the individual cannot be blamed for the disease, its symptoms, or its behavioral consequences. Whether for aggression, drug addiction, or psychopathy—the biological components of which are increasingly being elucidated (Blair 2003)—some scholars fear that individuals may now be seen as not being responsible for the behavioral problems they manifest. Problems arise in part since traits such as aggression or alcoholism are difficult, if not impossible, to define or quantify precisely (Alper 1998). Given the discovery of causes, pressures may increase to cure such patients. However, the notion that an etiology *de facto* generates a ready cure may in the end be illusory. Neuroimaging may alter perceptions and expectations of what patients can potentially do or not do to overcome their diagnosis.

## Privacy and disclosure

Given the intense stigma associated with cognitive and psychiatric symptoms, clinicians face major privacy concerns. Brain diseases carry particular stigma because they can decrease cognitive functioning, emotional stability, and behavioral control, all of which may lead to bias against the patient and precipitate explicit or implicit discrimination. Questions thus surface as to who should have access to a patient's neuroimaging or other test results. For example, if the ability to detect early dementias increases, what will be the implications in terms of a patient's future in the workplace? Should employers ever have a right to know a patient's diagnosis and, if so, how should this right be weighed against the patient's right to privacy? What if a physician, pharmacist, or airline pilot is found on an imaging study to have very early indications of dementia and insists that he wants to continue to work? What obligations will clinicians have and how should these be exercised?

In pediatric imaging, what if a child is found to have a minor abnormality? If disclosed to the parents, the parents might treat the child differently. If parents disclose these findings to the child's school, the school may treat the child differently. What if schools want to order tests or request results for students? Clinicians will be critical gatekeepers in ordering these tests and in determining who learns of the results.

## Genetics, ethics, and the brain

Increasingly, clinicians will face complex moral dilemmas about the use of not only neuroimaging technologies, but also genomic tests for neurological and psychiatric diseases. This next section focuses on the challenges of genomics in contrast with imaging, again with a particular emphasis on physician roles, privacy, and disclosure.

### Physicians and the ethics of genetic testing

Although genetic tests have been available for well over a decade, little research has been conducted on physician decision-making concerning genetic tests for brain or other diseases. In one of the few studies published, 71 percent of physicians reported that their knowledge of genetics and genetic testing was fair to poor (Menasha *et al.* 2000). A major determinant of whether physicians order genetic tests has been found to be patient interest (Wideroff *et al.* 2003). For example, 18 percent of doctors caring for patients with Alzheimer's disease have ordered at least one *APOE* test. Although this gene is associated with increased risk of Alzheimer's disease, it is neither necessary nor sufficient for the disease. Hence, its diagnostic significance remains unclear.

Diffusion of information about genetic testing is clearly very much needed to guide clinicians (Chase *et al.* 2002). Tests for these diseases will no doubt be marketed despite varying degrees of sensitivity and specificity. Just as a gene associated with Huntington's disease has been identified, researchers are now seeking genetic tests for epilepsy, multiple sclerosis, brain carcinomas, bipolar disorder, depression, and other brain disorders. Who should undergo genetic tests that may be developed in the future for these conditions? Should everyone at risk be tested? If so, how should such risk be defined? To which patients should providers offer or encourage testing? Patients will encounter hard decisions over whether and when to undergo testing, and about what these results mean. Physicians may seek to refer patients to genetic counselors, yet such counselors are in short supply. Hence physicians and patients are often confronting these ethical quandaries on their own.

Recent research conducted with individuals who have or are at risk for several different genetic diseases, including Huntington's disease, has explored many of these topics (R. Klitzman, unpublished data). For example, individuals who are at risk for a neurological or psychiatric disease may or may not see themselves as being at risk or be concerned about privacy. These two factors may also interact, creating four distinct scenarios: those who do and do not see themselves as being at risk, and those who are and are not worried about privacy. Each of these four possibilities can shape decisions in different ways that would best be addressed by clinicians proactively.

## Interpretation of genetic tests

We can reasonably expect that, in the future, new tests will be developed for genes that are associated with a range of neurological and psychiatric disorders but do not follow classical Mendelian patterns. Rather, these diseases will have complex or mixed etiologies involving gene–environment interactions. The statistics involved will no doubt be complicated. The presence of a particular gene may mean that an individual has, say, a 20 percent chance of developing a particular brain disease. What level of understanding will patients and clinicians have of such statistics? Physicians and patients may misunderstand what it means for an individual to have such a genetic predisposition for a neurological or psychiatric disease. On the one hand, many patients may feel that a positive genetic test result constitutes a fate that will profoundly and unalterably affect their lives. On the other hand, genetic diagnoses may provide helpful explanations for troubling symptoms (e.g. depression or psychosis), and alleviate blame for these symptoms. Should such complicated and ambiguous scenarios limit or bar the use of these tests? Who should make these decisions—the individual physician, the patient, policy-makers?

## Privacy and disclosure of genetic test results

With genetic tests, as with neuroimaging studies, clinicians and patients face challenges concerning disclosure of results. If a patient is found to have a genetic mutation for a neurological or psychiatric disease, who should be told? Here, analogies can be drawn from the experiences of individuals with HIV who are often forced to make difficult decisions about whether and how to tell relatives, friends, coworkers, employers, insurers, and others. Patients with positive genetic tests may only disclose partial information (e.g. being at risk of, rather than gene-positive for, Huntington's disease), or may ask a coworker to keep information a secret. If the information subsequently spreads, the patient may then feel angry and betrayed. Clearly, patients must gauge the trustworthiness and receptiveness of individuals with whom they interact concerning this information (Klitzman and Bayer 2003). Should a physician ever override the patient's decision not to disclose to a family member, even though that family member may be at risk for the disease as well? The lethality and treatability of a particular disease will no doubt be important in addressing these decisions.

Genetic information poses difficult choices related to privacy and confidentiality since this information represents permanent aspects of an individual, and can potentially be used in a discriminatory way. Clinicians and policy-makers have long debated genetic exceptionalism, i.e. whether genetic information should be treated differently than that concerning other diseases. Currently, in the United States, many states have enacted genetic privacy laws, but these policies vary widely in their scope, definitions, and enforcement. Thus a health care provider must be acutely aware of local policies relevant to this topic, and keep up to date with how they evolve over time. Nonetheless, patients are often wary of how effective privacy laws really are in preventing discrimination, given that information travels and employers could discriminate, even unconsciously, in subtle ways (Klitzman et al. 2004).

In many regards, genetic diseases have been viewed as constituting a single entity. But responses to various neurological and psychiatric diagnoses will no doubt vary, depending on factors such as availability and cost of treatment. A new sense of neuroexceptionalism may develop, whereby diagnostic information about neurological disorders is viewed and handled differently from that of certain other less stigmatized medical conditions.

## Difficult choices: bearing children

We can expect that patients with abnormal findings on genetic or other tests will increasingly consult physicians about whether or not to have children. Currently, pre-implantation genetic diagnosis (PGD) can lead to reduction of the transmission of certain genetically detectable diseases. It is entirely conceivable that patients may fear that if they avoid this expensive procedure, and subsequently have a child who has a disease, the child may later feel resentful. Yet, pre-implantation clinics that provide these diagnostic tests are the focus of substantial controversy, given questions about the moral status of an embryo and the ethics of selecting embryos for implantation based on diagnostic screening (Beyleveld 2000). As a result of these debates, these clinics are facing challenges from government regulators and an uncertain future. Even if PGD continues, at least in the near term, not all patients will have access to such procedures, and clinicians will be faced with difficult situations concerning who should undergo such testing.

## Other scenarios where neuroethics and clinical medicine meet
### Psychotherapy

Genomic and neuroimaging research on brain diseases may have critical implications for the selection and evaluation of treatments. For example, neuroimaging or genomics may one day predict which patients will benefit from psychotherapy *versus* pharmacotherapy, or from particular psychotherapies (e.g. Freudian *versus* cognitive–behavioral) for psychiatric disorders such as depression or anxiety. Already, research has claimed that psychotherapy leads to demonstrable changes in brain biology (Brody *et al.* 2001). How will insurance companies respond to such types of information? Will they challenge clinicians who provide psychotherapy as a sole treatment to a patient with depression or other disorders? Will community providers who are not able to order such tests, for whatever reason, become disenfranchised or unreimbursable? In addition, how will patients respond to genomic or imaging information that may give them a biological explanation for their disease and, even more meaningfully perhaps, how will these views affect attitudes and adherence concerning treatment?

## Coercive treatment

It is entirely reasonable to expect that neurotechnology and genetics may soon yield reliable predictive indicators for traits such as suicidality or homicidality. A patient in imminent and grave danger to himself or others can legally be treated involuntarily (Sadock and Sadock 2005). However, whether a patient meets criteria for imminent danger is not always clear (Cavanagh *et al.* 2003), and cultural and national differences in approaches to involuntary psychiatric hospitalization and treatment abound (Kjellin and Westrin 1998). When neurotechnology reaches the likely point of predicting dangerousness to self or others, such findings will have to be carefully weighed in the tenuous balance between protecting society and upholding individual free will.

## Pain management

Pain management has been a challenging and controversial area of medicine that will surely be affected by advances in neuroscience. Patients have been found to respond to and express pain differently depending on psychological and cultural factors (Encandela 1993). Clinicians often have fears, generally unfounded, of patients becoming addicted to opiate analgesics (Klitzman and Perry 1993). At the same time, new technologies are elucidating how the brain processes pain, and how cognitive mechanisms modulate this functioning. Neuroimaging has already documented the beneficial effects of hypnotic suggestion (Rainville *et al.* 1999, Chen 2000, Derbyshire *et al.* 2004), cognitive distraction (Petrovic and Ingvar 2002), and, most recently, neurofeedback (Mackey and Maeda 2004). This research holds much promise for pain management, and may support increased use of biofeedback and other alternative approaches to treatment. But even here, significant challenges arise. How individual differences in the expression or experience of pain will correlate with differences on neuroimaging, for example, and how these variations will be interpreted remain open questions at this time. Overall, the studies are still few in number. Cautions concerning interpretation must be strictly exerted (Illes and Racine 2005) so that physicians do not act on conclusions prematurely. Once again, education in both the practitioner and policy arenas will play pivotal roles (see also Chapter 15).

## Clinical neuroenhancement

What if clinicians can improve upon a person's baseline level of cognitive functioning? Should clinicians be limited in doing so in any way? Clinical psychiatrist Peter Kramer first wrote about 'cosmetic psychopharmacology' in his book *Listening to Prozac* (Kramer 1992), and helped to launch a broad debate about brain enhancement. Although society as a whole confronts these issues, clinicians will be prime gatekeepers in employing specific enhancement technologies. Increasingly, physicians may see patients who would not be considered to have a disease, but who still seek to enhance their cognition, mood, memory, or other traits. Such enhancements blur distinctions between clinical disease and normal variants, and it is not at all clear today how clinicians will grapple these issues. Aspects of these questions have already received attention (Rothman and Rothman 2003; Farah *et al.* 2004, see also Chapter 6), although much remains to be studied. Clinicians will face questions about the definition of disease and of their professional role. What clinical endpoints or outcomes should be used, if not the alleviation of suffering and disease?

Critics of neuroenhancement fear that the standard or threshold for acceptable behavior will be raised such that medicated states will come to be seen as the norm. In the end, adults can make their own decisions about these treatments. But the case is different for children. As minors, they cannot give consent and must have these decisions made for them. Physiologically and psychologically, they are more vulnerable as their brains are still highly plastic. As neuroenhancements become available and requested by patients, clinicians will need to be ready to address, and be poised to make, informed decisions. For example, how should clinicians respond to potential social dangers of such enhancements—injustices that may result from unequal availability of such interventions across sociodemographic groups? Do clinicians have a societal responsibility to take these larger social issues into account when making decisions about individual patients? Should the profession or the polity dictate that physicians focus on alleviating the suffering of many individuals before enhancing those few who are wealthy enough to afford these interventions? These questions will certainly continue to evolve in the coming years.

## Stem cells

Many scientists believe that a variety of neurodegenerative diseases will eventually be treatable using stem cells, yet ethical questions that clinicians will have to confront also emerge here. Potentially, stem cell research will lead to unique treatments for Parkinson's disease, multiple sclerosis, Alzheimer's disease, spinal cord injuries, and other conditions. Yet concerns exist about the proper implementation of these new technologies, including what information donors of embryos should be provided about future uses, and who should have access to such treatments once they are developed. Like transplant medicine and certain other technologies, conflicts may arise between those who can afford therapy and those most in need. In this emerging domain, clinicians may have to face difficult issues of meaning when patients are concerned about having another person's cells in their brain (or in the case of xenotransplanted tissues, cells from a non-human species). Already, difficult psychological issues exist with recipients of transplanted hearts and other organs, and about what burdens or responsibilities recipients bear (Fox and Swazey 1992). Voters in California recently decided to use state funds for stem cell research; other states may adopt similar policies. If private or non-federal funds are used to develop stem cell therapies, could these be employed in all clinical environments? Will Medicare and Medicaid reimburse for these treatments? If not, will large groups of patients be excluded from use of these interventions? Depending on the outcome of politically driven debates, clinicians may face the possibility of having to send patients abroad to receive certain stem cell treatments that may not be available in the United States. History would predict that, over time, the legalities of such a possibility will vary with changing public demand favoring or opposing it. In the meantime, however, clinicians will still have to be aware of their own moral views on this charged topic as they face innovative approaches to patient care.

## Infectious disease

Over upcoming years, understanding of the infectious components of certain brain diseases will surely increase and will pose special ethical problems for clinicians. For example, prions have been found to cause Creutzfeldt–Jakob disease (CJD), variant CJD (vCJD), which is contracted from ingestion of beef from cattle with bovine spongiform encephalopathy (BSE) ('mad cow' disease), scrapie in sheep, and kuru among the Fore group and their neighbors in Papua New Guinea. Investigators have been exploring whether prions may be involved in a variety of other disorders, including multiple sclerosis, Parkinson's disease, and certain forms of cancer (Klitzman 1998). Recently, vCJD has been transmitted through blood in two human cases (Hopkin 2004). It is possible that further such cases will be discovered, which may alarm the public, physicians, and the media. This transmissibility poses further challenges, especially with respect to maximizing the safety of blood supplies. As of now, there is no way to screen blood for prions. Should there be restrictions on who can donate blood? Over time, policy-makers in the United States have wavered on this question, and have gradually decreased the amount of time that a potential donor may have lived in the United Kingdom (Fischbach 2003). How much should individuals be protected from the risk of tainted or potentially tainted blood or beef?

Policy-makers throughout the world will no doubt continue to confront ethical and legal challenges: protecting critical blood supplies, testing cattle, banning herds if BSE is discovered, gauging the amount of information disseminated to the public, and maintaining appropriate transparency about decisions taken. Physicians will need to be attuned to policy-makers' decisions on these issues and prepared to discuss risks and benefits with patients. With increasing globalization and travel between areas that were previously separated, other infectious agents can be expected to spread, as did SARS, Legionnaire's disease, and HIV. Unprecedented neuroethical concerns will be evident in the face of wide uncertainty.

## End-of-life care

For some patients, neuroimaging technology emerging on the horizon may hold promise for clinical benefit even at the end of life. Recently, for example, in a limited research study, two patients in a minimally conscious state were reported to have brain activity similar to that of healthy controls in response to passive listening and tactile stimulation (Schiff *et al.* 2005). Will clinicians one day be able to detect reliably whether a patient in this state recognizes when a relative is speaking (Carey 2005)? This will be a significant stretch in terms of both resource allocation and population selection when, today, discussion is still ongoing about which patients with head trauma should undergo imaging studies (Dunning and Lecky 2004). While such research could surely have important clinical implications, the risk of false positives and false negatives is enormous. The impact of such studies on family decisions about 'do not resuscitate' orders poses potentially high levels of risk. A less dire but still highly sensitive scenario is one in which a patient does not show anticipated brain responses yet, unbeknown to family and health care workers, still retains an awareness of the presence of loved ones. An equally passionate challenge embodies the possibility that, while the technology may appear to provide an opportunity for family to express final words or talk meaningfully to a patient, no appreciation of those words is truly occurring or possible. Given the state of the art, it is essential that clinicians focus on fact and not fiction for family members involved in these desperate situations.

## Neuroethics, culture, and education

Concepts of selfhood, autonomy, disease, risk, and uncertainty vary around the world, and physicians will have to respond to neuroethical challenges in different and culturally appropriate ways. Ethical relativism, i.e. whether ethical principles are universal or culturally specific, has long been debated (Angell 1997). As neurotechnologies develop, attitudes and moral values both within and across national borders will be key factors for clinicians facing dilemmas about brain diseases, mental function, fate, and the future.

To respond to these challenges in clinical neuroethics, further scholarship, research, and education are essential. Heightened awareness of the complexities of these issues among neurologists, psychiatrists, psychologists, neuroscientists, social workers, ethicists, and other health care professionals is imperative. The intensely fast pace of neuroscience research is one of the greatest challenges to continuing medical education. We can fully anticipate that neurotechnology will shift perceptions and transform commonly held attitudes about disease etiology, prognosis, and treatment. Given new capabilities and new understandings of brain diseases, education focused on realistic expectations is key. Physicians and researchers must share the responsibility of information dissemination, communication, and partnership in the development of legislative responses to issues such as privacy, discrimination, and health insurance. In ways that we cannot even yet foresee, neurotechnology will challenge us—our understanding of disease, and of the self, of the mind, and of the brain. We have much to gain and learn, but also much to prepare as we further explore these new and exciting frontiers.

## References

Alper JS (1998). Genes, free will, and criminal responsibility. *Social Science and Medicine* 46, 1599–1611.

Angell M (1997). The ethics of clinical research in the Third World. *New England Journal of Medicine* 337, 847–9.

Applebaum PS, Lidz CW, Meisel A (1987). *Informed Consent: Legal Theory and Clinical Practice.* Oxford: Oxford University Press.

Beyleveld D (2000). Is embryo research and preimplantation genetic diagnosis ethical? *Forensic Science International* 113, 461–75.

Bigio IJ, Bown SG (2004). Spectroscopic sensing of cancer and cancer therapy: current status ofvtranslational research. *Cancer Biology and Therapy* 3, 259–67.

Blair JR (2003). Neurological basis of psychopathy. *British Journal of Psychiatry* 182, 5–7.

Bodkin A, Klitzman RL, Pope H (1995). Treatment orientation and associated characteristics among North American academic psychiatrists. *Journal of Nervous and Mental Disorders* 184, 729–35.

Bosk C (2003). *Forgive and Remember: Managing Medical Failure* (2nd edn). Chicago, IL: University of Chicago Press.

Brody A, Saxena S, Stoessel P, *et al.* (2001). Regional brain metabolic changes in patients with major depression treated with either paroxetine or interpersonal therapy. *Archives of General Psychiatry* 58, 631–40.

Carey B (2005). New signs of awareness seen in brain-injured patients. *New York Times* 8 February, A1.

Cavanagh JTO, Carson AJ, Sharpe M, Lawrie SM (2003). Psychological autopsy studies of suicide: a systematic review. *Psychological Medicine* 33, 395–405.

Chase GA, Geller G, Havstad SL, Holtzman NA, Bassett SS (2002). Physicians' propensity to offer genetic testing for Alzheimer's disease: results from a survey. *Genetics in Medicine* 4, 297–303.

Chen ACN (2000). New perspectives in EEG/MEG brain mapping and PET/fMRI neuroimaging of human pain. *International Journal of Psychopathology* 42, 147–59.

Christakis DA, Christakis NA, Feudtner C (1994). Do clinical clerks suffer ethical erosion? Students' perspectives of their ethical environment and personal development. *Academic Medicine* 69, 670–9.

Derbyshire SWG, Whalley MG, Stenger, VA *et al.* (2004). Cerebral activation during hypnotically indued and imagined pain. *NeuroImage* 23, 392–401.

Dunning J, Lecky F (2004) The NICE guidelines in the real world: a practical perspective. *British Medical Journal* 21, 404–407.

Encandela, JA (1993). Social science and the study of pain since Zborowski: a need for a new agenda. *Social Science and Medicine* 36, 783–91.

Farah M, Illes J, Cook-Deegan R, *et al.* (2004). Neurocognitive enhancement: What can we do? What should we do? *Nature Reviews Neuroscience* 5, 421–5.

Fischbach R (2003). Whether to present grave information in the face of uncertainty. Presented at: Annual Meeting of the American Society for Bioethics and Humanities: Bioethics Across Borders, 26 October 2003, Montreal, Canada.

Fox R, Swazey J (1992). *Spare Parts: Organ Replacement in American Society.* New York: Oxford University Press.

Hopkin M (2004). Fears grow as blood stocks pass on prions undetected. *Nature* 430, 712.

Illes J, Racine E (2005). Imaging or imagining? A neuroethics challenge informed by genetics. *American Journal of Bioethics* 5, 1–14.

Illes J, Fan E, Koenig B, Raffin TA, Kann D, Atlas SW (2003). Self-referred whole body imaging: current implications for health care consumers. *Radiology* 228, 346–351.

Johnson RL, Roter D, Powe NR, Cooper LA (2005). Patient race/ethnicity and quality of patient-physician communication during medical visits. *American Journal of Public Health* 94, 2084–90.

Kidd J, Patel V, Peile E, Carter Y (2005). Clinical and communication skills. *British Medical Journal* 330, 374–5.

Kjellin L, Westrin CG (1998). Involuntary admissions and coercive measures in psychiatric care. *International Journal of Law and Psychiatry* 21, 31–42.

Klitzman RL (1998). *The Trembling Mountain: A Personal Account of Kuru, Cannibals, and Mad Cow Disease.* New York: Plenum Trade.

Klitzman RL, Bayer R (2003). *Mortal Secrets: Truth and Lies in the Age of AIDS.* Baltimore, MD: Johns Hopkins University Press.

Klitzman RL, Perry SW (1993). Psychiatric complications in surgical intensive care. In: Barie PS, Shires, GT (eds) *Surgical Intensive Care.* Boston, MA: Little Brown 1247–1262.

Klitzman RL, Kirshenbaum SB, Kittel L, *et al.* (2004). Naming names: Perceptions of name-based HIV reporting, partner notification, and criminalization of non-disclosure among persons living with HIV. *Sexuality Research and Social Policy* 1, 38–57.

Kramer P (1993). *Listening to Prozac.* New York: Penguin Books.

Little P, Everitt H, Williamson I, *et al.* (2001). Observational study of effect of patient centredness and positive approach on outcomes of general practice consultations. *British Medical Journal* 323, 908–11.

Mackey SC, Maeda F (2004). Functional imaging and the neural systems of chronic pain. *Neurosurgery clinics of North America* 15, 269–88

McLean KL, Card SE (2004). Informed consent skills in internal medicine residency: how are residents taught, and what do they learn? *Academic Medicine* 79, 128–33.

Mechanic D (1998). The functions and limitations of trust in the provision of medical care. *Journal of Health Politics, Policy and Law* 23, 661–86.

Mechanic D, Meyer S (2000). Concepts of trust among patients with serious illness. *Social Science and Medicine* 51, 657–68.

Menasha JD, Schechter C, Willner J (2000). Genetic testing: a physician's perspective. *Mount Sinai Journal of Medicine* 67, 144–51.

Petrovic P, Ingvar M (2002). Imaging cognitive modulation of pain processing. *Pain,* 95, 1–5.

Rainville P, Hofbauer RK, Paus T, Duncan GH, Bushnell MC, Price DD (1999). Cerebral mechanisms of hypnotic induction and suggestion. *Journal of Cognitive Neuroscience* 11, 110–25.

Redelmeier D, Rozin P, Kanheman D (1993). Understanding patients' decisions: cognitive and emotional perspectives. *Journal of the American Medical Association* 270, 72–6.

Rothman D, Rothman SM (2003). *The Pursuit of Perfection: The Promise and Perils of Medical Enhancement.* New York: Pantheon Books.

Sadock BJ, Sadock VA (eds) (2005) *Kaplan & Sadock's Comprehensive Textbook of Psychiatry* (8th edn). Philadelphia, PA: Lippincott–Williams & Wilkins.

Schechter AN, Perlman RL, Rettig RA (2004). Why is revitalizing clinical research so important, yet so difficult? *Perspectives in Biology and Medicine* 47, 476–86.

Schiff ND, Rodriguez-Moreno D, Kamal A, *et al.* (2005). FMRI reveals large-scale network activation in minimally conscious patients. *Neurology* 64, 514–23.

Shiloh S, Sagi M (1989). Effect of framing on the perception of genetic recurrence risks. *American Journal of Medical Genetics* 33, 130–5.

Starfield B, Wray C, Hess K, *et al.* (1981). The influence of patient-practitioner agreement on outcome of care. *American Journal of Public Health* 71, 127–31.

Stone AA (1984). *Law Psychiatry and Morality: Essays and Analysis.* Washington, DC: American Psychiatric Press.

Suchman A, Markakis K, Beckman HB, Frankel R (1997). A model of empathic communication in the medical interview. *Journal of the American Medical Association* 277, 678–82.

Tulsky JA, Fischer GS, Rose M, Arnold R (1998). Opening the black box: how do physicians communicate about advance directives? *Annals of Internal Medicine* 129, 441–9.

Tversky A, Kahneman D (1981). The framing of decisions and the psychology of choice. *Science* 211, 453–8.

Welkenhuysen M, Evers-Kiebooms G, d'Ydewalle G (2000). The language of uncertainty in genetic risk communication: Framing and verbal versus numerical information. *Patient Education and Counseling* 43, 179–87.

Wideroff L, Freedman AN, Olson L, *et al.* (2003). Physician use of genetic testing for cancer susceptibility: results of a national survey. *Cancer Epidemiology Biomarkers and Prevention* 12, 295–303.

Part III

# Justice, social institutions, and neuroethics

# The social effects of advances in neuroscience: legal problems, legal perspectives

Henry T. Greely

Canst thou not minister to a mind diseased,
Pluck from the memory a rooted sorrow,
Raze out the written troubles of the brain,
And with some sweet oblivious antidote
Cleanse the stuffed bosom of that perilous stuff
Which weighs upon the heart?

    *Macbeth*, Act V, Scene 3

Shakepeare's Scottish play is drenched in blood, but is also suffused throughout by mind and brain. Macbeth chooses murder to reach his high ambition, his choice influenced both by his wife's will and the magical technology of the three witches. His choice ends up costing him everything: love and respect, his wife and his life.

Neuroscience offers us possible solutions to many of the human problems portrayed in *Macbeth*, but with those choices comes risk. Advances in neuroscience seem likely to cause major changes in our society in the next few decades, for better and for worse. And when society changes, the law must change—whether to guide those social changes or merely to respond to them. In roughly 100 years the automobile has changed much about life in the developed world and much about its laws—of traffic, insurance, accidents, pollution, franchising, land use, and many other issues. Social changes from neuroscience are likely to have even greater implications for the law, as they will change both the objects of the law and, in a very direct way, how the legal system functions. Those legal changes should make up one important part of the study of what has come to be called neuroethics.

The term 'neuroethics', popularized by William Safire, has been given several kinds of meanings. One use of neuroethics describes ethical problems arising directly from research in neuroscience; for example, what should researchers doing brain imaging tell research subjects about unusual findings of no known clinical significance? The term is also used to describe neuroscience (usually imaging) research into how humans resolve ethical or moral issues; for example, what parts of the brain are activated when subjects are wrestling with moral dilemmas? I will discuss a third area of neuroethics: the implications of new discoveries in, and capabilities of, neuroscience for our society and their consequences for the legal system. I will look specifically at three different ways in which neuroscience seems likely to change our society and our law: better prediction of future behavior or mental abilities, improved detection of current mental state, and increased ability to enhance the workings of the human brain directly. The discussion will focus on the society and the legal system of the United States, because they are what I know best, but the same basic issues will be found in all technologically advanced societies.

## Prediction

If you can look into the seeds of time,
And say which grain will grow and which will not,
Speak then to me

   *Macbeth*, Act I, Scene 3

Banquo and Macbeth seek predictions about the future from the three weird sisters. Neuroscience will provide less magical ways to predict some things, such as a person's behavior, neurological condition, or mental health. In a sense genetics has already led to increased neuroscience prediction: finding that a person has more than 36 CAG repeats in one of his two copies of a gene called huntingtin is a powerful predictor that he will be diagnosed with Huntington's disease; learning that a fetus carries an extra copy of chromosome 21 makes an eventual diagnosis of Down's syndrome highly likely, if not inevitable. Concerns about predictive genetics, which have been discussed, analyzed, and debated for over three decades, provide a useful template for thinking about neuroscience predictions (Andrews *et al.* 1994; Koenig *et al.* 1998). Today, imaging studies, both structural and functional, are offering further advances in prediction. Magnetic resonance imaging (MRI) can look for the build-up of amyloid plaque on neurons, perhaps predicting future Alzheimer's disease, or even its likely age of onset. Functional MRI (fMRI) is being used to try to show patterns of brain activation that can be used to predict future behavior such as violence.

Shakespeare's characters find the witches' predictions both accurate and misleading, helpful and deadly. Similarly, neuroscience-based prediction can be used, or misused, in many different ways. The criminal justice system, or the processes of civil commitment for sex offenders, may use such predictions to make decisions about imprisonment. Employers might want to know more about what kind of employees they are hiring; insurers may want to know more about the futures of their prospective and current policy-holders. Schools could use this kind of information to tailor programs to help their students succeed, or to help them select only students who will make the schools succeed. Businesses and advertisers might be able to improve sales by better prediction of how consumers' brains will respond to their products or advertisements.

Some of these, and other, possibilities for neuroscience prediction are explored in other chapters. This chapter examines what issues will arise as these predictions interact with our legal system. These interactions may take place in two contexts: through the use of such predictions within the courtroom itself, and by the legal system's efforts to regulate their use outside the courtroom. In both these locations, five factors are likely to be important to the law's reaction to such predictions.

- ◆ What are the consequences of the predictions?
- ◆ How accurate will these predictions be?
- ◆ How accurate will these predictions be perceived to be?
- ◆ How fair will it be to use these predictions?
- ◆ How well can limits on the use of such predictions be enforced?

In addition, prediction might raise another broader issue if neuroscientific predictions support generalizations about different human groups.

## Relevant factors in using neuroscience predictions

The response of the legal system to neuroscience will hinge in large part on the importance of the consequences of the predictions. Brain imaging that predicts a student's future schizophrenia should receive closer attention than imaging used for career counseling. A prediction about aggressiveness would deserve less scrutiny when used by professional sports teams than when used by a court in sentencing. The consequences for both sides must be examined: the one whose future is being predicted, and the one who wants to use that prediction. In general, the law will be more likely to restrict the use of predictions that could bring great harm to the tested party for small benefit to the user of the prediction and more likely to allow those that provide great benefits while risking only small harms.

The accuracy of the predictions will also be crucial. Accuracy will often need to be assessed in ways more complex than saying that the predictions are '92 percent accurate'. In determining whether someone should be civilly committed as a sex offender, the rates of both false positives and false negatives should be considered separately. If one were to screen adolescents in order to predict future mental illness, such as schizophrenia, the positive predictive value (the likelihood that, given the actual incidence of the condition, a positive test is likely to be a true positive) would also have to be calculated. One crucial question would become just how much accuracy, and of what kind, should be required before relying on such predictive tests. In addition, how to calculate these accuracy rates will raise their own difficult problems: we would not want to test the accuracy of tests for predicting pedophilia by releasing tested suspects to see how often they molest children. The possibility that accuracy will have to be measured indirectly, and perhaps poorly, makes the decision on whether to rely on such tests even harder.

Even if the accuracy of a predictive test accuracy has been thoroughly and accurately determined, another factor comes into play. How accurate will those using the prediction believe it to be? It seems likely that many neuroscience predictive tests, with their complicated and expensive machines and their dramatic false color images, may seem more accurate than they actually are. Confronted with a choice between a psychologist reading from his notes and a brain scan, jurors and judges, employers and school admissions officers, might grant unjustified accuracy to the more 'scientific' test, even in the face of weak accuracy statistics.

Using even accurate predictions of future behavior can raise questions of fairness. The criminal system punishes people for things that they have been convicted of doing. What if a neuroscience test could predict, with great accuracy, that someone was going to be a pedophile? Would it be fair to take action against the tested person before he had done anything? The question remains relevant even if the action taken is far short of protective detention. One could imagine requiring this pre-suspect to report regularly to the police or putting him under tight surveillance. His neighbors might be warned or he might be barred from jobs working with children. On the other hand, if there were strong evidence that the prediction was highly accurate, would it be fair to his future victims not to restrict him?

If we want to prevent, or restrict, some predictive uses of neuroscience, we must also consider how effectively those barriers can be enforced. Few legal rules can be enforced perfectly, or cheaply. Limits on the use of predictions in courtrooms would be among the easiest to enforce; private uses would be harder to control. As long as neuroscience predictions require complicated and intrusive interventions, control will be easier. Few people are likely to undergo an

MRI without their knowledge, and without a substantial record being left. (Even then, confidentiality provisions are important to keep the results of interventions made for a legitimate and consented purpose from being used for different and less benign ends.) Of course, if the interventions are less intrusive, controlling them becomes harder; if the predictive tests could be performed without the subject's knowledge, they could often avoid any enforceable regulation.

## Possible collective effects of neuroscience prediction

The issues discussed so far have revolved around the individuals who are the subjects of these predictions. Such predictions may also have broader implications for the groups to which those individuals belong. Consider a hypothetical neuroscience test that could accurately predict an infant's later ability at mathematics. Such a test might be used to try to provide special enrichment for talented children or remedial programs for those with less aptitude. But what if the test results purported to show that, on average or at the extremes, boys will be better than girls at mathematics? Or that, to a statistically significant extent, one-year-old Hungarians, Koreans, and Mayans are predicted to become better with numbers than Indonesians, Arabs, or Italians?

Today, mathematics tests given across the world measure knowledge at different ages, leading some nations to point with pride and others to view with alarm. But these are tests of schoolchildren, whom we assume are affected by their education and environments, now and when they were younger. The earlier the age of a predictive test, the less relevant environment and education will seem and the more natural the resulting disparities will appear. If the trait is considered important and if it varies significantly, on average, among culturally significant populations, such predictions could reinforce existing stereotypes or create new ones. This in turn might foreclose opportunities for some individuals in the 'less talented on average' group, and might stigmatize the entire group. We have no reason to believe that group variations exist in cognitive abilities for which such early tests might prove feasible, but we have extensive evidence from human history of a willingness, sometimes an eagerness, to classify some groups as inferior and others as superior. This possible use, and abuse, of tests for innate cognitive ability could be a problem.

## Conclusions on neuroscience predictive tests

None of the issues discussed above is new to neuroscience predictions. We make predictions all the time. Our society uses the SAT and similar tests to make predictions that are used to discriminate against, and for, prospective students; we use age and sex to predict a driver's liability risks. We already worry that juries will find some testimony more convincing than they should because it is scientific. The fairness of insurers' use of genetic tests remains controversial, with, thus far, largely different resolutions in the United States for health insurance and life insurance (Hudson *et al.* 1995; Diver and Cohen 2001; Greely 2001). To some extent, neuroscience is only expanding the fields in which, or the accuracy (real or perceived) with which, such predictions are possible. On the other hand, in some respects predictions based on the brain (predictions about an individual's cognitive abilities, future mental or neurological health, or likely future behavior) may be especially sensitive. Those predictions may strike closer to our sense of ourselves than predictions of our future driving record or of our college grades. Either way, the social implications of neuroscience predictions may well be substantial. If so, the legal system will change in response.

# Mind reading

There's no art
To find the mind's construction in the face;
He was a gentleman on whom I built
An absolute trust.

*Macbeth*, Act I, Scene 4

Because humans are social animals, discerning what other people *really* mean is one of the most important, and most difficult, tasks facing us all. From 'the check is in the mail' to 'I'll always love you', we cannot always count on others' outward expressions to be complete guides to their thoughts. Shakespeare's (and Scotland's) King Duncan bemoans having made this mistake with his treasonous noble the Thane of Cawdor, but immediately repeats it, this time fatally, with Cawdor's successor, Macbeth.

Neuroscience holds out the latest hope of knowing what someone really thinks or feels, or what their mental condition 'really' is. New technologies, particularly imaging technologies, can show us patterns of activity in the brain itself that may well prove to correlate strongly with states of mind, emotion, or thought. Thus studies show which regions of the brain, down to resolutions of under 2 mm$^3$, have slightly greater blood flow or slightly lower blood flow (and thus are 'activated' or 'deactivated') when a subject undergoing MRI senses, thinks, or does something. When the subjects, on average, show a statistically significant correlation between some mental activity or state and greater blood flow in particular brain regions, those regions are pronounced the sites of fear, of love (either romantic or maternal, which activate different but overlapping locations), or the feeling of mystical union with God. At this point, it is too early to know what these kinds of findings, being produced in thousands wherever MRI machines are available to researchers, will ultimately mean. But they might end up allowing us, in at least some cases, to 'read' someone's mental condition, emotional state, or even thoughts (see also Chapter 11).

The actual value of such technologies cannot be guessed at this point. We do not know what mental states, if any, could be accurately detected by such methods. Almost as important, we have no idea of the conditions that such testing would require. If testing required that each person whose mind was to be read be placed in an MRI machine similar to existing models for an hour, the costs and inconvenience of the technology would limit its uses to only the most important situations. If the technologies could be made miniature and portable—reduced, for example, to the size and shape of stereo headphones—the potential uses would be much broader.

Whether narrow or broad, any such mind-reading technologies could have enormous implications for the workings of the legal system. The law is often concerned about an individual's mental state or thoughts. Legal consequences of actions can vary depending on whether someone was acting as a result of mental illness or incompetence, or on whether someone responded on impulse or acted with careful premeditation. Neuroscience tests might provide useful, or possibly even definitive, information relevant to, for example, a criminal defendant's insanity defense, whether a convicted murderer was mentally retarded and hence could not constitutionally be executed, or whether an elderly person had been mentally competent when making a will. The truthfulness or the biases of parties, witnesses, jurors, and even judges can be important issues. A neuroscience technology that was a truly effective lie detector might see widespread courtroom use, as could a similar method of detecting bias.

Like the rest of us, judges and juries have had to assess a person's mental state by his actions—actions that may be, intentionally or otherwise, misleading.

These mind-reading technologies also have implications outside the courtroom. When and how should others, not under the immediate supervision or control of a judge, be allowed to use mind-reading technologies, with or without the consent of those whose minds are read? Governments will be interested in using this technology on the battlefield, in antiterrorist intelligence gathering, and in criminal investigation. Of course, enemy soldiers, terrorists, and organized crime will also have their uses for such technology, as might employers, educators, and parents. The legal system will inevitably be forced to try to sort out these conflicting claims.

To the extent that mind-reading technologies prove feasible, the law will face at least five major questions about their use.

♦ How accurate will the technologies be?
♦ How accurate will the technologies be perceived to be?
♦ Would it be proper to use even accurate mind-reading technologies in the courtroom?
♦ How should the use of these technologies outside the courtroom be regulated?
♦ How well can limits on the use of such technologies be enforced?

This chapter will follow some of my earlier work in using possible truth-testing technologies as a way to explore to those questions, but the same concerns will be relevant, perhaps in slightly different ways, for other mind-reading technologies (Greely 2004).

## Accuracy

The polygraph and its precursors have existed as lie detectors since the early 1920s. The polygraph measures several physiological reactions associated with nervousness: blood pressure, pulse, respiration rate, and skin conductivity (sweaty palms), among others. It has often been tested and it is more accurate than chance; a recent National Research Council report reviewed studies that showed a 85–90 percent accuracy for polygraphs (National Research Council 2003). That accuracy rate has not been sufficient to convince most courts in the United States that the technology is sufficiently reliable for its results to be introduced in evidence. All state and federal courts have generally prohibited polygraph evidence, except those of New Mexico. Some of these bans are as a result of statutes; most are the result of courts' application to polygraphs of the general rules governing admissibility of scientific evidence (although a few courts have begun to reconsider that question). On the other hand, polygraphs are widely used by the police, government investigators, and employers for non-judicial uses.

Assume that neuroscience produces a more accurate way of testing whether someone is telling the truth (or, at least, what that person believes is the truth) through the use of fMRI, electroencephalography, or other techniques. The true accuracy of such technology would be a crucial question. Careful measurement of accuracy would be even more important than in the context of predictive tests; some of those being truth tested will be strongly motivated to deceive the test and some may even be trained or practiced at doing so. One would want to know the rates of false-positive, false-negative, and inconclusive results as demonstrated on a broad and diverse cross-section of the population, including some who, with or without training, are trying to beat the test.

Courts in the United States currently use one of two standards for determining whether scientific evidence should be admitted. The older test, called the *Frye* test, actually arose from a 1923 case involving evidence from a precursor of the polygraph (*Frye* v. *United States* 1923).

It requires that the technology be 'sufficiently established to have gained general acceptance in the particular field in which it belongs'. Experts from the field testify as to whether the technology is generally accepted. The newer test, applicable in federal courts and in many state courts, comes from *Daubert* v. *Merrell Dow Pharmaceuticals*, a 1993 decision concerning a product liability suit. In *Daubert*, the Supreme Court instructed federal judges to replace the *Frye* test with a new standard. The judge must make a 'preliminary assessment of whether the reasoning or methodology underlying the testimony is scientifically valid and of whether the reasoning or methodology can be applied to the facts in issue'. The Court offered four considerations for judges in making such decisions: whether the theory or technique has been tested, whether it has been peer reviewed and published, what its known error rate is, and its degree of general acceptance.

Decisions under *Frye* or *Daubert* by a single judge seem a weak basis for admitting evidence from a technology with the potentially revolutionary implications of truth testing. A truth-testing procedure would not seem to be a drug or device regulated by the US Food and Drug Administration (FDA), as it would have neither the purpose of treating disease nor of affecting the structure or function of the human body. Nonetheless, it might well be appropriate to require intensive FDA-type clinical trials of such methods, involving controlled trials of thousands of diverse subjects, before allowing them to be admitted into evidence (Greely 2005). That kind of proof of accuracy would also be important as legislators and others try to decide how such technologies could be used out of court. Of course, pharmaceutical companies seeking profits can be counted on to spend the money for rigorous tests of promising drugs; it is not clear who would pay for extensive testing for mind-reading technologies.

## Perceived accuracy

A variation between the proven accuracy of a technique and its perceived accuracy would be particularly important for courtroom uses of truth testing. A jury might well place more weight on neuroscience testimony than it deserved, despite hearing evidence of its error rates. Nor can judges be presumed immune from the lure of scientific certainty. At the extreme, a consistent overweighing of this kind of evidence might require its exclusion. Short of that, if this does in fact prove to be problematic, the judicial system could experiment with required instructions to jurors about the limits of truth-testing methods. On the other hand, these arguments were made at the beginning of the forensic uses of DNA. The adversary system of justice, when applied by competent defense counsel, has been able, at least on occasion, to convince jurors or judges to disregard damning DNA evidence. It would be harder to counter overestimates of the strength of such technologies when used outside the courtroom. Warning labels on the devices seem unlikely to be much use.

## Propriety of uses within the courtroom

We might not want to use mind-reading technologies in the courtroom even if they were perfectly accurate. In 1998 four justices of the Supreme Court came to that conclusion about polygraphs in *United States* v. *Scheffer*.

Scheffer was an enlisted man in the Air Force. He had worked with the military police as an undercover informant in drug investigations; while he was undercover, the military police regularly gave him polygraph tests to try to ensure that he was not using illegal drugs. He successfully maintained under polygraph examination that he was not using such drugs, but his urine samples showed that he was taking methamphetamine. Scheffer wanted to introduce those polygraph test results, conducted before his arrest as a routine part of his role as a police informant, at his court martial. The evidence was excluded because Military Rule of Evidence 707 explicitly banned admission of the results of, or any reference to, a polygraph examination. Scheffer claimed that this flat ban violated his Sixth Amendment right to present a defense and the Court of Appeals for the Armed Forces agreed with him (*United States* v. *Scheffer* 1996).

The Supreme Court did not, and reversed the judgment. Justice Thomas wrote the main opinion for a fractured Court. Eight justices agreed that polygraph evidence was not sufficiently reliable for its admission to be required. Justice Thomas and three of his colleagues would also have reversed on another ground: the need to 'preserve the jury's core function of making credibility determinations in criminal trial'. This concern would seem to be even more powerful with our hypothesized perfectly accurate neuroscience truth detector. Justice Thomas's argument, with only four out of nine votes behind it, is not a binding precedent, at least not yet. Even if it never becomes a constitutional holding, the concern behind it could well sway courts forced to decide whether to allow such evidence to be presented to juries, or to legislatures regulating truth testing, or to forbid it. (It is not clear whether even Justice Thomas would exclude such evidence in non-jury trials.)

Other concerns beyond accuracy could limit other judicial uses of mind-reading technologies. One could imagine that some neuroscience evidence might demonstrate conclusively that a criminal defendant could not control his actions. Courts and legislatures might just disregard such evidence. We might choose to believe in free will, or act as if a defendant had free will, and thus refuse to excuse otherwise criminal conduct, whatever neuroscience told us.

Similarly, fMRI or other technologies might be able to show that a potential juror was biased against the defendant. The Sixth Amendment to the United States Constitution itself grants criminal defendants 'the right to a speedy and public trial, by an impartial jury...'. In practice, because of the limits of our ability to detect bias, an 'impartial jury' largely means 'not demonstrably biased jurors'. A juror who admits to being prejudiced against a party, because of race, religion, gender, or for any other reason, will be dismissed. If neuroscience allowed us to know that a potential juror felt a bias against a party even though that juror denied bias, we might end up changing the substantive rule rather than discharging more jurors. Thus the constitutional requirement might be reinterpreted as allowing jurors who were biased as long as they could overcome their biases and render a fair decision. For some defendants such a change might prove essential. For example, neuroscience tests for bias might find that all potential jurors were biased against large and scary-looking members of a motorcycle gang, except, perhaps, for other gang members, which might raise questions of bias in the other direction.

These kinds of questions ask whether, for one reason or another, we might not want to take into account neuroscience mind-reading evidence that would, under current standards, seem relevant. Courtroom uses of such technologies raise many other complex questions. Consider some of the other knotty constitutional issues involved in truth testing (Greely 2004). If voluntary truth-tested testimony were admissible, could a witness's credibility be enhanced by noting that he had been willing to undergo such testing? Could the witness's credibility be undercut by noting that he had refused to undergo that testing? The Fifth Amendment's ban on compelled self-incrimination might provide some protection against this kind of impeachment for criminal defendants who choose not to testify at all; it will not apply in other situations.

Could truth testing ever be compelled? At its narrowest, that might involve forcing a witness who had been truth tested by one side to undergo a similar examination by the other side's experts or devices. More broadly, except when the Fifth Amendment's privilege against self-incrimination applies, people can be forced, under penalty of law, to give testimony. In some cases, as when a medical condition is a material issue in a trial, they can be forced to undergo testing. Constitutional arguments against such compulsory truth testing might be made under at least the Fourth, Fifth, Fourteenth, and perhaps the First Amendments to the Constitution, but it is not clear that truth testing could not be similarly compelled from witnesses or, perhaps more powerfully, from parties who want to testify in their own behalf. All such constitutional questions might become more complicated if a witness claimed that his testimony was truthful, which might be viewed as waiving any rights to avoid truth testing. A legislature or a court might decide, on policy grounds, to forbid either voluntary or compulsory truth testing even if the Constitution did not prohibit it, but in some cases a defendant might establish that he had a constitutional right to use such testing. The Sixth Amendment argument that failed Airman Scheffer might work for other defendants; in *Rock* v. *Arkansas* (1987) the Supreme Court held that an Arkansas rule barring all testimony as to memories refreshed by hypnosis violated the right to put on a defense of a defendant who argued she could only present her case using such testimony.

It is not clear how any of these questions would be resolved. Good guesses are not even possible without knowing more about the details of the, so far, hypothetical technologies and cases. It is clear that a highly accurate technology for detecting whether witnesses were telling the truth could have enormous effects on the legal system. Not every law suit would disappear; for example, some turn not on what actually happened but on an assessment of those events (were the defendant's actions reasonable?) or on a disputed interpretation of the law. But many everyday criminal or civil cases would surely disappear if the court could be sure that a witness told the truth about the existence of a drug deal, or orally agreed-upon terms of a business deal. That kind of potential will make the judiciary both interested in, and nervous about, the potential for neuroscience mind reading.

## Uses outside the courtroom and invasion of privacy

Mind reading seems like the ultimate invasion of privacy. Since we first learned as children how to conceal our thoughts or feelings, we have known that, although others might make shrewd guesses, no one could know what was actually going on in our minds unless we told them. (And even then we might not be able to convey a full understanding.) Effective mind reading threatens to invade a last inviolate area of 'self'. Like removing the membrane from a living cell, removing our ability to withhold our mind's workings may threaten to eliminate, at least for some mental states, emotions, or thoughts, the difference between 'self' and 'other'. Even if we were to allow some such intrusions in the carefully controlled environment of the courtroom, mind-reading technologies might be used in many other contexts, by both the government and private parties. Those uses raise different issues, of both constitutional law and policy. Again, truth testing provides a useful example for exploring those issues.

When an American government (federal, state, or local) acts, it is bound by the Constitution whether or not the action takes place in a courtroom. A detective in a police station, a military officer on the battlefield, or a counter-intelligence agent in a foreign country will all be subject to some constitutional constraints, although those constraints may vary. Outside the courtroom, the voluntary application of truth testing to a mentally competent adult who had given his informed consent to the procedure would probably raise no constitutional issues. If the situation made the subject's agreement less than truly voluntary, such issues might arise. Consider, for example, a requirement that people answer truth-tested questions to in order to qualify for government jobs, government benefits, or government licenses. Today, one could imagine requiring applicants for government scholarships or government-guaranteed student loans to answer, under truth testing, questions about their possible illegal drug use. Yesterday, or tomorrow, the questions might be about their political views. Some questions might be ruled unconstitutionally intrusive, but even questions that are permissible when the subject has the power to lie might become impermissible if truth testing took away that form of self-help.

In other cases the government might just force someone to undergo truth testing. It might make sense to use such technologies to question a suspected member of an organized crime gang or of a terrorist organization about the group's plans or members even if the results could not be admitted in court, or even if the testing meant that that person could not be successfully prosecuted. Questions might well arise under at least the Fourth Amendment, which protects Americans against unreasonable searches and seizures, and the Fifth Amendment, which guarantees them due process and provides them with a privilege against self-incrimination. For state or local governments, the Fourteenth Amendment would also be implicated. Or consider surreptitious truth detection such as a miniaturized device built into airline security checkpoints. The Constitution does not protect travelers against mandatory metal detection and other screening at airports; would it protect against invasions of our minds?

The federal Constitution does not, for the most part, apply to non-governmental actors. Any protection against the voluntary or involuntary uses of truth testing by employers, parents, poker players, or others would usually be a legislative matter. [However, some states, such as California, do have constitutional protections for privacy that do apply to private actors (California Constitution, Article I, Section 1; *Hill* v. *National Collegiate Athletic Association* 1994)]. It would usually be difficult to a private party to force an unwilling subject into an MRI machine; it might be easier for an employer to offer an employee a choice—your cooperation or your job. Again, the development of technologies small and unobtrusive enough to be used without the subject's consent or even knowledge could greatly expand the plausible uses of truth testing.

Some private parties may well have legitimate reasons to want to use this technology and some innocent people may be eager to be able to clear up their boss's suspicions or their parents' worries by voluntarily undergoing this testing. Some governments have already passed legislation putting some limits on the use of polygraphs, most notably the federal government whose Employee Polygraph Protection Act of 1988 restricts most employers. Others have not. Faced with new, and possibly more accurate, mind-reading technologies, both groups will need to reconsider the issue. Deciding whether or when to allow frankly coerced, questionably voluntary, or enthusiastically accepted uses of truth testing, or of any other mind-reading technology, by private parties will pose complicated and difficult questions.

## Issues of enforcement

Assume that the uses of truth-testing methods are somehow limited. How well can such limits be enforced? Within the courtroom, enforcement should be easy. The adversary system should guarantee that one lawyer or the other will object to any improper use of such technologies. The courtroom comes equipped with a decision-maker, available and empowered to determine whether a use is proper—and with a clearly understood and delineated system for contesting that decision.

Outside the courtroom, the ability to enforce limits on the uses of these technologies will depend overwhelmingly on how the technologies are implemented. It would be relatively easy to exercise good, though not perfect, control of the uses to which multimillion dollar MRI scanners are put. Liability could be placed on the owners of the machines along with requirements for recording all their uses. Knowing where each machine was and identifying a party who could be held responsible (and, presumably, an organization like a hospital, clinic, or research university that would be responsible in other senses) would make it relatively easy to enforce civil or criminal prohibitions of some uses of the technologies.

On the other hand, a technology the size of headphones could not easily be controlled, especially if it were not very expensive or very difficult to manufacture. If the miniature version also had legitimate uses, controlling its distribution and uses would become even more difficult. (These problems would exist equally with pharmacological techniques, such as a truth pill or a truth serum.) With mind-reading devices, a regulatory scheme could try to build precautions into the machines themselves. For example, one might require registration of each machine and its owners, coupled with a system that broadcast the machine's location to the relevant authorities. Unauthorized users of the equipment might be detectable in that way, at least until they learned to defeat the locating system. In the long run, one would probably have to fall back on victims reporting illegal uses of these technologies to criminal or civil authorities. Prohibition, by itself or with sanctions, might deter misuse by some who might otherwise abuse the technologies, such as large employers. It would be far less effective among users unconcerned about following the law, particularly if the subjects of the mind-reading procedures underwent them voluntarily.

## Enhancement

I dare do all that become a man;
Who dares do more is none.

*Macbeth*, Act I, Scene 7

Our brains, and the powers they confer, are largely what separate us from the rest of life on this planet. The consciousness that springs from that brain defines us. We treat as humans those among us who have lost, or have never had, that consciousness, but we grieve that they are lacking this essential component of humanity. Tomorrow's neuroscience, and even today's, offers us the chance to enhance our consciousness, to change and improve our senses, our cognitive abilities, and the commanding power of our brains. Macbeth, despite his initial reluctance, ultimately did dare to kill Duncan; by daring more, he became less than human. Some fear that by daring to use neuroscience and other technologies to become more than we are, we may kill our own humanity. Neuroscience offers enhancement along at least two paths—through pharmacology and through neuroelectronic interfaces. Both have already begun (see also Chapter 6).

In 1998 the FDA approved Provigil® (the proprietary name for modafinil) as a treatment for excessive daytime sleepiness associated with narcolepsy; in 2003 it expanded the approved indications to daytime sleepiness associated with shift-work disorder and sleep apnea. Yet modafinil increases alertness and wakefulness not just in those with these medical conditions, but in healthy people. As a result, modafinil is now being used to enhance cognitive abilities by physicians on call, by academics going to overseas conferences, and, perhaps, by students 'pulling all-nighters'. Similarly, Ritalin® (the proprietary name for methylphenidate) and Adderall® (a complex mixture of amphetamines), prescribed mainly for attention-deficit disorder (ADD) or attention-deficit hyperactivity disorder (ADHD), are reportedly often used by students without ADD or ADHD to help them study or to concentrate on tests. If a drug were successfully developed to improve memory in patients with dementia and if it were shown to improve memory in non-demented people, it seems inevitable that many healthy people would seek it to improve their already normal memories.

Neuroelectronic interfaces seek to provide direct links between the central nervous system and electronic systems. These can involve electronic inputs to the brain or direct outputs from the brain to electronic systems. Both already exist in at least rudimentary form. Cochlear implants are FDA-approved medical devices for the treatment of some kinds of deafness. These devices use electronic sensors to detect and analyze sound arriving at the patient's ear, and then stimulate the appropriate parts of the auditory nerve, allowing the patient to hear. Electronic retinas are under development. These use photosensors to see and then electrically stimulate regions of the optic nerve to produce vision. Currently, these serve only to restore normal human function—very poorly for the experimental artificial retinas, but reasonably well for the cochlear implants. However, there is no reason why the sensors in either device are limited to abnormal human function. They could allow people to hear ultrasound or to see infrared radiation. Similarly, researchers can now detect neuronal firing patterns, either by microelectrodes or through electroencephalography, convert those detected patterns into electronic signals, and use these signals to control devices. Both monkeys and, more recently, human subjects have been trained to move a cursor on a computer screen by thought or, more accurately, by the electronic translation of their detected neuronal firing patterns (Carmena *et al.* 2003; Wolpaw and McFarland 2004; see also Chapter 13).

The issue of enhancement has been widely discussed in many contexts, from cosmetic surgery to germ-line gene therapy (Parens 1998; President's Council on Bioethics 1999; Buchanan *et al.* 2001; Elliott 2003; Rothman and Rothman 2003). It has not only ethical implications, but also legal ones. Specifically, efforts to regulate enhancement face legal challenges including the following.

◆ How should we regulate the safety of enhancements?
◆ How can we avoid coercive enhancement, express or implicit?
◆ Should we intervene to make sure enhancement is fairly distributed, and if so, how?
◆ How will enhancement affect the relationship between parents and children?
◆ Should the law intervene to 'preserve human nature'?
◆ How well can limits on neuroscience enhancement be enforced?

As with prediction and mind reading, these questions may have different answers depending on whether the legal system is using the enhancement or is trying to regulate its use by others.

## Regulating safety

The issue of the safety of neuroscience enhancements may seem straightforward, but it actually encompasses many complicated legal issues. The pharmacological enhancements discussed above look like drugs; the neuroelectronic interfaces would seem to be medical devices. Both are regulated by the FDA in the United States, and by roughly similar agencies in most rich countries. These neuroscience enhancements would appear largely, although not entirely, to require advance FDA approval after proof of safety and efficacy. (Whether they would be subject to similar regulation in other countries may hinge on the exact authority given to the regulators.)

The statute that gives the FDA the power to regulate drugs [Federal Food, Drug, and Cosmetic Act, Section 201(g)] defines them as follows:

(B) articles intended for use in the diagnosis, cure, mitigation, treatment, or prevention of disease in man or other animals; and

(C) articles (other than food) intended to affect the structure or any function of the body of many or other animals.

The same statute defines a medical 'device' as 'an instrument, apparatus, implement, machine, contrivance, implant, *in vitro* reagent, or other similar or related article' that is intended for either of the two uses that define drugs [Federal Food, Drug, and Cosmetic Act, Section 201(h)]. Enhancement uses would not qualify under the first of the two intended use provisions in the statute, but they do seem to fit under the category of 'intended to affect the structure or any function of the body'. All new drugs are subject to extensive regulation by the FDA, requiring controlled clinical trials that demonstrate, to the FDA's satisfaction, that the new drug is both safe and effective. The riskiest medical devices, those placed in Class III, are subject to similar, though somewhat weaker, requirements that they be shown to be safe and effective. However, under a procedure known as a Section 510(k) filing, even Class III devices that are 'substantially related' to previously marketed devices may avoid this testing. Some neuroelectronic devices, such as cochlear implants to 'hear' ultrasound, might be able to avoid stringent testing through this 510(k) procedure. It should be noted that the FDA does not regulate many things that fit the statutory definition of 'devices', such as clothes which, after all, 'affect the structure or any function' of the human body. Some cognitive enhancement technologies, including some currently marketed aural and visual stimulation methods, might not be regulated by the FDA simply because they are quite different from the kinds of medical devices the agency generally regulates (Halpern 2005).

Other pharmacological enhancements might qualify as 'dietary supplements', which have their own complex multipart definition in the statutes. After all, coffee, coca leaves, and chocolate all have neurological effects that might be considered enhancements. Dietary supplements are generally subject to the same regulation as new drugs if they make claims to treat disease, but they are subject to minimal regulation if they only make the so-called 'structure and function' claims that are likely for enhancement products.

Even if the enhancements are subject to strict FDA regulation, several safety issues remain. First, even the most stringent FDA testing requirements cannot guarantee that a drug will be safe. Clinical trials last for a few months to, at most, a few years, and a large Phase III trial might involve 4000 people. Slowly developing or rare risks simply cannot be detected in such trials. Diethylstilbestrol (DES), a drug prescribed from 1940 through 1971, was later shown to have caused reproductive system cancers, infertility, and other problems among some of the daughters of women who took the drug while pregnant. Rezulin, a very widely used diabetes drug withdrawn by the FDA amid safety controversy, appears to have caused severe liver problems in about one patient in 20 000. No clinical trial could plausibly have seen either of these problems. The potentially vast markets for enhancements, and the likelihood that the healthy people using the enhancement may well not be closely monitored by their doctors, increases the concern about their safety.

Secondly, some of these enhancements, such as modafinil or cochlear implants, will be approved for treating disease. Once approved by the FDA for one purpose, prescription drugs and their device equivalents (so-called restricted devices) can generally be prescribed by a physician for any purpose. Such off-label use has safety implications. A drug or device that has been tested mainly for safety in people with a particular illness and at defined doses can then be used at very different doses by healthy people. The safety of that kind of use of the drug will not have been tested in any substantial way.

Thirdly, it is not clear how the FDA would, or should, evaluate the safety of enhancement technologies. For drugs, the FDA tries to weigh the safety risks in light of the disease the drug is intended to treat. Highly toxic and dangerous drugs can be approved for the treatment of deadly cancers, while the FDA would require much greater safety for drugs to treat relatively minor ailments. How much risk should we allow in a drug that does not treat a disease but improves normal function? If it were to weigh the risks against the *health* benefits of the treatment, it might require almost complete safety. We regulate the safety of drugs and the riskier medical devices more closely than that of most other products. However, outside the world of medicine we allow people to take non-trivial risks without requiring the government to agree with consumers' cost–benefit assessments. In some cases, like the long-term safety of dietary choices, we scarcely regulate at all. Even when we regulate to prevent extreme safety risks, as in commercial air transportation or automobiles, we do not require perfect safety but allow consumers to make their own choices. Ultimately, the legal system will have to determine whether society should regulate this hypothetical memory enhancer like a drug, like an automobile, or like a choice of restaurant entrée.

## Coercion

Coercion is another important concern. It seems straightforward to say that the legal system should prohibit anyone from being compelled to use neuroscience enhancements, but implementing that goal may prove difficult. In some cases we may want to allow compelled enhancement. The Air Force might decide for good reason to require long-distance pilots to use modafinil or another alertness drug; hospitals might make the same decision with respects to physicians on night call in order to promote patient safety. Employers require employees to 'enhance themselves' through training courses; law schools require students to 'enhance themselves' through required first-year courses. The line between permissible requirements and impermissible intrusion may prove hard to draw.

Frank coercion may not be the most common way in which people are forced to use neuroscience enhancements. Assume that a drug is developed that improves a normal person's ability to memorize facts. Now consider an undergraduate introductory organic chemistry class, filled with premedical students who know that low grades in organic chemistry are a common barrier to medical school. Like bodybuilders who complain that they have to use steroids illegally in order to compete, students may feel that they have to use this memory-enhancing drug. The law might intervene by an effective ban on any use, by mandatory disclosure of drug use, by the establishment of separately graded sections of the organic chemistry class (drug and no-drug sections), or in other ways. This example also highlights a slightly different set of safety concerns about some forms of enhancement. If, for example, memory-enhancing drugs were effective, banning them might lead to somewhat less know-ledgeable, and possibly somewhat less safe, doctors. If, on the other hand, the drugs had only short-term effects, good for an examination but not for a career, permitting their use might lead to more doctors with less knowledge of organic chemistry who, as a result, might (or might not) be worse physicians.

The legal system's own use of enhancement technologies could raise questions of both express and implicit coercion, as they do with lie detection. Imagine a proven way of enhancing a witness's memory. A court might consider ordering a witness to use such an enhancing technology, where, for example, a criminal defendant argued persuasively that such an enhancement was essential to his defense. On the other hand, a party to litigation who was a witness in his own behalf might feel an implicit coercion to use the technology. His failure, or refusal, to use it might be construed as uncertainty on his part about the accuracy of his recollection. Of course, both these possibilities exist within the legal system but outside the courtroom, from police investigations to depositions. Hypnosis provides an example of an uncertainly effective memory enhancement technology; its uses in the legal system continue to be controversial (Webert 2003).

## Distributive justice

Effective enhancements raise questions of distributive justice. If enhancements cost money, those with more money will be more likely to be enhanced. At one extreme, some commentators have seen enhancement, particularly through genetic engineering, as leading to a self-perpetuating genobility, dividing humanity into different castes and possibly ultimately into different species (Mehlman 2003). More concretely, the organic chemistry class described above might seem unfair to the students who were not using the memory drug. Again, one could try to ban the drug entirely. Another option would be to make it equally available to all who wanted it, either by making it free to everyone or by providing subsidies to those who, by some standard, could not afford it. Even these solutions leave concerns about fairness to those individuals and groups who, for religious, philosophical, or other reasons, choose not to use the available enhancements.

Neuroscientific enhancements obviously do not create these problems; private schools (or well-funded public schools) and private tutors provide currently existing examples of the same kind of potential unfairness. Interventions to prevent that kind of unfairness exist, but are not thorough. One might still argue for banning neuroscience enhancements, either because they might be too effective or because new sources of unfairness should be prevented even if, for practical reasons, older ones cannot be eliminated.

## Parent–child relationships

The relationship between parent and child raises still other issues, some related to coercion and some that go far beyond it. Some enhancement interventions may well work best, or may only work, when used on young rapidly developing brains. (Note that the safety of pediatric uses of an intervention may be uncertain even after it has been approved for adult use; proving, or requiring proof of, such safety can be difficult.) In a sense, any parental decision applied to children, at least to young children, is coercive. A one-year-old cannot consent to an enhancement technology, whether it takes the form of a neuroelectronic interface device or an educational toy. An eight-year-old might be able to consent, but cannot usually give true informed consent. In most states of the United States, people cannot generally enter into binding contracts until they are 18, yet an enhancement technology might have major and irrevocable effects.

Of course, parents make such decisions for children all the time. Parents decide about their children's education, diet, entertainment options, and, except in extreme cases, health care. In extreme cases, such as where a parent's refusal to permit a blood transfusion might result in the child's death, the state may take custody of the child from the parent in order to protect the child, but normally we expect parents to act in their child's best interests. This parental control over children may even have constitutional protection in the United States. Governments can (and do) compel children to undergo the cognitive enhancement technology called education, but over 80 years ago the United States Supreme Court ruled that states cannot constitutionally forbid parents to educate their children in private schools (*Pierce* v. *Society of Sisters* 1925) nor can they prohibit children from learning particular foreign languages (*Meyer* v. *Nebraska* 1923). Society does prohibit children from doing some things, even with parental permission, that are legal for adults, such as driving, drinking alcohol, smoking, and so on. Whether it could, or should, intervene in the parent–child relationship to prevent parents from using enhancement technologies on their children is unclear.

Enhancement could affect the relationship between parent and child in another deeper way. Some worry that parents might react to enhancement technologies of various sorts by viewing their children more as a product to be manufactured, to parental specifications, than as a fully individual human being, to be cherished with all his or her quirks or flaws (President's Council on Bioethics 2003; Sandel 2004). Of course, parents seek to mold their children in many ways; trying to turn infants into responsible and successful adults is, after all, widely viewed as a parent's prime duty. Whether the law could be a sensitive and effective way to protect this vision of how parents should view children from technological advances is, at best, unclear.

## Banning the unnatural or the unholy

At the heart of many people's discomfort with neuroscience enhancement seems to be a fear of transcending some important limits God or Nature has placed on humanity. The idea of forbidden knowledge has deep roots that, in Western cultures at least, go back to the tree of knowledge of good and evil in Genesis. Are there ways in which humans should not enhance themselves? The law is not particularly helpful in answering that question. However, the law's desire to draw clear lines does lead directly to the issue of how one might define the limits of permissible enhancement. After all, civilization itself—from language, agriculture, and writing to the printing press, air travel, and the Internet—is arguably the product of a series of unnatural human enhancements. If one accepts that godliness or naturalness should limit the uses of neuroscience enhancement, determining how to write a statute distinguishing the permissible from the forbidden becomes a legal problem.

The legal system may have another role in this approach to regulating enhancement. One could make a plausible argument that laws banning neuroscience enhancement may be unconstitutional. First, in the unlikely event that such a ban were justified directly and solely as a religious matter, it might be struck down under the Constitution's First Amendment as an unconstitutional establishment of religion. More broadly, though, individuals may have a constitutionally protected interest in enhancement, at least if that enhancement causes no broader harms. The strength of this argument should not be exaggerated. The United States Constitution has not been construed to give competent and consulting adults a libertarian right to do anything that does not harm others. Yet in some areas, notably those involving repro-duction and sexual intimacy, the Supreme Court has provided some constitutional protections. The contraception and abortion cases could be viewed as providing a narrow, and intensely controversial, area of liberty (*Griswold* v. *Connecticut* 1965; *Roe* v. *Wade* 1973). However, in 2003, the Supreme Court ruled that a state may not criminalize certain sexual acts between consenting adults of the same sex (*Lawrence* v. *Texas* 2003). Although that decision may well end up applying only to sexual acts or intimate relationships, it could presage a broader ban on legislation that impairs a person's liberty based on a majority's moral principles (Charo 2004).

One might argue that control over one's cognitive abilities or mental functioning should be entitled to at least as much protection as sex acts. Such a broad reading of the case would have major consequences for American law (including bans on some 'recreational' drugs); one of those might be the invalidation of any constraints on enhancement technologies banned because they were unnatural or immoral. At this point, that kind of result seems unlikely, but not impossible.

## Enforcement issues

Finally, to be effective, limitations on neuroscience enhancement technologies have to be enforced, and thus enforceable. How easy or difficult such enforcement would prove will vary enormously with the enhancing intervention. The delicate surgery necessary to implant and connect neuroelectronic interfaces inside the skull is unlikely to be carried out secretly. On the other hand, the off-label use of drugs, approved for medical treatment, for enhancement purposes, even if made illegal, could be extremely difficult to enforce. From the perspectives of one student with a diagnosis of ADHD and a prescription for Ritalin and another who wants Ritalin to study for examinations, a transaction between them would seem, at most, a victimless crime. Enforcing laws against such offenses, like prostitution, drug abuse, and gambling, is very difficult because those most directly involved have, unlike the victims of robbery or assault, no reason to complain. Whether justified or not, the American 'War on Drugs' provides powerful evidence of the costs and difficulties of such an effort—in tens of billions of dollars spent and hundreds of thousands of citizens jailed each year.

Of course, no one country can control what happens throughout the world. A ban on, say, neuroelectronic interface enhancements in the United States might only lead interested Americans to seek the enhancement in countries that did not ban it. It could even lead to the creation of enhancement havens, like the small tax or banking shelter nations scattered around the world. Even worse, some countries might embrace the banned technologies, enhancing their own citizens or soldiers with 'weapons of mass enhancement'. International treaties might help to stem the spread of such enhancements, but such treaties are themselves not self-enforcing. The nearly universal membership of the Nuclear Non-Proliferation Treaty and the great expense and difficulty of developing nuclear weapons have not stopped several countries from illegally developing such weapons. One writer on genetic enhancement has gone so far as to advocate preventive war, when necessary, against countries that used such enhancements (Mehlman 2003) and has been criticized for it (Greely 2003). Whatever the wisdom of such an approach, it illustrates some of the difficulties of enforcement. But bans that have no teeth have little value and may be counterproductive. Bans on at least some enhancement technologies may well turn out to be futile.

## Conclusion

> If it were done when 'tis done, then 'twere well
> It were done quickly;
>
> *Macbeth*, Act I, Scene 7

Macbeth was wrong. Duncan's assassination was not 'done when 'tis done', nor was it 'well it were done quickly'. The consequences were neither short term nor predictable. More fore-thought and discussion, perhaps with a wider circle than just his wife, might have prevented the tragedy of Macbeth—and of many others. Forethought and discussion may also prove useful in implementing new technologies from neuroscience.

Negativity is an occupational hazard for those of us who work in bioethics. We write much more of concerns and problems than of benefits. The ongoing revolution in our understanding of the human brain will bring many great boons in the relief of human suffering and in the improvement of the human condition. But at the same time there are potential problems—and real fears. Legal perspectives are crucial to an accurate understanding of how those problems and fears might arise and how they might be addressed. Like many legal analyses, this chapter has been much better at raising questions than at providing answers. I am not confident that any set of legal answers, at this early stage of the development of these technologies, would be correct or even useful. I am hopeful that a set of law-influenced questions will prove useful as we strive to maximize the benefits of these emerging neuroscience technologies to humanity and minimize their harms.

# References

Andrews LB, Fullerton JB, Holtzman NH, *et al.* (1994). *Assessing Genetic Risks: Implications for Health and Social Policy.* Washington, DC: National Academy Press.

Buchanan A, Brock DW, Daniels N, Wikler D (2001). *From Chance To Choice: Genetics And Justice.* Cambridge, UK: Cambridge University Press.

Carmena JM, Lebedev MA, Crist RE, *et al.* (2003). Learning to control a brain–machine interface for reaching and grasping by primates. *Public Library of Science—Biology* 1. Available online at: http://biology.plosjournals.org/perlserv/?request=get-document&doi=10.1371/journal.pbio.0000042

Charo RA (2004). Political aspects. Presented at Conference on Unnatural Selection: Should California Regulate Preimplantation Genetic Diagnosis?, 27 February 2004, Stanford, CA. Audio recording of talk available online at http://www.law.stanford.edu/programs/academic/lst/bioscience/pgd/presentations.html

*Daubert v. Merrell Dow Pharmaceuticals* 516 U.S. 869 (1993).

Diver CS, Cohen JM (2001). What is wrong with genetic discrimination. *University of Pennsylvania Law Review* 149, 1439–79.

Elliott C (2003). *Better than Well: American Medicine Meets the American Dream.* New York: W.W. Norton.

Federal Food, Drug and Cosmetic Act, Section 201, codified at 21 U.S.C. 321.

*Frye v. United States* 54 App. D.C. 46, 293 F. 1013 (D.C. Cir. 1923).

Greely HT (2001). 'Genotype discrimination': the complex case for some legislative protection. *University of Pennsylvania Law Review* 149, 1483–1505.

Greely HT (2003). Human genetic enhancement, a lawyer's view: review of *Wondergenes: Genetic Enhancement and the Future of Society* by Maxwell J. Mehlman. *Medical Humanities Review* 17, 42–6.

Greely HT (2004). Prediction, litigation, privacy, and property: Some possible legal and social implications of advances in neuroscience. In: Garland B (ed) *Neuroscience and the Law: Brain, Mind, and the Scales of Justice.* New York: Dana Press, 114–56.

Greely HT (2005). Premarket approval for lie detection: an idea whose and time may be coming. *American Journal of Bioethics* 5(2), 50–52.

*Griswold v. Connecticut* 381 U.S. 479 (1965).

Halpern S (2005). You must remember this. Are there memory enhancing products that work? Available online at: http://www.slate.com/id/2111758/

*Hill v. National Collegiate Athletic Association,* 7 Cal.4th 1 (1994).

Hudson KL, Rothenberg KH, Andrews LB, Kahn MJE, Collins F (1995). Genetic discrimination and health insurance: an urgent need for reform. *Science* 270, 391–3.

Koenig BA, Greely HT, McConnell L, Silverberg H, Raffin TA (1998). PGES recommendations on genetic testing for breast cancer susceptibility. *Journal of Women's Health* 7, 531–45.

*Lawrence* v. *Texas* 539 U.S. 558 (2003).

Mehlman MJ (2003). *Wondergenes: Genetic Enhancement and the Future of Society.* Bloomington, IN: University of Indiana Press.

*Meyer* v. *Nebraska* 262 U.S. 390 (1923).

National Research Council Committee to Review the Scientific Evidence on the Polygraph (2003). *The Polygraph and Lie Detection.* Washington, DC: National Academy Press.

Parens E (ed) (1998). *Enhancing Human Traits: Ethical and Social Implications.* Washington, DC: Georgetown University Press.

*Pierce* v. *Society of Sisters* 269 U.S. 510 (1925).

President's Council on Bioethics (2003). *Beyond Therapy: Biotechnology and the Pursuit of Happiness.* New York: Regan Books.

*Rock* v. *Arkansas* 483 U.S. 44 (1987).

*Roe* v. *Wade* 410 U.S. 113 (1973).

Rothman S, Rothman D (2003). *The Pursuit of Perfection: The Promise and Perils of Medical Enhancement.* New York: Pantheon.

Sandel MJ (2004). The case against perfection. *Atlantic Monthly* 293.

*United States* v. *Scheffer* 44 M.J. 442 (U.S. Ct App Armed Forces 1996), reviewed 523 U.S. 303 (1998).

Webert DR (2003). Are the courts in a trance? Approaches to the admissibility of hypnotically enhanced witness testimony in light of empirical evidence. *American Criminal Law Review* 40, 1301–27.

Wolpaw JR, McFarland DJ (2004). Control of a two-dimensional movement signal by a noninvasive brain-computer interface in humans. *Proceedings of the National Academy of Sciences of the USA* 101, 17849–54.

Chapter 18

# Neuroethics in education

Kimberly Sheridan, Elena Zinchenko,
and Howard Gardner

## Introduction

In the coming years, educators and the general public will look increasingly to discoveries from the neurosciences for insights about how best to educate young people. To understand the ethical dilemmas posed by these advances, we first need to consider the nature of the education enterprise. Education is above all a value-laden profession, with its values in perpetual dispute. More so than most other professionals, educators experience competing demands from many stakeholders along with considerably less autonomy and status. Drawing on findings from the GoodWork Project, a study of how professionals cope with rapid change, we examine how neurocognitive advances may exacerbate these tensions in education. We then consider how educators might navigate the changes, challenges, and opportunities entailed in scientific discoveries. To this end, we propose the establishment of a class of professionals, 'neuroeducators'. The mission of these new professionals will be to guide the introduction of neurocognitive advances into education in a sensible and ethical manner.

Consider the following three possible scenarios set in 2010.

**Scenario 1** Ms E holds a parent–teacher conference with the parents of Daniel, a friendly hard-working second-grader. To prepare, she reviews his folder containing the routine items: his last year's grades and teachers' comments, standardized test scores, and a functional MRI (fMRI) report submitted by Daniel's parents. Many parents press their doctors for these fMRI reports of their child's brain functioning on basic visual and auditory processing as well as on school tasks such as reading and arithmetic. These can screen for dyslexia or other learning disabilities, thus allowing earlier intervention. Daniel has not been diagnosed with any specific learning disabilities, but his fMRI reports somewhat atypical auditory processing. His schoolwork has been adequate. When pressed by his parents about his auditory processing, Ms E remembers that on occasion Daniel has been inattentive during her lessons, and tends to do better on sight-reading familiar words than on sounding out unusual ones. These symptoms could be related to problems with auditory processing. She knows the importance of early intervention and has heard about 'critical periods' in brain development, and so she is wary of waiting until Daniel actually experiences difficulty in class. Some of her students with dyslexia utilize a program that addresses auditory processing deficits; she thinks it will help Daniel as well. She recommends the program to Daniel's parents who are eager to do something to help him with his processing issues before they become a serious problem. She is not sure if this is the 'right' thing to do, but believes that it is better than nothing.

**Scenario 2** For as long as fractions have been taught in elementary school they have proved difficult for many students. Recent research in a reputable peer-reviewed journal claims to have found a neurological basis for this difficulty. Scientists show a fairly linear relationship between understanding fractions and the strength of a particular neurological pathway. Buoyed by the educational potential of their findings, the neuroscientists consult with an educational software company to develop computer software that directly targets the neurological deficits. The software does not actually work on fraction problems. Instead it helps students practice the visualization of the relationships between parts and wholes. Early testing reveals that use of the software does indeed lessen the neurological differences between those who master fractions and those who do not. Impressed by this high-profile research and eager to embrace a new scientifically based approach to teaching fractions, heads of school districts are buying this 'silver bullet' software. Students will spend the first month of the fraction unit working on the software instead of traditional mathematics instruction, and then transfer back into regular class, once their neural pathways are 'built up'. Many teachers are wary about having their class miss so much mathematics instruction time. At the same time they acknowledge that traditional instruction in fractions has not been successful for many of their students.

**Scenario 3** In a review of the past several years' data on college admissions examinations, officials found a rapid rise in scores in the past 3 years alongside a widening gap between test scores of higher and lower socio-economic groups. Research into these surprising results, including anonymous surveys of students, reveals that the rise in scores is highly correlated with use of recently released prescription neurocognitive enhancers that improve memory and information-processing speed. While the use of neurocognitive enhancers during testing is officially forbidden, it is an ineffectual policy in the absence of a means of enforcement. Officials are also unsure where to draw the line on drug use as many test takers who are diagnosed with anxiety or attention deficit disorders routinely use drugs that are performance enhancing. Meanwhile, colleges wrestle with how to weight the inflated test scores and address the systematic disparity in scores between users and non-users of the drugs. Students and parents must choose between breaking the rules and using the drugs on the one hand, or competing on a high-stakes test at a disadvantage on the other. Ethical dilemmas around performance-enhancing drugs once limited to professional sports and the Olympic Games are now routine for most high school seniors, and policy makers have not considered the potential side effects and the little-researched long-term effects of using the drugs.

While these scenarios arise from technological advances in neuroscience, they also point to age-old dilemmas in education. Education is a value-laden enterprise that has always dealt with complex issues. At each level of the system, from working with an individual student to setting goals and policy at the national and international levels, educators encounter dilemmas of competing interests, innovations of uncertain potency, and disproportionate access to finite resources. To understand how cultural and technological change impacts education and creates novel ethical dilemmas, we need first to consider the signature characteristics of the existing profession.

# The enterprise of education

To reiterate, education is essentially about values. It is a system whereby we pass on knowledge and skills that we determine to be culturally important. Of course, all professions follow certain values: science embraces truth and integrity tied to its methods; medicine begins with the basic credo of 'do no harm'. But education stands out in light of the lack of common widely accepted values. Central decisions as to what knowledge, to which people, by which method, at what expense, and to what end, are perennially under debate. We can imagine (and discern across cultures and throughout history) a number of competing overarching goals for education: aiming to identify and pick out the elite students, equalizing the starting point, fulfilling each student's potential, and educating everyone just enough so that individuals do not become a burden on society, just to name a few. This choice among overarching goals cascades into a variety of other decisions: where to focus allocation of resources (e.g. gifted and talented programs, remediation programs, small class sizes), what to teach (e.g. calculus, media literacy, 'life skills'), and by what method (e.g. Socratic, lecture, drill).

While values and overarching goals may differ across contexts, educators have traditionally faced common dilemmas. No two students are alike, and these individual differences affect educational progress. Educators must decide what to do with burgeoning knowledge about individual differences in intellectual strengths, learning styles, temperament, motivation, and the like. Education is always done by some method, whether explicit or implicit, and competing methods are usually available. Educators must decide how they will assess and select new instructional methods. For example, if a new mathematics curriculum highlights basic but challenging numerical concepts like a 'set' and a 'function', educators must assess its pros and cons. At a population level, many forces lead to disparate access to quality education. Educators must face questions of what to do when one part of the population has an unfair advantage, for example students of affluent families who have easy access to Advanced Placement courses and skilled tutors.

Our own stance on these issues is that educators should pay careful attention to individual differences and use them to inform instruction, but not corral students into narrow tracks based on these differences. Methodologically, we see a progression in education beginning with basic literacies and then moving into disciplinary skills. We value instruction that yields deep understanding of fewer topics over superficial exposure to many topics. At the population level, we believe that every effort should be taken to minimize advantages for any part of the population. While this stance colors our analysis and recommendations, we hope that our account will prove useful across the profession.

## Neuroscience and education

While ethical dilemmas in education are not new, neurocognitive advances do pose unique ethical challenges. The dilemmas are sharpened and the stakes become higher as research blurs the boundaries between education, on the one hand, and medicine or neuroscience, on the other. While understanding brain function is relevant to both science and education, re-searchers and educators have different agendas. When looking at the same learning phenom-ena, researchers focus on the basic component processes of complex cognitive abilities, whereas educators want to understand how formal instruction can best utilize and develop these cognitive abilities in pursuit of specific educational accomplishments.

Researchers interested in the neural basis of learning have studied diverse phenomena such as long-term potentiation, phonological decoding, and genetic variance among people with learning disabilities. Their methods can be roughly divided into three levels of scope: cellular mechanisms (i.e. molecular biology), functional organization of the brain (i.e. neuroscience and brain imaging), and population-level analysis of genetic propensities (i.e. behavioral genetics). This body of research is vast and rapidly growing, and we highlight just a few of the recent areas to demonstrate how advances in neuroscience affect (and/or will soon affect) the educational enterprise.

One line of research attempts to recruit cellular mechanisms of memory formation in order to develop drugs that enhance learning performance on various tasks (Lynch 2002). Of course, pharmacological interventions for learning difficulties are now familiar to educators, particu-larly with the rise of diagnosis and treatment of disorders of attention. In contrast, this new class of neurocognitive enhancers aims at improving performance that is already adequate among the broad student population.

The development and use of neurocognitive enhancing drugs in the broad student population obviously raises many ethical issues (Farah *et al.* 2004). Tinkering with evolutionary developmental mechanisms in order to inflate an individual's performance on formal learning tasks should not be done lightly. For instance, there may be good developmental reasons for limits on short-term memory in children and adolescents, and these cannot easily be discerned in traditionally short-term neuroscientific studies. Even if such methodological concerns were completely addressed, the use of neurocognitive enhancers would still pose pedagogical questions for educators and ethical questions for society. Already there are front-page news reports of students inappropriately obtaining and using prescription drugs intended for attention disorders to boost their performance on college admissions tests (Zamiska 2004). We can only expect this practice to increase as more targeted drugs become available.

Another growth area in educationally relevant neuroscience involves mapping the functional organization of the brain. The connections to education are quite apparent since, at a basic level, education is about shaping our brain's functional organization. Learning to read, use calculus, or dance the tango all draw upon diverse neurological capacities, and instruction reshapes not only our behavior on these tasks but also the functional organization of the utilized portions of our brains. Advances in imaging techniques allow us to understand how various cognitive functions are represented spatially and temporally in the brain.

It has been argued that such information, while interesting scientifically, yields little that bears directly on education. However, the nascent field of functional neuroimaging has already yielded important educational insights into the neuronal organization of linguistic and other systems recruited for reading (especially when applied to research on reading disabilities). Neuroimaging research on dyslexia has documented the basic processes involved in graphic decoding that could not have been understood by behavioral studies alone. For instance, behavioral research in dyslexia did not allow us to discern the taxonomy of the disorder—whether it involves only a phonological processing deficit, only a deficiency in rapid naming tasks, or both. Neuroimaging experiments (Misra *et al.* 2004) have demonstrated that specific neuronal pathways dedicated to rapid naming of letters (rather than objects) do not overlap with brain areas whose activation is associated with phonological tasks. Similar behavioral manifestations of dyslexia can be caused by a combination of deficits in these independent systems. As a result, more focused interventions can be made at earlier ages for dyslexic children.

In another branch of neuroimaging research, researchers have examined the developmental trajectory for early versus late second-language exposure and acquisition using near-infrared spectroscopy (NIRS), evoked response potential (ERP), and fMRI. Here, brain imaging provides supporting evidence in favor of early second-language exposure. Various neuroimaging techniques provide convergent evidence that later bilingual exposure results in differential neuronal organization for language processing, while early exposure recruits areas similar for monolingual processing (Weber-Fox and Neville 1999; Wartenburger *et al.* 2003). Petitto and Dunbar (2004) note that, compared with late bilinguals, early bilinguals have a more efficient linguistic organization, earlier meta-linguistic awareness (which is important in reading acquisition), and no cognitive disadvantages. These findings indicate that earlier exposure to a second language recruits developing neuronal systems more effectively. In this case, neuroscience supports behavioral findings with implications for bilingual education and policy issues.

Finally, researchers in behavioral genetics have sought to identify genetic markers that express the probability of developing a learning disability. Large-scale twin studies combined with microarray (the 'gene chip') analysis are correlated with measures of environmental influence. Such techniques allow researchers to determine genetic markers that contribute to variance in learning difficulties in a given population (Butcher *et al.* 2004; Plomin and Kovas 2004). These analyses may eventually lead to establishing 'genetic risk factors', akin to the environmental risk factors (such as impoverished household) used currently for predicting learning difficulties at school. While such diagnostic measures may still be a long way off, educators will be faced with evaluating the intervention strategies based upon them.

Such advances raise a number of ethical questions for scientists, educators, and society as a whole.

♦ What is the quality of evidence purporting to be relevant to education, and by which standards of evaluation?

♦ What use should be made of new knowledge and advances? By whom and with what safeguards?

♦ How do we respond to unanticipated consequences of research? Who has responsibility?

## Professions, good work, and education

While neurocognitive advances undoubtedly affect the educational enterprise and create ethical dilemmas for educators, it is unclear who can and should provide answers to such questions. Education is a profession, and, like other professions, it has a particular mission, expertise, and sphere of action. Educators are neither doctors nor neuroscientists, and yet they are affected by findings and practices in these fields.

In pursuing these questions, we consider the nature of professions, and in particular the nature of the educational profession. Insight can be gained from the GoodWork project (http://www.goodworkproject.org). This interdisciplinary investigation looks at how members of a variety of different professions (e.g. genetics, journalism, law) navigate cultural and techno-logical changes in their respective professions as they strive to do 'good work', i.e. work that is both excellent and ethical (Fischman *et al.* 2004; Gardner *et al.* 2001). In what follows, we focus on the structures and practices that encourage or discourage good work in times of change, and consider how they might apply to educators facing challenges and opportunities posed by neurocognitive advances. Finally, we suggest how best to encourage good work in the emerging field of 'neuroeducation'.

As conceptualized by sociologists, a profession embodies an explicit or tacit agreement between the laity and a group of individuals with acknowledged expertise. In return for performing services of use to the community, and doing so in a disinterested (non-partisan) way, the professionals are accorded status and autonomy. Professionals are expected to use their judgment and to make complex decisions under conditions of uncertainty. In general profes-sions have explicit training and licensing mechanisms; professions police themselves and can remove delinquent members from their ranks.

In the most general terms, education involves a collection of individuals whose job it is to transmit the knowledge and skills that are most valued at the present time and to prepare young people to live in a world that may in crucial ways be different from the present one. With respect to the current educational system in the United States, university educators fit the above description of professionals more closely than pre-collegiate educators. While efforts are under way to professionalize all of education, numerous barriers remain. For example, there is excessive bureaucratic supervision of elementary and secondary school teachers. Such teachers have less formal training, and they are not given as much autonomy and status. (Of course, some pre-collegiate educators behave like high-level professionals, and many designated professionals in higher education and other domains do not behave like professionals.)

This lack of clear and strong professional status for pre-collegiate educators, combined with continual dispute about the fundamental values of the educational enterprise, creates additional barriers to 'good work' in education. Of course, like doctors and lawyers, educators have a mission that is agreed upon in general terms: passing on knowledge and developing skills. Once these bland generalities are proffered, the actual professional values educators hold are in much greater contention than that of most other professions. It is challenging to design and enforce effective and ethical standards of practice if there is little cohesion within the profession, little autonomy to make decisions, and little shared consensus in the broader community with respect to the values guiding education.

## Good work: alignment and the 'hat' problem

The GoodWork project focuses on the contexts and professional structures that either support or discourage 'good work', particularly during times of rapid cultural or technological change. We draw on findings from this work to consider how educators might best pursue good work in the light of dramatic neurocognitive advances.

One of the key findings of the study concerns the degree of alignment that obtains in a professional domain. Alignment within a profession is ascertained by determining whether the various relevant constituencies all desire the same thing from that profession. The degree of alignment is not fixed: market forces, changing societal demands, and new discoveries and technologies can all affect the extent of alignment or non-alignment in a profession at a given moment.

When the GoodWork project looked at the domain of genetics in the late 1990s, they found it to be well aligned. New technologies and discoveries allowed geneticists to pursue goals that were supported and valued by the broader society. Geneticists expressed much enjoyment in their work and were able to work in ways that served their values. Conversely, at the same time journalism was in a state of misalignment. Market forces and changing media structures pressured journalists to work in ways contradictory to the values of the traditional journalistic code (e.g. researching a story in painstaking detail, resisting pressures from advertisers and publishers). Long-standing members abandoned or considered abandoning the journalism profession because they could not do the work they valued. New inductees failed to connect traditional journalistic ideals with the actual practice that they observed and faced.

The study found, not surprisingly, that it was easier to do both excellent and ethical work when a domain or profession is in alignment. Without conflicting pressures, members find it easier to their best work and work congruent with their values. However, when a domain like genetics appears to be so well aligned, members may be less inclined to attend to signs of coming dangers. They may be inappropriately optimistic about the benefits of new technologies and discoveries. They may be not vigilant enough to police their members who, riding the wave of new advances and possibilities, drift from the standard code of ethics. Conversely, when a domain is misaligned, there may be greater reflection and self-examination among the ranks. While the negative experience of misalignment may spur some to leave the profession, it encourages others to change it from within, to realign. Journalistic outlets like C-Span and National Public Radio were responses to poorly aligned facets of the profession.

Whether or not there was ever a Golden Age of education in the United States, we believe that the profession of education is currently misaligned. Strong market and political pressures affect educators at all levels, and have proved especially jarring for school teachers. There is a general consensus among the public that pre-collegiate education is not strong enough to meet society's demands as well as vast disparities between population groups in terms of educational achievement and access to quality education. Education schools are faulted for not training teachers adequately. The field lacks sufficient research to justify many of its practices.

At the same time that these complaints are lodged, our expectations for educators are also increasing. We seek to educate a broader range of the populace to a higher level than ever before. As culture and technology rapidly shift, educators must continually re-evaluate whether they are adequately preparing their students for their future roles in society. As demands increase to create a knowledgeable and flexible citizenry and workforce, resources (material and human) are spread thin.

Recent national policies aim for a higher degree of accountability for educators. But policies such as tying funding to achievement on standardized testing have created turmoil for educators. Many educators feel pressured to work in ways contrary to their pedagogical standards or even their ethics. There have been well-publicized reports of school officials cheating on examinations. The misalignment of education reflects a situation where the professional status of many educators, particularly at the pre-collegiate level, has been under-mined.

Neurocognitive advances could conceivably serve as an aligning force within education. Amid the welter of competing value-laden claims, demands for resources, and political pressures, empirical facts about human cognitive functioning, especially when combined with targeted diagnosis and effective remediation, could help students learn. Drugs that improve students' memory, information processing, motivation, or attention could prove a boon to educators saddled with so many demands.

However, one cannot assume such a sanguine outcome. Of course, some research, such as the neurological research on dyslexia mentioned above, feeds into an already fairly well developed field of educational intervention. Most other neuroscientific research has less obvious connections. The tasks and scope of most studies are sufficiently narrow to render their relevance to educational situations questionable. Significant bridging research is needed in order for neuroscientific knowledge to become usable educational knowledge. Careful analysis needs to be done to determine whether this is the best use of limited educational resources.

As neuroimaging and genetic testing increase, there will probably be an increase in the number of individuals diagnosed with learning disabilities, as well as increases in prescriptions of neurocognitive medications. It will be a challenge for educators to adjust to the increase of individualization that is implied (see also Chapters 11 and 12). These forces are more likely to create further demands on educators for which they are inadequately trained. At least in the short term, advances will probably lead to further misalignment in the domain, rather than providing immediate help. For example, inconsistencies across governmental performance standards, teachers' personal value systems, the wishes of parents and teachers, medical precedents, and pressures are likely to exacerbate already frayed relations among the stake-holders.

While alignment focuses on the broad state of affairs in the domain, it is important to look specifically at how individuals are impacted by changes. Cultural and technological changes often create new interdisciplinary roles, new 'hats' to be worn, in a profession. Inevitably people feel pressured to take on more roles than they can responsibly handle or that have values or goals that are in conflict with one another.

A key finding of the GoodWork study is that people often get into ethical trouble when they wear too many hats or do too much switching between hats. For instance, advances in genetics led to new private sector opportunities in marketing drugs or techniques. Conflicts arise as academic geneticists accept public funds for basic research, and then create private biotechnology companies that operate in secret and profit illegitimately from this research. These spheres of science and business have different values and goals. For instance, businesses develop elaborate strategies to protect and limit access to research discoveries, while a primary goal of publicly funded work is to share it with others. Wearing these two hats may not necessarily be unethical, but the chances of irreconcilable value conflicts are far greater.

Similarly, neurocognitive advances provide conditions ripe for such confusion of roles in education, as educators start taking on aspects of roles of neuroscientists or medical professionals, and neuroscientists and drug researchers become part-time educators. Returning to our opening scenarios of hypothetical situations in the year 2010, we can identify different instances of this hat problem. In the first scenario, we see Ms E confronted with a variety of traditional assessments (e.g. standardized tests scores, last year's grades, current work) and a type of neurological report that will probably become standard in the near future. One of her core values as an educator is to help each student develop to the best of his or her potential, including seeking remediation for any learning disabilities. In an ideal case, a neurological evaluation yields a clear diagnosis to which an empirically valid remediation is yoked. However, it is likely that there will be many more like this hypothetical case—a report of atypical processing for which there is neither a clear diagnosis nor remediation.

In assessing the fMRI report, Ms E is expected to don a hat for which she is inadequately trained. In the face of her lack of expertise and the fMRI report's ambiguity, the report appears to reveal something 'true' about Daniel's functioning. She allows the biological finding to trump her observations as a teacher and Daniel's hitherto adequate performance in class. Drawing upon her classroom observations and educational training, Ms E may have given Daniel a positive report for his current progress and perhaps worked out some in-class or at-home strategies for his minor attention and reading issues. However, faced with this picture of his brain function, she feels out of her depth and considers remediation strategies that may not be appropriate for Daniel's needs.

Having one child complete a potentially unnecessary program may not seem like a major risk or source of ethical conflict. However, as the use of diagnostic tests becomes widespread, teachers will be pressured to put on the ill-fitting hat of neuroscientific clinician. As students, parents, and teachers seek individualized remediation for a wide range of neurological atypicalities, resources may be disproportionately allocated to remediation. Schools may struggle to allocate resources to those children who need remediation most, and for whom valid empirically tested interventions are available.

In the second scenario, we observe a different instance of hat confusion. Here, neuroscientists work with a software company to create a remediation program based on a hypothesized neurological basis for understanding fractions. While their findings may be scientifically sound, the neuroscientists have not demonstrated the educational merit of the product based upon them. Unfamiliar with the centuries-old history of mathematics pedagogy, disinclined or ill equipped to complete comprehensive educational evaluation studies, and ignorant of current classrooms and children, these hypothetical neuroscientists fail to embody the values and standards of the educational hat that they have chosen to wear. However, the fact that the school leaders also did not demonstrate skepticism in their assessment of the neuroscientists' intervention points out a gap; few, if any, educators are yet able to understand and assess the challenges and opportunities occurring at this border of neuroeducation.

## Neuroeducation

The emerging sphere of 'neuroeducation' provides opportunities for good work but requires professionals adequately trained to handle the challenges posed by neurocognitive advances. Heretofore we have taken a cautionary stance toward integrating neuroscience and education, but as members of this emerging interdisciplinary field we also recognize its promise. To help bridge the interdisciplinary effort, we argue for the establishment of a new class of professionals—neuroeducators. These individuals have been trained to wear the hats of both neuroscientist and educator and to guide the introduction of neurocognitive advances into education sensibly and ethically. The establishment of this new profession should help clarify the questions of responsibility raised above.

Much fruitful work can be done at this border of neuroscience and education. A variety of emerging professions can be envisioned, each with its own values and goals: neuroscientists who are guided by scientific values and work on basic research but are familiar with educational issues and collaborate with educators; businesspeople who collaborate with educators and scientists to make products based on the new research; policy-makers who work within the government to create organizations and enact regulations to accomplish this work; and educators specifically oriented to fostering the introduction of relevant neurocognitive advances into the educational system.

To do good work, neuroeducators will need to be knowledgeable about neuroscientific theories and findings for educationally relevant tasks and able to evaluate their validity and usefulness for education. Like other scientists, neuroeducators must assess how experimental paradigms used in neuroscientific studies are relevant to classroom applications and evaluate various intervention programs that claim to be so. But like other educators, neuroeducators also need an understanding of the heterogeneous values, methods, techniques, problems, and contexts of education.

Neuroeducators will need to assume a number of supervisory roles. First, they will anticipate and monitor how neurocognitive advances enter and affect the educational system, directly or obliquely. They will identify instances where neurocognitive advances may be leaking into the educational system without established policy for handling them. Neuroeducators will identify those neurocognitive advances that seem most promising with respect to specific educational goals. They will make research recommendations about how to translate these more basic scientific findings into usable knowledge and evaluate research and curricula. Finally, as a governing group of professionals, they will set guidelines or recommendations for policy on how neurocognitive advances should be applied (and not applied) in education.

In the light of our discussion of neuroeducators, let us revisit our opening scenarios.

In the first scenario, Ms E, an elementary school teacher, is faced with an fMRI report from a student showing minor neurological atypicalities. Since the student has not met any existing criteria to receive medical or learning disability intervention, Ms E is unsure of what to do. Probably feeling some pressure, she suggests to his parents the ad hoc solution of an intervention. We discussed some of the dilemmas associated with this in reference to the hat problem.

The advance of diagnostic fMRI tests brings knowledge that needs to be addressed. On the cautionary side, neuroeducators first need to monitor any inappropriate use of these (and other) tests. They need to set up controls, drawing on existing conventions and safeguards surrounding medical testing on minors, so that teachers are not in the situation of assessing findings of reports they do not understand. On the positive side, neuroeducators can guide research that uses fMRI diagnostic reports. Such research can help develop pedagogical strategies that work with common neurological atypicalities or dysfunctions, and contribute to the expanding knowledge base on differentiated instruction, learning disabilities, and individual differences.

In the second scenario, neuroscientists have teamed up with software designers to create a program that purports to help students master fractions. The key issue involved in this scenario is: What is the quality of evidence purporting to be relevant to education, and whose terms of evaluation are regnant? While the evidence for the underlying scientific findings is sound, little is known about its educational effectiveness. In this scenario, neuroeducators can be charged with assessing the evidence of the program's effectiveness and relevance to educational goals. In addition, neuroeducators can mine neurological research in a search for possible links to educational goals. One of their aims is to set up partnerships where scientists, curriculum developers, and educators would work together to create neurologically informed usable knowledge and products for education.

In the final scenario, we find a situation where the use of neurocognitive enhancing drugs has resulted in disparities in scores recorded on high-stakes college admissions examinations. Testing officials, college admissions officers, parents, and students are confused about what they should do. This scenario raises the questions: How do we handle unanticipated consequences of research? Who has the responsibility for handling them? While medical professionals address unanticipated physiological effect of new drugs, neuroeducators need to address educational side effects. They need to monitor the ways in which these drugs or other neurocognitive advances interfere with educational values (e.g. the goal of minimizing educational advantages for any segment of the population). They need to work with educational officials and the broader public to discuss possible options (e.g. allow the use of the drugs and provide them to anyone who wants them; disallow their use and set up effective enforcements; scrap high-stake college admissions tests altogether). Based on these discussions, neuroeducators in policy-making positions assume the role of designing and evaluating appropriate guidelines and controls.

The establishment of a new role of neuroeducator is not a panacea for the pressures facing education and the ethical dilemmas posed by scientific advances. Indeed, it may even create additional ethical challenges. Neuroeducators are likely to enter the field because they are drawn to the possibilities that these advances hold for education. They may be biased toward seeing the positive potential of research. There are probably more personal and professional rewards for successful implementation of research than for judicious caution. Because neuroeducators are more closely tied to education than traditional neuroscientists, they will have greater access to children and schools and greater opportunity to bring research into practical use. Without appropriate safeguards, they may import neurologically based findings prematurely. They may be less mindful of threats to educational values, thereby exacerbating systematic disparities in the population, marginalizing neurologically atypical students, channeling students too narrowly into educational modes guided by their neurologically revealed abilities, or interfering with essential developmental processes. To prevent this, neuroeducators need to be fully subject to the safeguards guiding the medical professions and research on human subjects (particularly children), and also responsible to a review system that safeguards educational values.

## Conclusion

Institutions of higher education are beginning to address the role neuroscience may have for education, with a few offering specific interdisciplinary programs in neuroscience in education (e.g. Harvard Graduate School of Education, Cambridge University, Dartmouth College). These programs are designed to address both research and policy issues of integrating neuro-science findings into education. In our Mind, Brain and Education program at Harvard, we explicitly introduce students to the roles of neuroscientist, cognitive scientist, and educator, and then give them practice in donning the respective hats. While the emerging roles and structures in neuroeducation are key to handling both the promises and the dilemmas posed by neurocognitive advances, it is essential that educational values remain at the core of this emerging interdisciplinary field. Good work in education requires addressing the issues raised by neuroscience, and good work in neuroeducation requires keeping educational values and goals at the center of the work. As we enter this new world, we need to be armed with cautious hope but appropriate skepticism.

## Acknowledgments

The studies reported in this paper were supported in part by the Atlantic Philanthropies, the Carnegie Corporation, the Ford Foundation, The Hewlett Foundation, The Christian Johnson Endeavor Foundation, The Louise and Claude Rosenberg Foundation, and Jeffrey Epstein.

## References

Butcher LM, Meaburn E, Liu L, *et al.* (2004). Genotyping pooled DNA on miscroarrays: A systematic genome screen of thousands of SNPs in large samples to detect QTLs for complex traits. *Behavior Genetics* 34, 549–55.

Farah MJ, Illes J, Cook-Deegan R, *et al.* (2004). Neurocognitive enhancement. What can we do and what should we do? *Nature Reviews Neuroscience* 5, 421–5.

FischmanW, Solomon B, Greenspan D, Gardner H (2004). *Making Good: How Young People Cope with Moral Dilemmas at Work.* Cambridge, MA: Harvard University Press.

Gardner H, Csikszentmihalyi M, Damon W (2001). *Good Work: When Excellence and Ethics Meet.* New York: Basic Books.

Lynch G (2002). Memory enhancement: the search for mechanism-based drugs. *Nature Neuroscience* 5 (Suppl), 1035–8.

Misra M, Katzir T, Wolf M, Poldrak, R (2004). Neural systems for rapid automatized naming in skilled readers: unraveling the RAN-reading relationship. *Scientific Studies of Reading* 8, 241–56.

Petitto LA, Dunbar K (2004). New findings from educational neuroscience on bilingual brains, scientific brains, and the educated mind. Paper presented at the Conference on Usable Knowledge in Mind, Brain and Education, Cambridge, MA.

Plomin R, Kovas Y (2004). Genetics and cognitive performance: genetic and developmental analysis of abilities. Paper presented at the Conference on Usable Knowledge in Mind, Brain and Education, Cambridge, MA.

Wartenburger I, Heekeren HR, Abutalebi J, Cappa SF, Villringer A, Perani D (2003). Early setting of grammatical processing in the bilingual brain. *Neuron* 37, 159–70.

Weber-Fox C, Neville H (1999). Functional neuronal subsystems are differentially affected by delays in second-language immersion: ERP and behavioral evidence in bilingual speakers. In: Birdsong D (ed) *New Perspectives on the Critical Periods for Second Language Acquisition.* Hillsdale, NJ: Erlbaum, 23–38.

Zamiska N (2004). Pressed to do well on admissions tests, students take drugs. *Wall Street Journal*, 8 November, p. A1.

Chapter 19

# Poverty, privilege, and brain development: empirical findings and ethical implications

Martha J. Farah, Kimberly G. Noble,
and Hallam Hurt

## Introduction

After my daughter was born people sometimes asked me (MJF): 'Has having a child gotten you interested in brain development?' My answer was 'No, not exactly, but having babysitters has'. More specifically, getting to know my daughter's babysitters and becoming close to some of them and their families called my attention to a set of complex social problems that are, I believe, partly related to brain development. Up until this time I had viewed cognitive neuroscience as an ivory tower pursuit, whose potential applications were few and far between (except, of course, in National Institutes of Health grant proposals). I now believe that cognitive neuroscience can provide a framework for understanding and even solving certain societal problems. One such problem is the persistence of poverty across generations. This chapter summarizes recent research I have undertaken with my co-authors on the relation between poverty and children's cognitive achievement, which is in turn related to their future socio-economic prospects.

My babysitters were mostly of low socio economic status (SES). These women had little education, little experience in jobs other than domestic work, and relied on state assistance supplemented by cash babysitting wages to support themselves and their children. Although they had one foot in the middle-class world through their babysitting jobs, the differences between their lives and my middle-class existence were nevertheless immense. Nowhere were the differences more dramatic than in the realm of child development. Their daughters and sons and nieces and nephews began life with the same evident promise as my daughter and her friends. Yet as the years went on, I saw their paths diverge.

On our side of the tracks, preschoolers know their letters and numbers, elementary school children are familiar with different neighborhoods and different cities, and middle school children read newspaper headlines and ask their parents about them. Not so with the children I met on their side of the tracks. However, the low SES children did show a kind of sad precocity compared with middle-class children in their first-hand experience of violence, death, and the criminal justice system. Preschoolers growing up in the inner city learn to fear the neighbors from the local crack house. By elementary school they recognize the sound of gunshots, and by middle school they know about prison because a relative has been there. It seemed to me that children's experience of the world is very different in low and middle SES environments. Most middle SES children have abundant opportunities to explore the world, literally, in terms of people met and places seen, and figuratively, in terms of the world of ideas. In contrast, low SES children generally have fewer interactions with the wider world and much of what they do experience is stressful. Basic research with animals has established the powerful effects of both environmental impoverishment and stress on the developing brain.

The research reported in this chapter is an attempt to relate findings on SES and brain development. The ultimate goals of this work are to inform practical decisions concerning child policy, and to reveal the neuroethical dimensions of the problem of childhood poverty.

## Socio economic status and child development

There is a gulf between low and middle SES children in their performance on just about every test of cognitive development, from the Bayley Infant Behavior Scales to IQ and school achievement tests. Furthermore, these SES disparities are not subtle. For example, in one study we conducted, the average IQ of a group of healthy low SES 6-year-olds was 81. Only 20 percent of the sample scored in the normal range, defined as 90 or above (Hurt *et al.* 1998). Looking further ahead in the developmental trajectories of poor and middle class children, a $10 000 increment in family income was associated with a 16 percent increase in high school graduation rates for children of middle income families, but a *600 percent* increase in high school graduation for low income and poor children (Duncan *et al.* 1998).

The gap in cognitive achievement between children of low and middle SES suggests one possible answer to the question of why poverty persists. This question has occupied sociologists since their field began, and has been answered in many ways. Marx (1867) emphasized purely economic factors that create and maintain social stratification. Functionalist accounts highlight the many ways in which society as a whole is served by the enduring presence of a lower class (Weber 1923). The concept of a culture of poverty (Lewis 1965) emphasizes causes within individuals and their subculture, rather than external societal forces, in perpetuating poverty across generations. Each account undoubtedly captures some truth about the complex and multifactorial processes that confine children born of poor parents to lifelong poverty. Cognitive neuroscience offers yet another perspective on the problem. Without good intellectual development and educational attainment, people are denied all manner of economic and social opportunities. If cognitive neuroscience can help us understand the SES gap in cognitive achievement, it will have provided an important new perspective on the problem of poverty.

In order to explore the cognitive neuroscience perspective on transgenerational poverty and to discover what, if anything, it can contribute to correcting socio economic inequality, the first order of business is to ask whether socio economic status bears any straightforward relation to brain development. On the face of things it might seem unlikely that characteristics such as income, education, and job status, which are typically used to estimate SES, would bear any systematic relationship to physiological processes such as those involved in brain development. However, it is well established that SES affects physical health through a number of different causal pathways (Adler *et al.* 1994), many of which could play a role in brain development. It is also clear that poverty is associated with differences in brain function on the basis of the differences in standardized test performance cited earlier, as cognitive tests reflect the function of the brain. However, for a cognitive neuroscience approach to be helpful, the relations between SES and the brain must be relatively straightforward and generalizable. Therefore the first question that we addressed was: Can we generalize about the neurocognitive correlates of SES? Once we have established the neurocognitive profile of childhood poverty, we can begin to test more specific hypotheses about causal mechanisms.

# The neurocognitive profile of childhood poverty: three studies

In an initial study we compared the neurocognitive performance of 30 low and 30 middle SES African American Philadelphia public school kindergarteners (Noble *et al.* 2005a). The children were tested on a battery of tasks adapted from the cognitive neuroscience literature, designed to assess the functioning of five key neurocognitive systems. These systems are described briefly below.

- The **prefrontal/executive system** enables flexible responding in situations where the appropriate response may not be the most routine or attractive one, or where it requires maintenance or updating of information concerning recent events. It is dependent on prefrontal cortex, a late-maturing brain region that is disproportionately developed in humans compared to other species.
- The **left peri Sylvian/language system** is a complex distributed system encompassing semantic, syntactic, and phonological aspects of language and dependent predominantly on the temporal and frontal areas of the left hemisphere that surround the Sylvian fissure.
- The **medial temporal/memory system** is responsible for one-trial learning, the ability to retain a representation of a stimulus after a single exposure to it (which contrasts with the ability to gradually strengthen a representation through conditioning-like mechanisms), and is dependent on the hippocampus and related structures of the medial temporal lobe.
- The **parietal/spatial cognition system** underlies our ability to mentally represent and manipulate the spatial relations among objects, and is primarily dependent upon posterior parietal cortex.
- The **occipitotemporal/visual cognition system** is responsible for pattern recognition and visual mental imagery, translating image format visual representations into more abstract representations of object shape and identity, and reciprocally translating visual memory knowledge into image format representations (mental images).

Not surprisingly, in view of the literature on SES and standardized cognitive tests, the middle SES children performed better than the low SES children on the battery of tasks as a whole. For some systems, most notably the left peri Sylvian/language system and the prefrontal/executive system, the disparity between low and middle SES kindergarteners was both large and statistically significant. Indeed, the groups differed by over a standard deviation in their performance composite on language tests, and by over two-thirds of a standard deviation in the executive function composite. The other systems did not differ significantly between low and middle SES children, and in fact differed significantly less than the first two.

In a subsequent study we attempted to replicate and extend these findings in a larger group of children: 150 first graders of varying ethnicities whose SES spanned a range from low through middle (Noble *et al.* 2005b). These children completed a different set of tests designed to tap the same neurocognitive systems as the previous study, but with two main differences: First, instead of considering 'prefrontal/executive' to be a single system, we subdivided it into three subsystems each with its own tests.

- The **lateral prefrontal/working memory system** enables us to hold information 'on line' to maintain it over an interval and manipulate it, and is primarily dependent on the lateral surface of the prefrontal lobes. (Note that this is distinct from the ability to commit information to *long-term* memory, which is dependent on the medial temporal cortex.)

◆ The **anterior cingulate/cognitive control system** is required when we must resist the most routine or easily available response in favor of a more task-appropriate response, and is dependent on a network of regions within prefrontal cortex including the anterior cingulate gyrus.

◆ The **ventromedial prefrontal/reward processing system** is responsible for regulating our responses in the face of rewarding stimuli, allowing us to resist the immediate pull of a attractive stimulus in order to maximize longer-term gains.

A second noteworthy difference between this and the previous study concerned the tests of the medial temporal/memory system. In both of the tasks used to assess memory in the previous study, the test phase followed immediately after the initial exposure to the stimuli and memory *per se* may not have been the limiting factor in performance. The tasks that we used in the second study included a longer delay between initial exposure to the stimuli to be remembered and later test.

As before, the language system showed a highly significant relationship to SES, as did executive functions including lateral prefrontal/working memory and anterior cingulate/cognitive control components and the parietal/spatial cognition system. With a more demanding delay between exposure and test in the memory tasks, we also found a difference in the medial temporal/memory system.

Finally, we assessed these same neurocognitive systems in older children. We tested 60 middle school students, half of low and half of middle SES, matched for age, gender. and ethnicity (Farah *et al.* 2004). Again, sizeable and significant SES disparities were observed for language and the two executive subsystems, working memory and cognitive control, as well as for memory. SES was not associated with significant differences in the parietal/spatial cognition system, the occipitotemporal/visual cognition system, or the ventromedial prefrontal/reward processing system.

In sum, although the outcome of each study was different, there were also commonalities among them despite different tasks and different children tested at different ages. The most robust neurocognitive correlates of SES appear to involve the left peri Sylvian/language system, the medial temporal/memory system (insofar as SES effects were found in both studies that tested memory with an adequate delay) and the prefrontal/executive system, in particular its lateral prefrontal/working memory and anterior cingulate/cognitive control components. Children growing up in low SES environments perform less well on tests that tax the functioning of these specific systems.

The profile of SES disparities, with greatest disparity in systems needed for language, memory, working memory and cognitive control, would be expected to affect children's life trajectories. The importance of language and memory is obvious, from the social sphere to the world of school and work. Less obvious is the impact of working memory and cognitive control on real-world success, but studies have linked individual differences in these systems to individual differences in children's behavioral self-regulation and adult intelligence and problem-solving ability (Duncan *et al.* 2002; Engle *et al.* 2002; Davis *et al.* 2002; Gray *et al.* 2003).

## Disentangling cause and effect in the neurocognitive correlates of SES

Do these associations reflect the effects of SES on brain development, or the opposite direction of causality? Perhaps families with higher innate language, executive, and memory abilities tend to acquire and maintain a higher SES. Such a mechanism seems likely, a priori, as it would be surprising if genetic influences on cognitive ability did not, in the aggregate, contribute to individual and family SES. However, it also seems likely that causality operates in the opposite direction as well, with SES influencing cognitive ability through childhood environment. Note that the direction of causality is an empirical, not an ethical, issue. The issue of whether and to what extent SES differences cause neurocognitive differences or vice versa should not be confused with the issue of whether we have an obligation to help children of any background become educated productive citizens.

Given that the direction of causality is an empirical issue, what data bear on it? The methods of behavioral genetics research can, in principle, tell us about the direction of causality in the association between SES and the development of specific neurocognitive functions. However, these methods have yet to be applied to that question. They have been applied to a related question, namely the heritability of IQ and SES. Cross-fostering studies of within- and between-SES adoption suggest that roughly half the IQ disparity in children is experiential (Schiff and Lewontin 1986; Capron and Duyme 1989). If anything, these studies are likely to err in the direction of underestimating the influence of environment because the effects of prenatal and early postnatal environment are included in the estimates of genetic influences in adoption studies. A recent twin study by Turkheimer *et al.* (2003) showed that, within low SES families, IQ variation is far less genetic than environmental in origin. Additional evidence comes from studies of when, in a child's life, poverty was experienced. Within a given family that experiences a period of poverty, the effects are greater on siblings who were young during that period (Duncan *et al.* 1994), an effect that cannot be explained by genetics. In sum, multiple sources of evidence indicate that SES does indeed have an effect on cognitive development, although its role in the specific types of neurocognitive system development investigated here is not yet known.

## Potential causes: physical and psychological

What aspects of the environment might be responsible for the differences in neurocognitive development between low and middle SES children? A large set of possibilities exist, some affecting brain development by their direct effects on the body and some by less direct psychological mechanisms. Three somatic factors have been identified as significant risk factors for low cognitive achievement by the Center for Children and Poverty (1999): inadequate nutrition, substance abuse (particularly prenatal exposure), and lead exposure.

American children living in urban poverty are at risk for iron deficiency and mild to moderate protein energy malnutrition (PEM), which involves shortages of both protein and calories. The neurocognitive impact of these deficiencies is not well established [see Ricciuti (1993) and Sigman (1995) for opposing viewpoints]. The Center on Hunger, Poverty and Nutrition Policy (1998) has suggested that mild to moderate PEM probably has little effect on its own. Iron deficiency anemia, which is known to impair brain development when severe, afflicts about a quarter of low-income children in the United States (Center on Hunger, Poverty and Nutrition Policy 1998). The role of nutrition in SES disparities in brain development has been difficult to resolve because nutritional status is so strongly correlated with a host of other family and environmental variables likely to impact neurocognitive development, including all the potential mechanisms of causation to be reviewed here. Although nutritional supplementation programs could in principle be used as an 'experimental manipulation' of nutritional status alone, in practice these programs are often coupled with other non-nutritional forms of enrichment or affect children's lives in non-nutritional ways which perpetuate the confound (e.g. children given school breakfast are absent and late less often). The consensus regarding the role of nutrition in the cognitive outcomes of poor children has shifted over the past few decades from primary cause to a factor that contributes indirectly and through synergies with other environmental disadvantages (Center on Hunger, Poverty and Nutrition Policy 1998).

Lead is a neurotoxin released by peeling paint, and accumulates in the bodies of low SES children who are more likely to live in old and poorly maintained housing stock. A meta-analysis of low-level lead exposure on IQ showed a deleterious effect of lead even at low levels (Lanphear *et al.* 2005). As with nutrition, the effect of lead synergizes with other environmental factors and is more pronounced in low SES children (Bellinger *et al.* 1987). For example, low iron stores render children more susceptible to environmental lead (Center on Hunger, Poverty and Nutrition Policy 1998).

Prenatal substance exposure is a third factor that affects children of all SES levels, but is disproportionately experienced by the poor. Maternal use of alcohol, tobacco, marijuana, and other drugs of abuse has been associated with adverse cognitive outcomes in children (Chasnoff *et al.* 1998). Although the highly publicized phenomenon of 'crack babies' led to predictions of a generation of irreparably brain-damaged children growing up in the inner city, in retrospect this was over-reaction. Indeed epidemiological studies have found the effects on cognitive performance to be subtle (Hurt *et al.* 1995; Mayes 2002; Vidaeff and Mastrobattista 2003). For example, the low SES 4-year-olds of Hurt's cohort, whose average IQ was 81, served as control subjects for a cohort with prenatal cocaine exposure whose average IQ was a statistically indistinguishable 79. This lack of difference contrasts with the substantial difference between the scores of the low SES group scores and those of typical middle SES children.

The set of potentially causative somatic factors just reviewed is far from complete. There are SES gradients in a wide variety of physical health measures, many of which could affect children's neurocognitive development through a variety of different mechanisms (Adler *et al.* 1994). Having briefly reviewed the most frequently discussed factors, we now turn to a consideration of the psychological differences between the experiences of low and middle SES children that could also affect neurocognitive development.

As with potential physical causes, the set of potential psychological causes for the SES gap in cognitive achievement is large, and the causes are likely to exert their effects synergistically. Here we will review research on differences in cognitive stimulation and stress.

One difference between low and middle SES families that seems predictable, even in the absence of any other information, is that low SES children are likely to receive less cognitive stimulation than middle SES children. Their economic status alone predicts that they will have fewer toys and books and less exposure to zoos, museums, and other cultural institutions because of the expense of such items and activities. This is indeed the case (Bradley *et al.* 2001), and has been identified as a mediator between SES and measures of cognitive achievement (Brooks-Gunn and Duncan 1997; McLoyd 1998; Bradley and Corwyn 1999). Such a mediating role is consistent with the results of neuroscience research with animals. Starting many decades ago (Volkmar and Greenough 1972) researchers began to observe the powerful effects of environmental stimulation on brain development. Animals reared in barren laboratory cages showed less well developed brains, by a number of different anatomical and physiological measures, compared with those reared in more complex environments with opportunities to climb, burrow, and socialize (reviewed by van Praag *et al.* 2000).

Other types of cognitive stimulation are also less common in low SES homes, for example parental speech designed to engage the child in conversation (Adams 1998). The average number of hours of one-to-one picture-book reading experienced by children prior to kindergarten entry has been estimated at 25 for low SES children and between 1000 and 1700 for middle SES children (Adams 1990). Thus, in addition to material limitations, differing parental behaviors and concerns also contribute to differences in the amount of cognitive stimulation experienced by low and middle SES children.

The lives of low SES individuals tend to be more stressful for a variety of reasons, some of which are obvious: concern about providing for basic family needs, dangerous neighborhoods, and little control over one's work life. Again, research bears out this intuition: Turner and Avison (2003) confirmed that lower SES is associated with more stressful life events by a number of different measures. The same appears to be true for children as well as adults, and is apparent in salivary levels of the stress hormone cortisol (Lupien *et al.* 2001).

Why is stress an important consideration for neurocognitive development? Psychological stress causes the secretion of cortisol and other stress hormones, which affect the brain in numerous ways (McEwen 2000). The immature brain is particularly sensitive to these effects. In basic research studies of rat brain development, rat pups are subjected to the severe stress of prolonged separation from the mother and stress hormone levels predictably climb. The later anatomy and function of the brain is altered by this early neuroendocrine phenomenon. The brain area most affected is the medial temporal area needed for memory, although prefrontal systems involved in the regulation of the stress response are also impacted (Meaney *et al.* 1996).

## In search of mechanisms: a preliminary study

The three studies summarized earlier show an association between SES and the development of specific neurocognitive systems, namely language, memory, and executive function. Whereas we previously knew that SES was associated with cognitive achievement as measured by broad-spectrum tests of cognitive ability such as IQ and school achievement tests, our results re-describe this relationship in terms of the theoretically more meaningful components of cognitive function specified by cognitive neuroscience. However, we are still left with a description rather than an explanation.

Nevertheless, appropriately describing a phenomenon can be a crucial step in understanding it. Explanations are facilitated when the phenomenon to be explained is described in terms corresponding to the natural kinds involved in potential mechanisms. Knowing that SES effects are manifest in IQ and high school graduation rates tells us little about the possible brain mechanisms of SES effects on cognitive achievement. In contrast, knowing that SES effects are found in specific neurocognitive systems enables us to harness what we know about the development of those systems to frame hypotheses about the origins of the effects. An important corollary of this point is that different mechanisms may be responsible for SES effects on different neurocognitive systems. By resolving the SES disparity into its multiple underlying components, we can disentangle multiple causal pathways and test hypotheses about each separately. This is important, because such separation allows more selective, and hence more powerful, tests of mechanism.

The latest phase of our research is an attempt to make use of the description of the SES disparities in neurocognitive development in testing hypotheses about the causal pathways. Drawing on our previous research that identified three neurocognitive systems as having the most robust differences as a function of SES (peri Sylvian/language, medial temporal/memory, and prefrontal/executive), we are now testing hypotheses concerning the determinants of individual differences in the development of these systems in children of low SES. Specifically, we are investigating the role of childhood cognitive stimulation and social/emotional nurturance (Farah *et al.* 2005a).

The participants in this research are 50 low SES middle school students from a cohort of children enrolled at birth in a study of the effects of prenatal cocaine exposure (Hurt *et al.* 1995). Approximately half the children have been exposed to cocaine prenatally and half have not. Maternal use of cocaine, as well as amphetamines, opiates, barbiturates, benzodiazepines, marijuana, alcohol, and tobacco, is ascertained by interview and medical record review at time of birth and, for all but the last three, maternal and infant urine specimens.

As part of the ongoing study of these children, a research assistant visited the home of each child at ages 4 and 8 years and administered the Home Observation and Measurement of Environment (HOME) (Caldwell and Bradley 1984). The HOME includes an interview with the mother about family life and observations of the interactions between mother and child. The HOME has a number of different subscales relevant to different aspects of the child's experience. We combined a number of different subscales indicative of the amount of cognitive stimulation provided to the child to make a composite measure of cognitive stimulation, and a number of different subscales indicative of the amount of social/emotional nurturance provided to the child to make a composite measure of social/emotional nurturance. The subscales used for each composite, together with representative items, were as follows.

◆ The **Cognitive Stimulation Composite** for 4-year-olds was composed of *learning stimulation* ('child has toys which teach color', 'at least 10 books are visible in the apartment'), *language stimulation* ('child has toys that help teach the names of animals', 'mother uses correct grammar and pronunciation,'), *academic stimulation* ('child is encouraged to learn colors', 'child is encouraged to learn to read a few words'), *modeling* ('some delay of food gratification is expected', 'parent introduces visitor to child'), and *variety of experience* ('child has real or toy musical instrument', 'child's art work is displayed some place in house'). For 8-year-olds, the subscales used for the cognitive stimulation composite were *growth fostering materials and experiences* ('child has free access to at least 10 appropriate books', 'house has at least two pictures of some type of art work on the walls'), *provision for active stimulation* ('family has a television, and it is used judiciously, not left on continuously', 'family member has taken child, or arranged for child to go, to a scientific, historical or art museum within the past year'), and *family participation in developmentally stimulating experiences* ('family visits or receives visits from relatives or friends at least once every other week', 'family member has taken child, or arranged for child to go, on a trip of more than 50 miles from his home').

◆ The **Social/Emotional Nurturance Composite** for 4-year-olds was composed of *warmth and affection* ('parent holds child close 10–15 minutes per day', 'parent converses with child at least twice during visit') and *acceptance* ('parent does not scold or derogate child more than once', 'parent neither slaps nor spanks child during visit'). For 8-year-olds, the subscales used were *emotional and verbal responsivity* ('child has been praised at least twice during past week for doing something', 'parent responds to child's questions during interview'), *encouragement of maturity* ('family requires child to carry out certain self care routines', 'parents set limits for child and generally enforce them'), *emotional climate* ('parent has not lost temper with child more than once during previous week', 'parent uses some term of endearment or some diminutive for child's name when talking about child at least twice during visit'), and *paternal involvement*.

◆ Two other variables with the potential to account for differences in neurocognitive development included in our analyses were maternal intelligence and prenatal substance exposure. The former was measured by the Weschler Adult Intelligence Scale—Revised (WAIS-R). Maternal IQ could influence child neurocognitive outcome by genetic mechanisms or by its effect on the environment and experiences provided by the mother for the child. Prenatal substance exposure was coded for analysis on an integer scale of 0–4, with one point for each of the following substances: tobacco, alcohol, marijuana, and cocaine. Use of other substances was an exclusionary criterion.

We used statistical regression to examine the relations between the neurocognitive outcome measures and the predictor variables cognitive stimulation, social/emotional nurturance, maternal IQ, and polysubstance use, as well as the child's gender and age at time of neurocognitive testing. Our results indicate that the development of different neurocognitive systems is affected by different variables.

Children's performance on the tests of left peri Sylvian/language was predicted by average cognitive stimulation. This was the sole factor identified as predicting language ability by forward stepwise regression, and one of three factors identified by backward stepwise regression, together with the child's gender and the mother's IQ. In contrast, performance on tests of medial temporal/memory ability was predicted by average social/emotional nurturance. This was the sole factor identified as predicting memory ability by forward stepwise regression and one of three factors identified by backward stepwise regression, together with the child's age and cognitive stimulation. The relation between memory and early emotional experience is consistent with the animal research cited earlier, showing a deleterious effect of stress hormones on hippocampal development. Our analyses did not reveal any systematic relation of the predictor variables considered here with lateral prefrontal/working memory or anterior cingulate/cognitive control function. In conclusion, different aspects of early experience affect different systems of the developing brain. Cognitive stimulation influences the development of language, whereas social/emotional nurturance affects the development of memory but not language.

## Conclusions: brain plasticity and human potential

Change, continuity, and personal identity are core problems in bioethics. They arise when we ask at what stage of human development the organism is a person, whether to respect the current or prior wishes of a demented individual (see Chapter 7), and whether drugs like Ritalin or Prozac undermine the 'authenticity' of healthy people using them for enhancement (see Chapter 6). What each of these examples has in common is that a biological process—development, disease, or drug action—results in a corresponding mental change. We are left pondering how to apply the fundamentally static categorical concepts of person, competency, and identity following these physical shifts.

The research summarized here concerns another manifestation of this core neuroethical conundrum. It reminds us that who we are is determined not only by genetically programmed development, neurodegenerative disease, and psychoactive drugs, as in the familiar neuroethical examples just noted, but also by the socio-economic circumstances of our childhood in equivalently physical mechanistic ways. Neuroethicists have rightly called attention to the ethically complex ability of drugs to change who we are, for example giving us increased self-esteem or self-control by the effects of certain molecules on certain receptors (Fukuyama 2002; Kass 2003). It is metaphysically just as perplexing, and socially at least as distressing, that an impoverished and stressful childhood can diminish us by equally concrete physical mechanisms, such as the impact of early life stress on medial temporal memory ability through neuroendocrine mechanisms.

What are the implications for society of a more mechanistic understanding of the effects of childhood poverty on brain development? To different degrees, and in different ways, we regard children as the responsibility of both parents and society. Parental responsibility begins before birth and encompasses virtually every aspect of the child's life. Society's responsibility is more circumscribed. In the United States, for example, society's contribution to the cognitive development of children begins at the age of 5 or 6 years, depending on whether public kindergarten is offered. However, the physical health and safety of all infants and children is a social imperative well before school age. Laws requiring lead abatement in homes occupied by children exemplify our societal commitment to protect them from the neurological damage caused by this neurotoxin. Research on the effects of early life stress and limited cognitive stimulation has begun to show that these concomitants of poverty also have negative effects on neurological development, by mechanisms no less concrete and real. Thus neuroscience may recast the disadvantages of childhood poverty as a bioethical issue rather than merely one of economic opportunity.

# References

Adams BN (1998). *The Family: A Sociological Interpretation*. New York: Harcourt Brace.

Adams MJ (1990). *Learning to Read: Thinking and Learning About Print*. Cambridge, MA MIT Press.

Adler NE, Boyce T, Chesney MA, *et al.* (1994). Socioeconomic status and health: the challenge of the gradient. *American Psychologist* 49, 15–24.

Bellinger D, Leviton A, Waternaux C *et al.* (1987). Longitudinal analyses of prenatal and postnatal lead exposure and early cognitive development. *New England Journal of Medicine* 316, 1037–43.

Bradley RH, Corwyn RF (1999). Parenting. In: Tamis-Lemonda CLB (ed), *Child Psychology: A Handbook of Contemporary Issues*. New York: Psychology Press, 339–62.

Bradley RH, Corwyn RF, McAdoo HP *et al.* (2001) The home environments of children in the United States. Part 1: Variations by age, ethnicity, and poverty-status. *Child Development* 72, 1844–67.

Brooks-Gunn J, Duncan GJ (1997). The effects of poverty on children. *Future of Children* 7, 55–71.

Caldwell BM, Bradley RH (1984). *Home Observation for Measurement of the Environment (HOME)*. Little Rock, AR: University of Arkansas.

Capron C, Duyme M (1989). Assessment of effects of socio-economic status on IQ in a full cross-fostering study. *Nature* 340, 552–4.

Chasnoff IJ, Anson A, Hatcher R *et al.* (1998). Prenatal exposure to cocaine and other drugs. Outcome at four to six years. *Annals of the New York Academy of Sciences* 846, 314–28.

Center for Children and Poverty (1999) http://www.nccp.org/pub-pbd 99. html

Center on Hunger, Poverty and Nutrition Policy (1998) http://www.centeronhunger.org/cognitive. html

Davis EP, Bruce J, Gunnar MR (2002). The anterior attention network: associations with temperament and neuroendocrine activity in 6-year-old children. *Developmental Psychobiology* 40, 43–56.

Duncan GJ, Brooks-Gunn J, Klebanov PK (1994). Economic deprivation and early-childhood development. *Child Development* 65, 296–318.

Duncan GJ, Yeung WJ, Brooks-Gunn J *et al.* (1998). How much does childhood poverty affect the life chances of children? *American Sociological Review* 63, 426–423.

Duncan J, Burgess P, Emslie H (2002). Fluid intelligence after frontal lobe lesions. *Neuropsychologia*. 33,261–8.

Engle RW, Tuholski SW, Laughlin JE, *et al.* (1999). Working memory, short-term memory, and general fluid intelligence: a latent-variable approach. *Journal of Experimental Psychology: General* 128, 309–31.

Farah MJ, Savage J, Brodsky NL, *et al.* (2004). Association of socioeconomic status with neurocognitive development. *Pediatric Research Suppl.*

Farah MJ, *et al.* (2005a). Childhood experience and neurocognitive development: dissociation of cognitive and emotional influences. Submitted for publication.

Farah MJ, Savage J, Shera D, *et al.* (2005b) Childhood poverty: selective correlations with neurocognitive development. Submitted for publication.

Fukuyama F (2002). *Our Posthuman Future: Consequences of the Biotechnology Revolution.* New York: Farrar, Straus and Giroux.

Gray JR, Chabris CF, Braver TS (2003). Neural mechanisms of general fluid intelligence. *Nature Neuroscience* 6, 316–22.

Hurt H, Brodsky NL, Betancourt L, *et al.* (1995). Cocaine exposed children: follow-up at 30 months. *Developmental and Behavioral Pediatrics* 16, 29–35.

Hurt H, Malmud E, Braitman L, *et al.* (1998). Inner-city achievers: who are they? *Archives of Pediatric and Adolescent Medicine* 152, 993–7.

Kass L (2003). *Beyond Therapy: Biotechnology and the Pursuit of Happiness.* New York: HarperCollins.

Lanphear BP, Homung R, Khoury *et al.* (2005). Low-level environmental lead exposure and children's intellectual function: An international pooled analysis. *Environ. Health Perspect.*, 113, 894–9.

Lewis O (1965). *La Vida.* New York: Random House.

Lupien SJ, King S *et al.* (2001). Can poverty get under your skin? Basal cortisol levels and cognitive function in children from low and high socioeconomic status. *Development and Psychopathology* 13, 653–76.

McEwen BS (2000). The neurobiology of stress: from serendipity to clinical relevance. *Brain Research* 886, 172–189.

McLoyd VC (1998). Socioeconomic disadvantage and child development. *American Psychologist* 53, 185–204.

Marx K (1867). *Capital,* Vol. 1. New York: Penguin, 1976.

Mayes LC (2002). A behavioral teratogenic model of the impact of prenatal cocaine exposure on arousal regulatory systems. *Neurotoxicology and Teratology* 24, 385–95.

Meaney MJ, Diorio J, Francis D, *et al.* (1996). Early environmental regulation of forebrain glucocoricoid receptor gene expression: implications for adrenocortical responses to stress. *Developmental Neuroscience* 18, 49–72.

Noble KG, Norman MF, Farah MJ (2005a). Neurocognitive correlates of socioeconomic status in kindergarten children. *Developmental Science* 8, 74–87.

Noble KG, McCondliss B & Farah MJ (2005b). Socioeconomic gradients predict individual differences in neurocognitive abilities. Submitted for publication.

Ricciuti HN (1993). Nutrition and mental development. *Current Directions in Psychological Science* 2, 43–6.

Schiff M, Lewontin R (1986). *Education and Class: The Irrelevance of IQ Genetic Studies.* Oxford: Clarendon Press.

Sigman M (1995). Nutrition and child development. *Current Directions in Psychological Science* 4, 52–5.

Turkheimer E, Haley A, Waldron M, *et al.* (2003). Socioeconomic status modifies heritability of IQ in young children. *Psychological Science* 14, 623–8.

Turner RJ, Avison WR (2003). Status variations in stress exposure: implications for the interpretation of research on race, socioeconomic status, and gender. *Journal of Health and Social Behavior* 44, 488–505.

van Praag H, Kempermann G. Gage FH (2000). Neural consequences of environmental enrichment. *Nature Reviews Neuroscience* 1, 191–8.

Vidaeff AC, Mastrobattista JM (2003). *In utero* cocaine exposure: a thorny mix of science and mythology. *American Journal of Perinatalogy* 20, 165–72.

Volkmar FR, Greenough WT (1972). Rearing complexity affects branching of dendrites in the visual cortex of the rat. *Science* 176, 1145–7.

Weber M (1923). *General Economic History.* New York: Collier, 1961.

## Chapter 20

# Religious responses to neuroscientific questions

Paul Root Wolpe

## Introduction

Religion is one of the basic and most pervasive of human experiences, as well as one of the most enigmatic. There is scarcely a relevant academic discipline that has not puzzled over the existence of religion; in fact, it is not an exaggeration to suggest that modern anthropology, sociology, and, to a lesser degree, psychology were all founded on written works contemplating the nature and origins of religion. Therefore it is not surprising that the powerful new technologies available to neuroscience would eventually be employed to try and understand the neural nature of religious experience.

The paradox of human religious belief makes tempting the suggestion that it is somehow hard-wired into the brain. Why is religion, in all its forms, ubiquitous? Why is humankind so willing to drop its need for concrete evidence in the face of its belief in the invisible, omnipotent, omniscient, and supernatural? If an organ of belief were found in the brain, it would be tempting to explain these tendencies away by crediting the paradox to some innate structural proclivity, and therefore reduce the phenomenon to a by-product of our brain's functioning.

As a recent editorial in *Nature* suggests (Anonymous 2004), science and religion are often at odds today, as in times past. The tension between the two need not be destructive; science can reinforce or illuminate religion as well as refute it. However, when science does challenge religion, it is usually with one of three kinds of activities or claims. First, science can propose lines of research or goals that religious traditions oppose or believe should be infused with certain values, as in the stem cell, anti-aging, or cloning debates. Secondly, it can challenge religious dogma or belief by, for example, countering a creationist interpretation of the origins of the world with an evolutionary one. Finally, science can also challenge the nature of religious impulses or beliefs themselves. Freud did, for example, by suggesting that religious experience is inspired by an Oedipal desire for an omnipotent and omniscient father.

Modern neuroscientists have engaged religious thinkers on all three fronts. They have developed new means of enhancing brain function that have implications for religious values about selfhood. They have suggested that the soul is an illusion, and that all human experiences are reducible to the functioning of the brain (Pinker 2002a). The newly minted field of neurotheology has begun to locate the centers of religious experience in the brain, suggesting to some that religious experience is reducible to neurological phenomena without the need for supernatural or divine elements.

It is not surprising that advances in neuroscience should engage religious scholars. In ways similar to the ongoing dialogue about genetics, neuroscience examines fundamental aspects of human existence—who we are and why we behave as we do; the nature of human thought and free will; the appropriate limits of human enhancement; and our rights to the inviolability of our innermost thoughts and feelings. However, unlike genetics, where many of the issues (such as the moral status of the embryo) are well-trodden in religious thought, neuroethics brings up questions that can be somewhat murkier. The function of the brain was a source of confusion historically. The ancient Egyptians, for example, prescribed elaborate rituals to prepare the heart for burial, while the brain was treated as a minor organ. Aristotle thought that the brain was an organ to cool the heart. In the sixteenth and early seventeenth century, when the anatomy of the brain was being described with greater and greater precision, the function of the brain was still obscure.

Historically, therefore, little systematic thought developed in religious quarters on the nature of the brain itself. However, a substantial amount of thought has been devoted to the human qualities that (presumably) reside therein—emotion, thought, intellect, spirit. Modern neuroethics concerns itself largely with how neurotechnologies and the insights of neuroscience might impact just these human qualities. Therefore, the questions confronting religious thought as our understanding of the brain expands are not so much about religion's views on this or that ethical issue, but rather an understanding of exactly what the religious questions are that neuroscientific findings pose. When the questions posed by the Human Genome Project (see also Chapter 8) and genetic technologies were encountered by the various faith traditions, the resulting dialogue was, and continues to be, rich and illuminating. So, too, with neuroethics; while the field is too new to have generated a rich literature among religious scholars, the process is already beginning. Conferences with names like 'Neuroscience and the Soul' (Woodstock Theological Center, Washington, DC, 1998) and 'Neuroscience, Religious Experience, and the Self' (Montreal 2001) have begun to define the field and suggest approaches that religious traditions might take to the kinds of questions neuroethics is beginning to confront.

Science and religion are not always in conflict, as mentioned, and science can often be used to understand, confirm, or enrich religious thought. Some find in the complexity and nuance of the brain itself a reinfusing of religious meaning, and find fodder for a deeper understanding of human religiosity in many of the findings of neuroscience. For example, Ashbrook and Albright (1997) contemplate what they call a 'neurobiology of meaning', exploring the nature of the brain as both the focus of our understanding of the world (the brain is designed, they claim, to focus on and seek out the human element in the world) and the mirror of the Divine. Therefore religion need not only be reactive to the challenges posed by neuroscience; it can also mold science to its needs, and use the discoveries of neuroscience as data in pursuit of religious insight into the human condition.

In this chapter I will explore the three areas where neuroscience challenges religion as described above: first, in religion's ethical response to neuroscientific findings; secondly, how religion responds to the claims of some neuroscientists that current research refutes ideas such as ensoulment; and finally, through the field that has come to be known as neurotheology, the neuroscientific study of the religious impulse itself.

## Neuroethics and religion

The major religions, almost without exception, include codes of ethical behavior, and being ethical is itself a universally praised religious standard. While religious ethicists use their traditions to gain insight into almost any ethical issue, the contributions of religious scholarship may vary, depending on the particular set of issues at stake. Some of the challenges raised by neuroethics are more amenable to religious analysis than others.

For example, one clear result of increasingly sophisticated brain imaging technologies is the threat to personal privacy. Should we realize the potential to derive information directly from brain processes, we would, for the first time, bypass the peripheral nervous system, which is the gatekeeper on our communication with others. If information can be gleaned directly from the brain, we may lose the ability to filter it, deny it to the listener, or communicate it in the manner we desire. How should we think about the right to privacy if we are able to extract personal information directly from individuals' brains, perhaps even without their consent or knowledge? Who has the right to such information?

Judaism, Christianity, and Islam have all developed ideas of privacy and confidentiality over the centuries. Clearly, the idea of absolute privacy does not exist in any system that believes in an omniscient God. My subjective thoughts may forever be hidden from my fellow man, but part of the control mechanism of all three religions is the idea that God is always watching, always has access to thought and action. However, it is precisely because it is understood that only God can know our thoughts, for example, that the act of sharing one's private sins through confession holds the priest to such inviolable standards of confidentiality.

The long history of religious consideration of privacy and confidentiality can help us to think about emerging ethical issues such as the threat to privacy posed by brain imaging. While it is up to religious thinkers in each tradition to develop their own interpretation of the challenges posed by brain imaging, some suggestions might be illustrative. In Judaism, for example, the Talmud has extensive discussions about what kind of information should properly be sought and communicated, particularly about a person's family background that may be relevant to marriageability, or duties related to priestly descent. The Talmudic discussion is highly nuanced and has already been employed to elucidate issues in genetic privacy. Christianity, as another example, has a long history of concern about confidentiality in medicine; the Hippocratic Oath was adopted in a Christian version before the third century CE (Carrick 1985). The model of confessional confidentiality has been a hallmark of the Roman Catholic Church, and the balance of protecting individual privacy versus the public good has a long history of consideration in the church. As another example, in some Islamic cultures, *qurba*, the webs of obligations and relations between family members, lead to complex sets of obligations about confidentiality. In that tradition, the family unit as a whole can take the place of the individual as the recipient of confidential disclosure and non-disclosure.

While these three examples are in some sense arbitrary, and many others could be used, they highlight the ways in which different faith traditions have discussions reaching back centuries about the kinds of challenges to privacy that brain imaging may some day pose. Mining those traditions for insights into the issue may enrich the discussions of neuroethics in the same way as they have in genetics.

The same is true in other areas of neuroethics. For example, after the publication of *Listening to Prozac* (Kramer 1993) started a nationwide discussion of the use of pharmaceuticals to alter affect and perhaps personality, a number of religious writers contributed views on what their faith traditions had to say about depression, drug treatment, and pharmaceutical enhancement. Some Christian writers defended treatment of depression as fully compatible with a Christian spiritual path, citing medicine as part of God's plan for healing (Barshinger *et al.* 1995). Others lamented the substitution of Prozac for seeking true spiritual enlightenment (Gordon 2003). In that sense, the religious literature mimicked the secular literature, which was going through a similar discussion of the proper roles of psychopharmaceuticals although, perhaps, with fewer religious metaphors. The President's Council on Bioethics is not constituted as a religious body. Yet, its report *Beyond Therapy* (President's Council on Bioethics 2003), although suffused with secular disclaimers and reinterpretations of religious terms like 'soul', is clearly inspired in its critique of enhancement by religious arguments and sensibilities. That is not necessarily inappropriate, in the sense that ultimate questions should be informed by the traditions that have contemplated them for centuries. It is appropriate that religious scholars contribute to discussions of the neuroethical issues that confront society, and that society consider those arguments seriously in its assessment of bioethical issues. However, in a pluralistic society that has an avowed separation of church and state, the biases and presuppositions of all contributors to public discourse must be made clear. Religious arguments should be clearly labeled as such, as should arguments coming from particular philosophical or political positions.

## Neuroscience and the soul

The history of modern Western religion has been one of steady retreat from science. Before empirical science began its rise, the Church was the source of both moral knowledge and knowledge of a world designed by God. While religion in general no longer claims jurisdiction over the realm of empirical fact, and contentious areas such as the 'intelligent design' theory still exist, it is willing to mount a challenge when science seems to be treading on territory that religion claims.

It seems that neuroscience may develop into a primary battleground of claims and counterclaims between science and religion. For example, Steven Pinker, an evolutionary psychologist and popular author, claims (Pinker 2002a) that there are three 'myths' in modern thinking about the brain: 'the blank slate', the mind has no inherent structure and so is malleable to social forces; 'the noble savage', violence is a learned behavior, humans are naturally good; and 'the ghost in the machine', the existence of an immaterial soul. One can see the challenge that refutations of the latter two claims in particular make to at least some religious doctrines. Pinker's refutation of the noble savage claim may challenge Christian ideas such as the fall from grace, at least in some conceptualizations. Conversely, it may provide support to religious traditions that support the idea that the will to violence is an innate part of our nature. Judaism, for example, postulates a *yetzer ha'ra*, an innate 'evil inclination'.

Perhaps most controversial to religious thinking is Pinker's explicit rejection of the idea of a soul as an entity independent of brain structures. He claims that neuroscience supports the materialistic view of the soul:

> Neuroscience is showing that all aspects of mental life—every emotion, every thought pattern, every memory—can be tied to the physiological activity or structure of the brain. Cognitive science has shown that feats that were formerly thought to be doable by mental stuff alone can be duplicated by machines, that motives and goals can be understood in terms of feedback and cybernetic mechanisms, and that thinking can be understood as a kind of computation. (Pinker 2002b)

Thus neuroscience is said to shrink the possible set of human activities that can plausibly be attributed to the soul. As Brown (2004) puts it, 'If all our thoughts, actions, and experiences are functions that emerge from the complex interactive processes of our nervous system, then of what value is the concept of a separate soul?'.

The claim that neuroscience itself can tell us something about the existence or non-existence of the soul is precisely the kind of claim that makes religious thinkers nervous. Ultimately, science cannot adjudicate on the supernatural or metaphysical claims of religion. Let us imagine for a moment that there is an immaterial soul. Is there a scientific experiment that would detect it? Does the neural nature of emotion, thought, memory, disprove a soul? Even though neuroscience ultimately cannot disprove a metaphysical soul, there are also religious thinkers who have to some degree given up the idea of a metaphysical soul altogether, and have redefined the soul in practical neuroscientific terms. Ashbrook and Albright (1997) equate soul with memory; using Augustine's concept of soul, they argue that memory expresses the meaning of soul most deeply:

> Human beings are made to seek a center of meaning and power inside themselves, that is within yet beyond consciousness... Within consciousness, meaning involves memory. In the vast palaces of memory, to continue Augustine's imagery, people confront themselves with themselves: when, where and what we have done and under what feeling and with what meaning.

Similarly, Brown (2004) suggests that one can understand spirituality and soul in the light of our new understandings of the brain in terms of 'nonreductive physicalism', which maintains that while higher-level capacities like thinking are dependent on lower-level neural processes, they are still causal in their own right, i.e. they also have top-down influences on lower-level processes. In that sense, they are more than the sum of their contributing neural parts, and in that emergent property is room for a sense of the spiritual. It is a time-tested and integral part of modern religious thought to revise and reinterpret in light of changing times and new scientific knowledge. Thus the consequence of the neuroscience challenge to the soul may not be its refutation, but its reinvigoration.

The soul is not the only idea that neuroscience is exploring that might influence religious thought on the matter; neuroscience is also researching, and sometimes questioning traditional views of human traits like free will, responsibility, and agency. For example, Greene *et al.* (2001) used functional MRI to study moral reasoning, a subject of great interest to religion. They employed a classic ethics vignette that has often been pondered by philosophers: most people report that they would pull a lever redirecting a train onto a track where one person would be killed rather than allow it to remain on a track where five people would be killed. However, they say they would not physically push a single person in front of the train to stop it from killing five others. Yet, both cases involve killing one to save five, and so, speaking consequentially, they both result in saving four extra lives. Why then will people use one technique to save four lives, and not the other? Green and his colleagues found that emotional centers of the brain were much more active when considering physically pushing someone onto the track (a moral–personal scenario) than when simply pulling a switch (a moral–impersonal scenario). The role of emotionality in moral decision-making can be a useful insight for religious ethics.

Neuroscientists are also looking at the neural correlates of forgiveness (Newberg *et al.* 2000), empathy (Singer *et al.* 2004), and other religiously relevant human actions. For example, Singer and colleagues discovered that the feeling of empathy originates in the same part of the brain as does pain itself. In that sense, empathy really does have something to do with one's own experience of pain. Research like that of Singer and Greene can teach us about the nature of the very kinds of emotional responses that religion tends to encourage, and therefore can be a source of insight for religions in their teaching of moral behavior.

## Finding religion in the brain

Perhaps no area of neuroscience and religion has received as much attention as the field that has come to be known as neurotheology. Books like *Why God Won't Go Away* (Newberg and

D'Aquili 2001) and *The God Gene* (Hamer 2004) have highlighted the question: Where in our brain does religion live? The paradox of human religious belief makes it tempting to look for its secrets in the structure of the brain. Religion is a universal human phenomenon, found in every culture and time. It is not therefore probable that the brain's structure would reflect such a basic, ubiquitous human trait? And if we indeed do find such a structure what whould be its implications for religion as an institution or for individual religious practice?

To try and determine where religious experience resides in the brain, researchers have put meditators, nuns, and monks in scanners as they prayed and meditated. They have mapped the neurophysiology of spiritual experience. During religious or meditative experience, the brain displays increased activity in the posterior superior parietal lobe, which orients a person in physical space and which Newberg and D'Aquili (2001) have dubbed the 'orientation association area, or OAA'. 'To perform this crucial function, [the OAA] must first generate a clear, consistent cognition of the physical limits of the self. In simple terms, it must draw a sharp distinction between the individual and everything else; to sort out the you from the infinite not-you that makes up the rest of the universe'. It is this area that, as one meditator put it, gives you '. . . a sense of timelessness and infinity. It feels like I am part of everyone and everything in existence'.

The achievement of this state requires a coordinated set of brain functions. According to Austin (1988), the amygdala, which is the site of fear and anxiety, must be quieted, while activity in the parietal lobes that orients us to space and environment, and separates our sense of ourselves from the rest of the world, must be minimized. The areas of the frontal and temporal lobes that mark time and generate self-awareness also must be quiescent. Austin suggests that then 'what we think of as our "higher" functions of selfhood appear briefly to "drop out", "dissolve", or be "deleted from consciousness"' (Austin 2000). Newberg and Iverson (2003) performed brain imaging studies of skilled meditators. The neurophysiological effects observed in these studies point to a consistent pattern of changes in cerebral structures in conjunction with autonomic and hormonal changes, as well as neurochemical changes involving the endogenous opioid GABA, norephinephrine, and serotonin receptor systems.

Another kind of evidence comes from the use of transcranial magnetic stimulation (TMS), a technology that sends magnetic or electrical impulses across the skull that can disrupt brain function in discrete areas of the brain (see also Chapter 14). Persinger (1987) has used TMS to try and understand the nature of human consciousness and religious and mystical experience. He has experimented for over a decade with ways to induce religious experience, including using LSD. Recently, his work has concentrated on TMS, where he induces a small pulsating magnetic field in the temporal lobes of his subjects. The result is potentially transformative, and Persinger reports that his technique produces sensations that volunteers describe as supernatural or spiritual (Begley 2001). He claims that he can modify hypnotizability, consolidate 'quasi experiences' that are reconstructed by the subject as autobiographical memory, and induce changes in the self (Tiller and Persinger 1994). There are already products on the market claiming to use electrical or magnetic impulses to try and induce spiritual experiences in users (e.g. www.innerworlds.50megs.com/shakti/shakti_proposal.htm).

If we can find the areas of the brain that express religious feeling, have we, in fact, 'explained' the human need for religion? Perhaps not surprisingly, the question was addressed over 100 years ago by William James (1902):

> . . . when other people criticize our own more exalted soul-flights by calling them 'nothing but' expressions of our organic disposition, we feel outraged and hurt, for we know that, whatever be our

organism's peculiarities, our mental states have their substantive value as revelations of the living truth; and we wish that all this medical materialism could be made to hold its tongue... According to the general postulate of psychology just referred to, there is not a single one of our states of mind, high or low, healthy or morbid, that has not some organic process as its condition... To plead the organic causation of a religious state of mind, then, in refutation of its claim to possess superior spiritual value, is quite illogical and arbitrary, unless one has already worked out in advance some psycho-physical theory connecting spiritual values in general with determinate sorts of physiological change.

It is precisely that psychophysical theory that is the goal of modern neurotheology. However, the existence of organs of religion or spirituality in the brain does not itself disprove their connection to, or perceptions of, higher spiritual truths. In the end, neuroscience will do little to dissuade the spiritual of the truth of their experience or the believer of the existence of God.

## Conclusion

The goals of neuroscience are to understand the function and structure of the brain and its relation to human behavior in general. As religion is a fundamental ubiquitous human activity, it is natural that neuroscientists would be interested in exploring how the brain expresses religious belief and experience. Yet religion sees itself as tying the neurological into something greater. Religion celebrates the human desire to make meaning of the world, finding in it a sense of sacredness that is innate to existence and nurturing that sense through adopting specific beliefs or behaviors such as spiritual experience. In that sense neuroscience may teach religion something about the neurological nature of religious experience or give it insight into moral decision-making, but it will never challenge the basic assumptions of religion.

Albert Einstein once said:

The most beautiful and profound emotion we can experience is the sensation of the mystical. It is the foundation of all true science. He to whom this emotion is a stranger, who can no longer stand rapt in awe, is as good as dead. To know that what is inconceivable to us really exists, manifesting itself as the highest wisdom, as the most radiant beauty which our dull faculties can comprehend only in their most primitive form this knowledge, this feeling, is at the center of true religiousness. (Bucky 1992)

Perhaps that is the true connection of neuroscience to religion; both embrace a sense of awe in a quest to understand the nature of the human condition.

## References

Anonymous (2004). Where theology matters (Editorial). *Nature* 432, 657.
Ashbrook JB, Albright CE (1997). *The Humanizing Brain*. Cleveland, OH: Pilgrim Press.
Austin JH (1988). *Zen and the Brain: Toward an Understanding of Meditation and Consciousness*. Cambridge, MA: MIT Press.
Austin JH (2000). Consciousness evolves when the self dissolves. *Journal of Consciousness Studies* 7, 209–30.
Barshinger CE, LaRowe LE, Andres T (1995). The gospel according to Prozac. *Christianity Today*, 14 August.
Begley S (2001). Your brain on religion: mystic visions or brain circuits at work? *Newsweek*, 7 May.
Brown WS (2004). Neurobiological embodiment of spirituality and soul. In: Jeeves M (ed) *From Cells to Souls—And Beyond*. Grand Rapids, MI: William B. Eerdmans.
Bucky P (1992). *The Private Albert Einstein*. Kansas City, MO: Andrews McMeel, 85–7.

Carrick P (1985). *Medical Ethics in Antiquity.* Dordrecht, The Netherlands: Reidel.

Gordon M (2003). Job on Prozac: the pharmaceutical option. *The Christian Century,* 9 August.

Greene JD, Sommerville BR, Nystrom LE, Darley JM, Cohen JD (2001). An fMRI investigation of emotional engagement in moral judgment. *Science* 293, 2105–8.

Hamer D (2004). *The God Gene.* New York: Doubleday.

James W (1902). *The Varieties of Religious Experience.* Cambridge, MA: Harvard University Press, 1985.

Kramer P (1993). *Listening to Prozac.* New York: Viking.

Newberg AB, D'Aquili EG (2001). *Why God Won't Go Away: Brain Science and the Biology of Belief.* New York: Ballantine.

Newberg AB, Iversen J (2003). The neural basis of the complex mental task of meditation: neurotransmitter and neurochemical considerations. *Medical Hypotheses* 61, 282–91

Newberg AB, D'Aquili EG, Newberg SK, deMarici V (2000). The neuropsychological correlates of forgiveness. In: McCullough ME, Pargament KI, Thoresen CE (eds) *Forgiveness: Theory, Research and Practice.* New York: Guilford Press.

Persinger M (1987). *Neuropsychological Bases of God Beliefs.* New York: Praeger.

Pinker S (2002a). *The Blank Slate: The Modern Denial of Human Nature.* New York: Penguin Books.

Pinker S (2002b). Biology and the blank slate (Interview). Available online at: http://reason.com/0210/fe.rb.biology.shtml (accessed 8 May 2005).

President's Council on Bioethics (2003). *Beyond Therapy.* New York: HarperCollins.

Singer T, Seymour B, O'Doherty J, Kaube H, Dolan RJ, Frith CD (2004) Empathy for pain involves the affective but not sensory components of pain. *Science* 303, 1157–62.

Tiller S, Persinger M (1994). Enhanced hypnotizability by cerebrally applied magnetic fields depends upon the order of hemispheric presentation: an anisotropic effect. *International Journal of Neuroscience* 79, 157–63.

## Chapter 21

# The mind in the movies: a neuroethical analysis of the portrayal of the mind in popular media

Maren Grainger-Monsen and Kim Karetsky

## Introduction

The media has a profound influence on our society. While there may be debate about the extent of the media's influence on societal attitudes, values, and behavior, there really can be no argument that it exerts an impact on everything from public tolerance for violence to changing sexual mores and creating desire for material goods. People are increasingly aware of the media's growing influence on the public's understanding of health issues. The pharmaceutical industry spends more than 3 billion dollars on direct-to-consumer advertisements each year—because it has been shown to affect people's behavior (Kaiser Family Foundation 2003). Coverage of health topics is more pervasive, and, in turn, the public is seeking more information about health from media sources. In 1998, health stories constituted the fifth most common topic in local American television news (Kaiser Family Foundation 1998). Another study of commercials found that in 1998, American television showed more than 17 commercials per hour containing health information (Byrd-Bredbenner and Grasso 2000). Seventy-five percent of adults surveyed in a National Health Council Report said they pay either a 'moderate' or 'great deal' of attention to medical and health news reported by the media. They went on to say they obtained more medical information from the media than from their own doctors. Fifty-eight percent said they had changed their behavior or taken some kind of action as a result of having read, seen, or heard a medical or health news story in the media (National Health Council 1997). Therefore it is clear that the media are powerful forces in the public's perception of issues of medicine and health. How have the media specifically influenced the public's understanding of health and the neurosciences? In this chapter we will focus on one aspect of the media, the film industry, and look at its effect on the public's perception of how the mind works, both in mental illness and in the neuroscience enhancement technologies that the future holds.

Given that stereotypes created by the media can have tremendous influence on public perception, one can argue that those created by narrative films are even more powerful, since they touch people emotionally and thus leave a more enduring image. The psychotherapist A. Hollander writes that film is an interesting medium for depicting stereotypes, as 'the visual elements in film are similar to music, in the way they transmit emotive material without calling attention to it... In this way, a lot of visual movie material has been swallowed whole, seen without being remarked, responded to without consciousness...' (Hollander 1991, pp. 449–50). As a result, many of the negative stereotypes of mental illness, which are deeply rooted in historical pictorial media and portrayed in current popular films, possess great power to reflect and shape audience perceptions with great poignancy and directness (Gilman 1982), leaving viewers with sometimes inaccurate and unwarranted beliefs about mental disabilities. We will document the use of the mind and images of the altered mind in popular entertainment media, focusing on motion pictures. We have outlined some of the stereotypes of psychiatric illness revealed in popular Hollywood films and hope to highlight the impact that these stereotypes have on both the public and the mentally ill. What message do these films send to the public? Do these films fairly and ethically portray the challenges faced by an altered mind? Are mentally ill individuals justly represented?

We will also examine some of the new independent documentary films addressing mental illness that have been successful in breaking down some of these stereotypes by showing more realistic portrayals of mentally ill patients and families. These films are particularly important, in that they are able to open up the image of patients with mental illness within the world of storytelling, which is fundamentally different from factual news-based documentaries. Films, including documentaries that tell stories and build characters, have more potential to combat stereotypes because they touch people in a more profound and emotional way. To this end we will look at the expanding genre of independent documentary films exploring the area of mental illness that seek to break down the stereotypes created in the Hollywood mass media. Finally, we will examine how the new frontiers of neuroscience are being portrayed in motion pictures and explore the neuroethical issues that are brought up, as well as questioning the impact that science fiction films have on the public consciousness. These are just some of the many poignant neuroethical questions and dilemmas raised by modern motion pictures that deserve our attention and discussion. It is incumbent upon us in the health field to teach the public to look critically at and analyze the media, as opposed to being merely passive consumers.

## Portrayal of mental illness by the media

Stereotypes of psychiatric disability are often conveyed to the general population through the mass media including literature, television, and especially film. Popular Hollywood movies reach vast audiences in theaters and continue to do so over time through constant television replay. Movies provide an opportunity for viewers to empathize with characters suffering from mental illness, yet they also can create distortions and misperceptions about what mental illness really is.

In 2001, the Australian government published a large-scale literature review examining how mental health is portrayed in the media (Francis *et al.* 2001), which revealed that media representations of mental illness promote negative stereotypes—specifically, the false connection between mental illness and violence. Other studies have shown a connection between negative media portrayals of mental illness and the public's negative attitudes toward the mentally ill (Wahl and Roth 1982; Wahl 1995; Diefenbach 1997; Rose 1998; Wilson *et al.* 1999; Cutcliffe and Hannigan 2001; Coverdale *et al.* 2002; Olstead 2002). A 1996 Department of Health study in the United Kingdom found that media representations of mental illness have a negative effect on public perception (Rose 1998). A study conducted by the Glasgow University Media Group also found that the belief in a link between mental illness and violence was derived, in large part, from the media, and that the media's representation of the mentally ill is powerful enough to alter people's own personal experiences with mental illness (Philo 1993).

In 1997, the National Mental Health Association conducted a study entitled 'Stigma Matters: Assessing the Media's Impact on Public Perceptions of Mental Illness'. This study revealed that

**Table 21.1** Sources from which the public receives information about mental illness (From Hottentot 2002)

| | |
|---|---|
| TV newsmagazine shows | 70% |
| Newspapers | 58% |
| TV news | 51% |
| News magazines | 34% |
| TV talk shows | 31% |
| Radio news | 26% |
| Internet | 25% |
| Non-fiction books | 25% |
| Radio talk shows | 18% |
| Women's magazines | 18% |

the public generally receives its information about mental illness from the following sources as shown in Table 21.1 (Hottentot 2000).

According to a report from the Canadian Mental Health Association in Ontario (Edney 2004), over the past 30 years numerous studies have been completed to determine the effect that the mass media have on the public's perceptions. These studies reveal how the degree to which people are exposed to media representations and media's power to influence common beliefs make the mass media one of the most significant forces in society. It is evident that the media plays a critical role in influencing society about psychiatric disorders; however, research has indicated that media portrayals of mental illness are often inaccurate and overly negative (Diefenbach 1997 and references cited therein).

Gilman's (1982) survey of the iconography of 'madness' in the older visual arts reveals a set of deviancy icons of 'insanity' and major thematic stereotypes of disability present in the print and visual media (Biklen and Bogdan 1977; Institute for Information Studies 1979). However, little has been written about how stereotypes of psychiatric disability are communicated in film. This is a significant weakness, since film is one of the most important media sources (Sless 1981; Hollander 1991), which quite often deals with issues of psychiatric disability, and communication in film has significant social and political power to generate misleading stereotypes (Nichols 1981; Andrew 1984; Thomas 1982). Other than Gilman's work, very little research has been conducted on the symbolic representation of 'mental illness' in film (Winick 1978; Fleming and Manvell 1985).

## History of 'madness' in film: change over time

Beginning in 1934, the Hollywood Production Code, a set of rules governing the production of films, began prohibiting the use of 'insanity' as a major theme in films (Roffman and Purdy 1981). It was not until 1968 that the Production Code was discarded and mental illness was permitted to be a theme of motion pictures (Winick 1978). Therefore, during the years between 1934 and 1968 mental illness could not be dealt with in any naturalistic way in films. The presentations of protagonists were highly stylized depictions of how a director, film-maker, or actor interpreted the subject. In pre-1968 films, these highly stylized protagonists were often shown in juxtaposition to their horrific environments. Elizabeth Taylor in *Suddenly Last Summer* remains beautiful, poised, and without a hair out of place throughout the film and stands out in stark contrast to the appalling surroundings of the mental asylum (Levers 2001). However, after 1968, when the ban was lifted, there was an attempt to portray mental illness in a socially conscious and accurate manner (Roffman and Purdy 1981) and films began to be produced that depicted mental health patients as more clearly ill and suffering. Levers points out that the filmic depiction of hospital environments changed over time, reflecting the changing social policy about mental illness. In the pre-1968 films, mental institutions were generally portrayed by darkness and shadows, mirroring the current social policy of uninformed and secretive treatment of mental illness, and this shifted toward a depiction of mental institutions in bright white sterility in the post-1968 films.

## Mental illness in the media

Stigmatization of people with mental illness has been thoroughly researched (Siller 1976; Goffman 1963; Finkelstein 1980; Altman 1981; Roth 1983), and the extent to which negative attitudes have been conveyed by the media is well documented (Biklen and Bogdan 1977; Institute for Information Studies 1979; Byrd and Pipes 1981; Bogdan *et al.* 1982; Elliot and Byrd 1982; Gartner 1982; Kriegel 1982; Quart and Auster 1982; Byrd and Elliott 1985; Byrd 1989). Research has revealed that stigmatizing portrayals of people with mental illness have had a direct effect on the viewers' attitudes toward people with disabilities (Elliott and Byrd 1982; Domino 1983; Bywater and Sobchack 1989; Wahl and Lefkowits 1989).

Prior literature regarding media portrayal of disability (Biklen and Bogdan 1977; Institute for Information Studies 1979) identified the following 10 stereotypes of persons with psychiatric disabilities as they appear in the media: as dangerous; as objects of violence; as atmosphere; as pitiable and pathetic; as asexual or sexually deviant; as incapable; as comic figures; as their own worst enemy or only enemy; as 'super-crips' or helpless cripples; as burdens.

Over the past four decades the most common illustrations of mental illness in the media have involved the mentally ill engaging in some criminal or violent behavior (Cutcliffe and Hannigan 2001; Olstead 2002 and references cited therein; Wahl and Roth 1982; Wilson *et al.* 1999). It has been argued by Rose (1998) that the media portrays psychosis as an 'unclassifiable experience' which poses a threat. Mental illness is depicted as being incomprehensible, unpredictable, and unstable. In addition, mentally ill people are often seen as extremely violent, unsafe and dangerous.

## Mental illness in film

Levers (2001) conducted research pertaining specifically to the stereotypes of psychiatric disability in film. She used the study by Gilman (1982) as a base to create a list of icons, associated with the historic portrayal of 'madness', to discover whether similar representations could be found in film. The icons included images such as objects near to or held by the 'insane' subject, clothing worn, facial expressions, physical characteristics, physical posturing and gesturing, and environments in which those deemed 'mentally ill' are placed. Levers analyzed the frequency of icons in a carefully determined list of 21 films. The results of the study revealed that all of the 10 stereotypes identified by Gilman's research were found in the films and two additional stereotypes emerged, including psychiatric disability as 'artistic or creative genius' and psychiatric disability as 'pathological' or 'medicalized'. Levers' study revealed that people with psychiatric disabilities are often depicted in film in several distinct ways, including as dangerous, as passive objects of violence, as medically pathological, and as pathetic or comical beings. Most of the frequently recurring icons demonstrate the dangerous aggressor or the object of violence. Although these portrayals of 'madness' are not necessarily representative of the reality of the psychiatric impairment, they are significant considering the powerful impact that film images have on the viewer.

According to Hyler (2003), negative stereotypes of patients with mental illness have a long history in Hollywood. Inaccurate portrayals have a critical and underestimated negative effect on the perception of the mentally ill by the public, legislators, families, and patients themselves. Some of the common stereotypes seen in Hollywood film include: the mentally ill as the 'homicidal maniac', the 'narcissistic parasite', the 'rebellious free spirit', and the 'specially gifted', and the female patient as 'the seductress'.

The stereotype of homicidal maniac is one of the earliest negative stereotypes pertaining to the mentally ill. Several years before *Birth of a Nation* (1915), D.W. Griffith created *The Maniac Cook* (1909), which depicted a 'deranged' mental patient who is excessively violent and therefore requires incarceration to avoid wreaking havoc on society. The 1960s horror films, including *Psycho* (1960), and later films, such as *Halloween* (1978) and the *Friday the 13th* series (1980 and later), continued to display characters with this stereotype. More recently, the psychiatrist in *Silence of the Lambs* (1991) continues this stereotype by murdering his victims and, in one case, eating his liver 'with some fava beans and a nice Chianti'. Other films of this genre include *American Psycho* (2000), a film that never resolves whether the protagonist is actually committing the gruesome murders or whether they exist solely in his imagination, thereby conveying the message to viewers that psychosis is equivalent to homicidal mania. *Summer of Sam* (1999) depicts the protagonist in the midst of his psychosis, howling at the moon and wrecking his room. Other films that illustrate the incorrect stereotype of the mentally ill equalling violent maniacs include *Primal Fear* (1996) and *The Bone Collector* (1999).

In reality, individuals with mental disorders are no more likely to commit violent crimes than members of the general public (with the possible exception of substance-induced mental illness) (Hyler *et al.* 1991). What is the cumulative effect on audiences who see mental patients depicted as violent maniacs? Are viewers likely to sympathize with people with mental illnesses? Will the public feel comfortable welcoming or supporting halfway houses or community centers? What effect might the public's perception of mental illness have on the vote to allocate limited funds to mental health research (Hyler 2003)?

Many popular films including Woody Allen's *Annie Hall* (1977), *Lovesick* (1983), *Love at First Bite* (1979), and *High Anxiety* (1978) feature mentally ill patients characterized as self-centered attention seekers who are involved in narcissistic relationships with their therapists (Hyler 2003). *Down and Out in Beverly Hills* (1986) portrays a psychotherapist who even treats neurotic dogs. This stereotype stigmatizes the mentally ill by ridiculing and trivializing their problems, making it far more difficult for such patients to reveal their disability and seek treatment.

A final stereotype of mental illness found in Hollywood film is that of the female psychiatric patient as a seductress or nymphomaniac. *Spellbound* (1945), *The Caretakers* (1963), *Lilith* (1964), and *Girl Interrupted* (1999) all portray female mental patients as seductresses who try to seduce their therapists. Hyler argues that this stereotype could be quite harmful to a woman with emotional problems or a history of abuse who is trying to decide whether or not to seek help for a clinically significant mental illness, such as depression, anxiety disorder, or post-traumatic stress disorder.

## Mental illness in prime time television

In an analysis of prime time television programming, Wilson *et al.* (1999) found that 43 percent of mentally disabled characters on television lacked understanding of everyday procedures and processes and often appeared confused and lost. Such characters frequently appeared disheveled and used simplistic childlike language. In many cases, the mentally ill character was poor, homeless, or being detained by police for a crime which he or she had little recollection or understanding of having committed. Wilson *et al.* (1999) also concluded that 67 percent of prime time television's mentally ill characters were depicted as unproductive failures, who were unemployed and had ineffective or non-existent relationships with family or friends. While this may be the case for patients suffering from severe mental illness, this is clearly a vast overstatement for patients with mild to moderate mental illness. This is significant, because 15 percent of the population suffers from depression or anxiety (Blaxter 1990; Goldberg and Huxley 1992; Meltzer *et al.* 1995), and it is stigmatizing to present them as unable to hold a job or have relationships with family and friends. Olstead (2002) describes the mentally ill as often lacking 'in markers of social identity', such as family, friends, roots or history. He contends that when mental illness is presented as a person's only characteristic, that individual becomes 100 percent defined by the illness and is inherently different from others.

## Class differences in media reporting of mental illness

Olstead (2002) examined Canadian newspaper articles and analyzed representations of mental illness and how they relate to violence and class. He found that when the mentally ill person was middle class, 14 percent of the stories reported details of the person's specific behaviors. The focus was on their occupations, socio-economic status, and influential families and associations. However, when the mentally ill individual was considered to be poor or lower class, 62 percent of articles emphasized his poverty as a significant factor attributing to his behavior. Of these articles, 89 percent detailed the behaviors of the individual and highlighted specific incidents of criminality, violence, and dangerousness. In addition, references were made to homelessness, begging, and the use of soup kitchens and shelters. Olstead's study reveals that newspaper articles are written in such a way that readers are left to assume a link between mental illness and violence, criminality, and poverty. This assumption further stigmatizes the mentally ill.

## Why media portrayals of mental illness matter

Despite recent increases in the social acceptance of seeking professional help for mental illness, a great deal of stigma continues to be attached to psychiatric disability (Gilman 1985). According to the US Department of Health and Human Services (1999), fewer than 50 percent of those who experience mental disorders actually seek treatment. It is perhaps not surprising that so few individuals seek therapy, since the popular stereotype of mental health practitioners coins them as exploitative, mentally unstable, unethical, and likely to cause irreparable harm to patients. It is no wonder that patients are so hesitant to seek treatment for mental illness symptoms; the prospect of seeing a therapist is widely depicted as fear inducing and, the treatment itself as ineffective (Freeman *et al.* 2001; *Healthweek* 2003).

Grinfeld (1998) cites Glen Gabbard, author of *Psychiatry and the Cinema*, stating that since the mid-1960s, only three films, [*Good Will Hunting* (1997) *Ordinary People* (1980) *I Never Promised You a Rose Garden* (1977)], and have portrayed therapists sympathetically. In other instances, mental health practitioners were portrayed in one or more of the following ways: neurotic, unable to maintain professional boundaries, drug or alcohol addicted, rigid, controlling, ineffectual, mentally ill themselves, comically inept, uncaring, self-absorbed, having ulterior motives, easily tricked and manipulated, foolish, and idiotic. Grinfeld (1998) concludes that such portrayals reinforce the idea that helping the mentally ill is a profession requiring little or no expertise or skill.

In Woody Allen's film *Deconstructing Harry* a therapist is depicted as neurotic, boundary-breaking, and emotionally unstable. The character is played by Kirstie Alley, who proudly stated in a *USA Today* article that she 'doesn't like psychiatry. And I don't believe it works. And I believe psychotherapists are neurotic or psychotic, for the most part. I wanted to play her that way...I wanted to be taking Prozac or drugs during the session with the patient. I wanted to show that this woman is so twerked out that she has to take drugs, too...' Adding fuel to the already hot negative stereotype of therapists, in the same article Woody Allen bragged, 'I didn't have to give her [Kirstie Alley] even one direction. I never had to. Her instincts were right on from the start' (*USA Today*, 11 December 1997, cited by Grinfeld 1998).

Although stereotypical depictions of the mentally ill may seem like harmless Hollywood distortions, it is important to note that media images have a way of working themselves into the society's subconscious, thereby affecting and influencing the way we perceive the world we live in. While negative inaccurate stereotypes do the most damage, positive inaccurate depictions can also be quite harmful (Edney 2004). Wahl (1995) argues that inaccurate information in the media about mental illness, even if that information is positive, results in public misunderstanding. If, for example, a family suspects that a relative shows signs of schizophrenia, but the family is misinformed about the exact symptoms (in many cases, the media confuses schizophrenia with multiple personality disorder), recognition and treatment for the patient may be dismissed or delayed.

According to Hyler (2003), there are several strategies that might be effective in combating the negative stereotypes that stigmatize mental patients. One such strategy would be a letter-writing campaign to producers of films and television programs and advertisers of such programs that depict these stereotypes. Promoting public information campaigns, such as Mental Health Awareness Week, encouraging public testimonials by respected celebrities with mental illnesses, and enhancing communication between mental health professionals and clinicians in other medical fields are additional methods of alleviating some of the stigma of psychiatric disability.

The evidence that media portrayals of the mentally ill are inaccurate and stigmatizing is overwhelming. This has a significant impact when seen in the context that people suffering from mental illness frequently do not seek treatment. So what can we in the health field do? The most important thing is to discuss and analyze stereotypes that are presented in the media. Being aware of these stereotypes—and making an effort to determine which attributes are accurate portrayals of mental illness and which are unhelpful fabrications—goes a long way toward reducing the impact that media imagery can have. It is essential that we move beyond being mere consumers of media and actually play an active role in dissecting it. Then our obligation is to educate our students, our patients, and the public in these skills.

## Documentary film as a means of breaking down stigmatization

There has been a movement in contemporary film to provide a more realistic portrayal of mental illness. This has primarily been in the realm of independent documentary films that have taken on the issue of representing mental illness through the personal experience of either the patients themselves or family members close to them. The goal is to break down stereotypes of mental illness and present psychiatric disorders in a more realistic and humane manner. This has coincided with the development of a new genre of film-making, where the film-making process is revealed, thereby dismantling the illusion that the events unfolding on camera are real and uninfluenced by the presence of the camera. This is often done by incorporating the film-maker's own personal account of the events and the experience of making the film into the film itself.

*Complaints of a Dutiful Daughter*, the 1994 film by Deborah Hoffmann, is one of the best examples of this kind of personal film-making. Hoffmann gives a first-person account of caring for her mother and coming to terms with her progressive Alzheimer's disease. The film won substantial critical acclaim, including an Academy Award nomination, and was broadcast on the highly acclaimed PBS series POV, where it won a national Emmy Award. The film chronicles the film-maker's desire to cure the incurable—to set right her mother's confusion and forgetfulness, to temper her mother's obsessiveness—and finally gives way to an acceptance, which is liberating for both daughter and mother. She does this with tremendous humor and insight throughout the film. Hoffmann uses a series of on-camera interviews in which she talks candidly to the camera about her experiences. What is intriguing in the film is the evolution that Hoffmann as the film-maker goes through in her ability to understand and cope with her mother's loss of memory, sense of reality, and ultimately identity. The film uses home movie clips to show her mother of the past—a vibrant and intellectual woman. This is contrasted with conversations between the film-maker and her mother as an 84-year-old, when she asks Hoffmann who her mother is and reveals her belief that the two of them had just met. The result is at once a devastating and riveting depiction of one type of mental illness.

*Twitch and Shout*, the 1994 documentary film by Laurel Chiten exploring the world of Tourette's syndrome, is another example of personal film-making. Tourette's syndrome is a genetic disorder that causes a bizarre range of involuntary movements and tics, obscene vocalizations, and compulsions. Yet in this case, instead of the film-maker giving a personal account of her own illness, she collaborates with a photojournalist who is living with this disorder and follows him as he narrates the film in a first-person portrayal of the illness. He introduces the audience to a wide range of other individuals (note that they are not referred to as patients) living with Tourette's syndrome, such as a professional basketball player, an actress, an artist, and a Mennonite lumberjack. These people describe how they finally discovered the name of their illness and how they have come to terms with it. They share their experiences about coping with a society that often sees them as insane or mentally ill and with a body or mind that often will not do as it is told. The film also takes us to a Tourette's syndrome convention where, for a weekend, it is normal to have the syndrome since everyone there does. One woman says that even though they spend the whole weekend talking about it, it is the only time in her life where she has been able to forget about the illness, because she feels normal for the first time in her life—a powerful statement.

The film played successfully on the film festival circuit and was broadcast on the well-known PBS series POV, where it was nominated for an Emmy. It also received an award from the American Psychiatric Association because of its realistic and humane portrayal of people suffering from a misunderstood mental illness. The film allows the viewer to make contact with and ultimately understand some of the people living with the disease, and thus it goes a long way toward breaking down stereotypes of people with mental illness.

*A Beautiful Mind*, the 2001 film by Ron Howard, portrays the struggle of Nobel Prize winning mathematician, John Forbes Nash, to maintain his sanity while working to develop groundbreaking new mathematical theories. By his early thirties Nash, who possessed one of the most extraordinary mathematical talents in the world, became overwhelmed by his creative powers after accomplishing important work in several fields of mathematics. After three decades of struggling with schizophrenia, in 1994 he was awarded the Nobel Memorial Prize in economic science for work he completed in the 1940s.

As viewers of the film, we find ourselves unable to distinguish truth and fiction, or reality and distortion in Nash's life. An interesting aspect of the portrayal of mental illness is that the character is not introduced as ill from the outset. Thus it is only little by little that the viewer begins to realize that perhaps Nash's vision of reality is not the same as that of the people around him. This is a compelling filmic device that creates an experience for the audience that is much the same as that of the characters in the story. Schizophrenia develops slowly and it often takes time before people around the patient actually realize there is a disease involved, and even longer before the patient believes this to be true. The National Alliance for the Mentally Ill (NAMI) has promoted *A Beautiful Mind* as a powerful teaching tool for schizophrenic patients and their families, claiming that despite its 'Hollywoodesque' qualities, the film avoids clichés and unrealistic endings that are often a flaw of other mental illness films. However, the film does depict Nash as having mainly visual schizophrenic hallucinations, rather than the more frequent and common auditory hallucinations (Rosenstock 2003).

Nash's illness caused him to think in ways that are incomprehensible to the ordinary individual. Most would say that his thinking was way beyond the norm. However, it is interesting to question just how competent Nash was in relating to the world around him. Was he ever able to discern truth from reality? At what point did he begin to lose that ability? The movie illustrates his wife, Alicia, committing him to an institution and his treatment with insulin. We never see Nash officially agreeing to any treatment for his condition, which raises ethical questions of its own. Even if he had agreed to the insulin, was he competent enough to give his informed consent? The key neuroethical questions of autonomy and free will are highlighted throughout Nash's plight with schizophrenia.

*A Beautiful Mind* gives a fair and responsible representation of mental illness. It portrays Nash's life with schizophrenia as accurately as cinematically possible and allows the viewer to see the world from his perspective. The audience comes away with a realistic understanding of the disease, but not with a sense of false hope for an immediate cure.

Films such as *A Beautiful Mind*, *Complaints of A Dutiful Daughter*, and *Twitch and Shout* are important in breaking down stereotypes by creating memorable characters and narrative storylines that touch viewers emotionally. The characters are subconsciously integrated and referenced in one's daily experience and therefore are more powerful forces in changing public perception of mental illness than fact-driven news stories. For example, a friend of one of the authors related that the first image that came to mind when his child was diagnosed with autism was Raymond Bobbitt, the character played by Dustin Hoffman in *Rain Man*. This character had stayed with him for 10 years after he had seen the film, whereas all the news documentaries on autism had slipped from his mind. Yet *Rain Man*, while being a remarkably accurate and sensitive portrayal of savant syndrome, is not a realistic portrayal of the experience of the majority of people suffering from autism. Only one in 10 autistic persons has any savant abilities, let alone the remarkable skills of the character Raymond Bobbitt (Treffert 2004). The National Autistic Society developed an advertising campaign to dispel the 'Rain Man myth'—the common perception that people with autism possess extraordinary talents.

The National Autistic Society's position is that continued media misrepresentation has led many people to see autism as more of an eccentricity than the very real disability that it is.

## The portrayal of frontier neurotechnologies in the movies

While the media's representation of mental illness has been well researched and documented, little has been written about the portrayal of frontier neurotechnologies in the movies, or the impact this has on the public. Recent innovative neurotechnological advancements sound like a science fiction film. It is quite possible that in the future 'thought maps' will be used to determine truth in the courtroom, profile prospective employers, screen for potential terrorists in airports, evaluate students for learning capacity in the classroom, or even choose lifetime partners based on compatible brain profiles for personality, interests, and desires (Illes and Racine 2005).

So the relevant question becomes: What is the impact on public consciousness of hi-tech sci-fi thrillers that push the boundaries of new neurotechnological development? These sci-fi films both exoticize and glamorize new technology, while evoking a sense of fear in these innovations. This represents the duality of values in our culture. Can the constant exposure to fantasy technologies in these films serve to dull the public's ability to be critical and thoughtful of actual new developments? As television news increasingly focuses on entertainment, the line between new technologies in the news and those in the movies becomes blurred. How does this affect the public?

Steven Spielberg's *Minority Report*, released in 2002, is a futuristic film with timely themes relevant to the country's drastic increases in national security. As a result of the terrorist attacks of 11 September 2001, law enforcement agencies have been working harder than ever to create electronic profiles of nearly all individuals. *Minority Report*, which is loosely based on a 1956 science fiction short story by Philip K. Dick, is set in the year 2054, when the mere intent to murder is considered a blameworthy offense. The set is an intriguing blend of the familiar and the futuristic. People still live in the same charming brick houses, listen to the same boring elevator music in shopping malls, and wear clothes that look like those worn in 2002. However, cars have become magnetic vehicles able to travel both horizontally and vertically, advertisers recognize and target consumers by scanning their eyes, and blackmarket doctors sell identity changes with a switch of the eyeballs.

'Pre-cogs' (precognitive human beings, who drift in a flotation tank with their brains linked to complex computers) have the ability to pick up thoughts of premeditated murders and send signals to law enforcement officers who in turn seek to stop the crimes before they are committed. The plot of *Minority Report* centers on a fault in the visions of one of the pre-cogs. The pre-cogs claim never to be wrong; however, sometimes they disagree and the dissenting pre-cog's vision is said to be a 'minority report'.

*Minority Report* raises critical questions about civil liberties. In the film, individuals are targeted and stopped from committing their crime based solely upon the vision of the pre-cogs. There is no due process or appeals—only accusations by what are assumed to be 'credible sources', followed by punishment. And all this happens even before a crime is committed.

Although completed before 11 September 2001, *Minority Report* displays significant similarities to present day national security. The film illustrates a world in which retinal scanning is common, not only for glimpses into one's personality and inner soul, but also into one's security clearance, legal status, and consumer preferences. According to Ann Hornday of the *Washington Post*, 'One of the most sophisticated notions posited by *Minority Report* is that personal privacy will be violated and exploited by marketers far sooner than by the government' (Hornday 2002).

In addition to the question of the privacy of human thought, *Minority Report* raises the ethical questions of predictive intelligence. Scott Kirsner of the *Boston Globe* writes about the pivotal debate within the technology world centering on the ability to use software running on powerful computers to analyze information about behavior (and prior behavior). Kirsner (2002) goes on to describe Navy Admiral John Poindexter's creation of a system called Total Information Awareness, which seeks to identify terrorists, before they commit crimes, on the basis of a series of suspicious transactions. In the private sector, companies are already using predictive intelligence to analyze individual's data profiles to determine whether they are likely to feign illness in order to take time off work for leisure activities. Kirsner believes, 'This is terrible stuff. It invades our privacy, and reduces us all to data models rather than human beings' (Kirsner 2002). Will Poindexter's system evolve into a system that subjects all innocent people to extreme scrutiny? Or will people be willing to have 'our every bank withdrawal, car rental, and phone call scoured by a sophisticated piece of software . . .' in the hopes that one day it might be able to tell us which individuals are likely to be involved in dangerous terrorist plots? Critics of Poindexter's system feel that this is an unconstitutional system of public surveillance. Although a highly political issue, predictive intelligence is one that will only grow more intense as the technology improves—it is already a theme in Hollywood and is becoming a reality which all of us will face.

The release of *Minority Report* and similar science fiction films poses critical ethical questions: What are the risks of science fiction meeting reality? When do we begin to worry that audiences of such films will begin to believe that everything they see in the movies will soon become a reality in our society? What is the impact of watching films based on extreme examples of predictive intelligence, and then reading in the newspaper about the use of predictive intelligence by the government in the name of national security? What is the public's response to films that both glamorize and spread fear about these new technologies?

*Charly*, the 1968 film based upon Daniel Keyes' novel *Flowers for Algernon*, deals with another pertinent neuroethical issue—brain enhancement. Charly, the main character in the film, is born with an IQ of 68, yet has limitless goodwill and enthusiasm for learning. Recruited by his teacher for a scientific experiment, Charly becomes the first human to undergo a brain operation in an attempt to increase his learning capacity. Charly's operation transforms him from a mentally challenged individual into a genius, and allows him to progress from his menial job in a bakery to study science, literature, and multiple languages. Charly's transformation, although something he always dreamed about, turns out not to be an altogether positive experience. Once he gains intelligence and perspective of the world around him, Charly comes to the painful realization that not everyone is as nice as he had once thought, and that his 'friends' were not laughing *with* him but *at* him (Reynolds 2000).

*Charly* seems to be even more relevant today than it was in the 1960s with the recent development of brain enhancements and common use of organ transplants. The film addresses important ethical issues that come into play when human beings are involved in scientific research.

Despite Charly's postoperation ability to learn several new languages at a time, his brain cannot compensate for years of social maladjustment, and he finds himself more lost and lonely than ever (Rich 1980). Charly observes, 'When I was retarded, I had lots of friends. Now I have none' (Nagai 2001). Charly is a prime example of why it is so critical for scientists to consider the benefit of conducting an experiment on a human subject. What is the neuroethical definition of benefit? In Charly's case, his increased intelligence is considered a benefit clinically, but socially it is not at all a benefit. Charly is no longer happy and carefree, but lonely and depressed because he no longer fits in with the world. The impact of an experiment such as this on the subject should be of utmost important to the investigators, yet in Charly's case it was of minimal importance.

Among the many ethical questions that Charly poses, the most obvious is whether or not Charly had the competency to give his informed consent to participate in the experiment. Although we are told that Charly's estranged sister provided her consent to his participation, it seems that very little information about the procedure and possible negative effects were mentioned to either Charly or his sister.

Furthermore, consent in the realm of research ethics should inform individuals of any risks involved with the research (Beauchamp and Childress 2001). Although we observe the scientists warning Charly that the experiment might not work and that he might go back to being retarded at some point in the future, they never convey to him the risks associated with the success of the experiment. The isolation, frustration, and anger that Charly experiences because of the success of the experiment are surprises—he is never warned that he might not like being so smart. Full disclosure of the risks would include both the positive and negative aspects of the success and failure of the experiment.

While the neurocognitive enhancement represented in *Charly* is an exaggeration of the capabilities of modern technology, reality is not far behind. Currently, the enhancement of normal neurocognitive function by pharmacological means is already a fact of life in many schools. Furthermore, non-invasive transcranial magnetic stimulation of targeted brain areas is currently being used for treatment of depression and other psychopathology (Illes and Raffin 2002; see also Chapter 14). Thus the ethical issues addressed in these films go beyond mere fantasy, and are important ethical dilemmas to be addressed and taken seriously.

## Conclusion

The mind is complex and fascinating. It is even more intriguing when altered in some way—whether its natural abilities are reduced or enhanced. In this chapter we have focused on the film industry and its influence on public understanding of how the mind works, both in mental illness and in the neuroscience enhancement technologies that the future holds. We argued that the stereotypes created by the media have tremendous influence on public perception, and those created by narrative films are even more powerful since they touch people emotionally and thus leave an image that stays with them throughout their lives. It has been clearly documented that the film industry has created inaccurate and negative depictions of people with mental illness, often leaving viewers with erroneous and unwarranted beliefs about mental disabilities.

We discussed some of the new independent documentary films that have been successful in breaking down some of these stereotypes about mental illness by showing more realistic portrayals of mentally ill patients and families. Films such as *Complaints of a Dutiful Daughter* and *Twitch and Shout* are particularly important in that they portray mental illness from the first-person perspective of the people and their families who suffer from it.

Finally, we examined how the new frontiers of neuroscience are being portrayed in motion pictures, and we explored the neuroethical issues that they bring up. *A Beautiful Mind*, on the one hand, portrays impaired and confused mental capacity, while *Minority Report* and *Charly* depict enhanced cognitive abilities. Research has revealed that the general public obtains much of its information from popular media sources, including Hollywood films. Major motion pictures, such as the three analyzed in this chapter, attract vast audiences, and therefore it is critical that portrayals in the films be accurate and responsible. Most importantly, those of us who are educated in the health field have a responsibility to teach the public how to critically analyze and deconstruct the media. Passive consumerism will only perpetuate injustices to the beneficiaries of significant and continuous neuroscientific advances.

## References

Altman BM (1981). Studies of attitudes toward the handicapped: the need for new direction. *Social Problems* 28, 321–3.

Andrew D (1984). *Concepts in Film Theory.* New York: Oxford University Press.

Beauchamp GL, Childress JF (2001). *Principles of Biomedical Ethics* (5th edn). New York: Oxford University Press.

Biklen D, Bogdan R (1977). Media portrayals of disabled people: a study in stereotypes. *Interracial Books for Children Bulletin* 8, 4–9.

Blaxter M (1990). *Health and Lifestyles.* London: Routledge.

Bogdan R, Biklen D, Shapiro A, Spelkoman D (1982). The disabled: media's monster. *Social Policy* 13, 32–35.

Byrd EK (1989). A study of depiction of specific characteristics of characters with disability in film. *Journal of Applied Rehabilitation Counseling* 20, 43–5.

Byrd EK, Elliott TR (1985). Feature films and disability: a descriptive study. *Rehabilitation Psychology* 30, 47–51.

Byrd EK, Pipes RB (1981). Feature films and disability. *Journal of Rehabilitation* 47, 51–53, 80.

Byrd-Bredbenner C, Grasso D (2000). Health, medicine, and food messages in television commercials during 1992 and 1998. *Journal of School Health* 70, 61–6.

Bywater T, Sobchack T (1989). *An Introduction to Film Criticism.* New York: Longman.

Coverdale J, Nairn R, Claasen D (2002). Depictions of mental illness in print media: a prospective national sample. *Australian and New Zealand Journal of Psychiatry* 36, 697–700.

Cutcliffe JR, Hannigan B (2001). Mass media, 'monsters' and mental health clients: the need for increased lobbying. *Journal of Psychiatric and Mental Health Nursing* 8, 315–21.

Diefenbach DL (1997). The portrayal of mental illness on prime-time television. *Journal of Community Psychology* 25, 289–302. Available online at: http://www3.interscience.wiley.com

Domino G (1983). Impact of the film *One Flew Over the Cuckoo's Nest* on attitudes toward mental illness. *Psychological Reports* 53, 179–82.

Edney DR (2004). *Mass Media and Mental Illness: A Literature Review.* Ontario: Canadian Mental Health Association.

Elliott T, Byrd EK (1982). Media and disability. *Rehabilitation Literature* 43, 348–55.

Finkelstein V (1980). *Attitudes and Disabled People: Issues for Discussion.* International Exchange of Information in Rehabilitation Monograph No. 5. New York: World Rehabilitation Fund.

Fleming M, Manvell R (1985). *Images of Madness.* Cranbury, NJ: Associated University Presses.

Francis C, Pirkis J, Dunt D, Blood RW (2001). *Mental Health and Illness in the Media: A Review of the Literature.* Canberra: Mental Health and Special Programs Branch, Department of Health and Aging, Australia.

Freeman H, Wahl O, Jakab I, Linden TR, Guimón J, Bollorino F (2001). Forum—Mass media and psychiatry: commentaries. *Current Opinion in Psychiatry* 14, 529–35.

Gartner A (1982). Images of the disabled/disabling images. *Social Policy* 13, 15.

Gilman SL (1982). *Seeing the Insane.* New York: Wiley–Brunner/Mazel.

Gilman SL (1985). *Difference and Pathology: Stereotypes of Sexuality, Race and Madness.* Ithaca, NY: Cornell University Press.

Goffman E (1963) *Stigma: Notes on the Management of Spoiled Identity.* Engelwood Cliffs, NJ: Prentice-Hall

Goldberg D, Huxley P (1992). *Common Mental Disorders: A Bio-Social Model.* London: Routledge.

Grinfeld MJ (1998). Psychiatry and mental illness: are they mass media targets? http://www.psychiatrictimes.com/p980301a.html *Psychiatric Times* **15.**

*Healthweek* (2003). *Behind the headlines. Mental illness and the media.*

Hollander A (1991). *Moving Pictures.* Cambridge, MA: Harvard University Press.

Hornday A (2002). Steven Spielberg gazes into a future with no pleasant fantasies. *Washington Post,* 21 June, p. C01.

Hottentot EI (2000). *Print Media Portrayal of Mental Illness: An Alberta Study.* Edmonton: Alberta Mental Health Board Consumer Advisory Council.

Hyler SH (2003). Stigma continues in Hollywood. *Psychiatric Times,* **33.** http://www.psychiatrictimes.com/p030633.html

Hyler SE, Gabbard GO, Schneider I (1991). Homicidal maniacs and narcissistic parasites: stigmatization of mentally ill persons in the movies. *Hospital and Community Psychiatry* **42,** 1044–8.

Illes J, Racine E (2005). Imaging or imagining? *American Journal of Bioethics* **5,** 1–14.

Illes J, Raffin T (2002). Neuroethics: an emerging new discipline in the study of brain and cognition. *Brain and Cognition* **50,** 341–4.

Institute for Information Studies (1979). *How to Make Friends and Influence the Media.* Washington, DC: Institute for Information Studies.

Kaiser Family Foundation (2003). Impact of direct-to-consumer advertising on prescription drug spending. Available online at: http://www.kff.org/rxdrugs/market.cfm (accessed 2 November 2004).

Kaiser Family Foundation (1998). Crime most common story on local television news. Available online at: http://www.kff.org/mediapartnerships/upload/14618_1.pdf (accessed 2 November 2004).

Kirsner S (2002). Getting smart about predictive behavior. *Boston Globe,* 20 December, p. C1.

Kriegel L (1982). The wolf in the pit in the zoo. *Social Policy* **13,** 16–23.

Levers LL (2001). Representations of psychiatric disability in fifty years of Hollywood film: an ethnographic content analysis. *Theory & Science.* Available online at: http://theoryandscience.icaap.org/content/vol002.002/lopezlevers.html (accessed 9 May 2005).

Meltzer H, Gill B, Petticrew M (1995). *OPCS Surveys of Psychiatric Morbidity in Great Britain. Report 1. The Prevalence of Psychiatric Morbidity Among Adults Aged 16–64 Living in Private Households in Great Britain.* London: HMSO.

Nagai A (2001). Young people ponder meaning of 'Algernon'. *Daily Yomiuri,* 26 July, p. 13.

National Health Council 1997. 21st Century Housecall: The link between medicine and the media (This report examines where people get their health information and the impact of health news on the actions of consumers. The report is based on the proceedings of a National Health Council Symposium held in December 1997. (October 1998).

Nichols B (1981). *Ideology and the Image.* Bloomington, IN: Indiana University Press.

Olstead R (2002). Contesting the text: Canadian media depictions of the conflation of mental illness and criminality. *Sociology of Health and Illness* **24,** 621–43.

Philo G (1993). *Mass Media Representations of Mental Health: A Study of Media Content.* Glasgow: Glasgow University Media Group.

Quart L, Auster A (1982). The wounded vet in post-war film. *Social Policy* **13,** 24–31.

Reynolds I (2000). Captivating TV tale of a man and a mouse. *Daily Yomiuri,* 5 October, p. 10.

Rich F (1980). Theater: Musical *Charlie and Algernon. New York Times,* 15 September, Section C, p. 17.

Roffman P, Purdy J (1981). *The Hollywood Social Problems Film.* Bloomington, IN: Indiana University Press.

Rose D (1998). Television, madness and community care. *Journal of Community and Applied Social Psychology* **8,** 213–28.

Rosenstock J (2003). Beyond *A Beautiful Mind:* film choices for teaching schizophrenia. *Academic Psychiatry* **27** 117–22.

Roth W (1983). Handicap as a social construct. *Society* **3,** 56–61.

**Siller J** (1976). Attitudes toward disability. In: Rusalen H, Malikin D *Contemporary Vocational Rehabilitation.* New York: New York University Press.

**Sless D** (1981). *Learning and Visual Communication.* New York: John Wiley.

**Thomas S** (ed) (1982). *Film/Culture.* Metuchen, NJ: Scarecrow Press.

**Treffert D** (2004). '*Rain Man' The Movie/Rain Man, Real Life.* Available online at: http:www.wisconsinmedicalsociety.org/savant/rainman/cfm. (accessed 11 November 2004).

**US Department of Health and Human Services** (1999). *Mental Health: A Report of the Surgeon General.* Washington, DC: US Department of Health and Human Services. Available online at: http://www.surgeongeneral.gov

**Wahl O** (1995). *Media Madness: Public Images of Mental Illness.* New Brunswick, NJ: Rutgers University Press.

**Wahl O, Lefkowits JY** (1989). Impact of a television film on attitudes toward mental illness. *American Journal of Community Psychology* **17**, 521–8.

**Wahl O, Roth R** (1982). Television images of mental illness: Results of a metropolitan Washington media watch. *Journal of Broadcasting* **26**, 599–605.

**Wilson C, Nairn R, Coverdale J, Panapa A** (1999). Mental illness depictions in prime-time drama: identifying the discursive resources. *Australian and New Zealand Journal of Psychiatry* **33**, 232–39. Available online at: http://www.blackwell-synergy.com

**Winick C** (1978). Mental illness and psychiatrists in movies. In Winick C (ed) *Deviance and Mass Media.* Beverly Hills, CA: Sage, 45–77.

# Neuroethics: mapping a new interdiscipline

## Donald Kennedy

My colleague at Stanford Law School, Hank Greely, is the author of a chapter in this volume (Chapter 17). He has never recorded from a brain nor done neurochemistry; he is an academic lawyer with lengthy experience in evaluating the dilemmas presented by the use of genetic data. Thus he has a strong familiarity with the domain in which ethics and biology really connect. At the meeting held in San Francisco in 2002 sponsored by the Dana Foundation that mapped the terrain for neuroethics (Marcus 2002), he had this to say about the use of information gained from individuals by means of neuroimaging techniques:

> Essentialism is a more interesting issue in neuroscience than in genetics... I am more than my genes. The genes are an important part of me, but I can be certain that they are not my essence; they are not my soul. When we shift that notion to the neuroscience area, though, I am not so confident. Is my consciousness—is my brain—me? I am tempted to think it is.

That thoughtful comment illuminates one piece of the intellectual terrain that we encounter as we ponder 'neuroethics'—a term in which I mean to include the ethical basis of conducting certain experiments in neuroscience, as well as the distribution and use of information and materials gathered in the course of performing neurophysiological research. The issue Professor Greely isolates involves privacy: How comfortable are we with sharing information about the specific, often individual, ways in which our brains work? To put it more directly, should society be limited in the degree to which it can appropriately make use of such information in evaluating individuals in regulatory, legal, medical, or commercial contexts (see Chapter 8)? Here I plan to consider some present or possible future efforts to apply functional MRI (fMRI) or other techniques for a variety of purposes: psychiatric diagnosis (see Chapters 15, 16), forensic analysis, behavior prediction in an employment situation, marketing studies, cognitive enhancement, and the like.

A second region of the neuroethical terrain involves the conduct of the experiments themselves (see Chapter 9). Ethical questions may arise about whether we ought to undertake certain kinds of neuroscience experiments in view of possible misuse of the results. Should consideration be given to regulating particular kinds of investigation because of questions about end-use? Or, instead, should regulation be limited to process issues?

The third domain is occupied by questions of neurobiological intervention. Increasingly, it is becoming possible to modify behavior or capacity by pharmacological or other means (see Chapters 6, 13, 14). The issue often boils down to an attempt to discriminate between treatment (e.g. medication to combat clinical depression) and enhancement (e.g. consumption of a drug expected to improve cognition by a person of normal intelligence).

There is a fourth region, more difficult to define, in which new neurobiological knowledge may have positive or negative effects. On the positive side, there may be ways in which we can use our science so as to clarify our own humanity, deepening and broadening our own ethical sense. Might we encounter new understandings about the degree to which our brains really do contain, by their wiring and chemistry, our nature? That could be rewarding—but it might present new challenges to our concept of free will (see Chapters 1–5, 7, 10, 20). Indeed, a deeper knowledge of our brains might serve either to conserve our sense of human uniqueness, or to expand our knowledge in a way that makes us conscious of being more clearly a part of the rest of the natural world?

These different domains coincide with different historical experiences of my own, as I moved from a career in laboratory science into one that has involved the social uses to which science is put. I became more acutely aware of the first—the problem of research and its regulation on ethical grounds with respect to prospective end-use—during 12 years as a university president. It was not infrequently argued to me that certain kinds of research should not be allowed to go on, because one or more anticipated end-products of that work would be unacceptable. In the early 1980s, research that could conceivably be used in weapons development was sometimes the focus of such claims. On the other side we often heard the argument that information is value free, that it may be normatively good, and that we should never hesitate to get more of it. Projects that harm subjects or subject experimental animals to severe and unnecessary pain are morally unacceptable; we of course acceded to reasonable demands that they be subject to process regulation.

But regulation by potential end-use is quite a different matter. What about projects that might, with reasonably high plausibility, be turned to harmful purposes—but which might also yield significant benefits? We regularly rejected arguments that we should ban such work, out of a conviction that research really is a form of speech, and that prior restraint is not any more appropriate for the next experiment underway in the laboratory than it is with respect to the publication of an investigator's own views. Therefore we generally resolved those issues in favor of leaving the ethical decisions in the hands of the researchers themselves. This approach has been well tolerated, although not universally applauded, and I leave this problem there with some relief

## New ways of knowing the brain

The neurosciences have entered a period of extraordinary, possibly unprecedented, promise. Let me just sketch some of the new capacities that are allowing us to enter experimental domains that were inaccessible to us when I left the field a quarter of a century ago. I will start with modern magnetic resonance technology, which is making it possible to undertake a whole new level of exploration in functional architectonics. In a way, this capacity is the unexpected fulfillment of a development that began in animal experiments more than 30 years ago. In the early 1950s, Vernon Mountcastle and Ed Evarts used to talk about the value of being able to 'Get the monkey up off the table'. The implication, sometimes even impolitely stated, was that much of what we knew about the details of brain function consisted of single unit recording from doped-up anaesthetized animals lashed to a table. Once indwelling electrodes could be used with upright behaving primates, the game really changed. Thanks to the pioneers, it became possible to investigate far more complex behaviors than we ever thought could be studied. Much of that is possible because investigators and computer-driven technologies have been able to train primates to perform extraordinary tasks, so that the experimenters can explore heretofore unapproachable capacities—including, for example, the evaluation of expected reward. The monkeys in William Newsome's laboratory at Stanford, for example, are about as different from your average monkey as baseball player Barry Bonds is from the average neurophysiologist. They are world-class athletes at whatever complicated difficult task the investigator sets for them: making saccades to a spot of this color in that part of the receptive field, for example, so as to indicate a choice. They are trained to this level so that we can explore the neural loci for expectation of reward, or the sites for holding short-term memories, or for the recognition of complex topologies—or the divide that separates the watershed for perception from that of action.

Given the success of these developments, it was only natural for neurophysiologists to ask: Why not us? Of course we could not fit ourselves with indwelling electrodes the way we fit macaques—at least, we would not *want* to—but there is fMRI, a non-invasive way of looking at localized brain activity while people are behaving. This exploding technology has now moved from a straightforward analysis—of what part or parts are active during $x$, $y$, or $z$ behavior—to pose a far more sophisticated and interesting set of questions. Are there regions in which predicted rewards appear to be encoded? As debated elsewhere in this volume, are there signals that can be reliably associated with economic judgments, or difficult moral choices made by subjects as they encounter scenarios in virtual reality: if you move the lever to the left, the careening streetcar kills three strangers; if you move it to the right it spares them but kills your best friend (see Chapters 11 and 12). Can it be that even as we prepare to think about neuroethics, we are developing a neural connectivity map for other kinds of ethics? Compassion? Altruism? You pick one. Before returning to some ethical issues raised by the imaging techniques, I want to explore those that arise in the pharmacological area.

## Neuropharmacology, treatment, and enhancement

The biochemistry of neural signaling in embryonic development and in the modulation of plastic changes—learning, memory, motivation—has moved along at least as rapidly as electrophysiology and neuroimaging. We now know, for example, that mood disorders may be influenced for better or worse by pharmacological intervention. In the case of depression, it is now clear that the major classes of antidepressants probably work by permitting neurogenesis to occur in the hippocampus. We know that stress in early adult life amplifies a particular genetic predisposition to depression. As to learning and memory, we are nearing an understanding of the underlying chemistry and molecular biology that may soon permit targeted intervention in that process. Work in progress in several small for-profit ventures is promising to create a new generation of 'precognitive' therapies. Meanwhile, not surprisingly, part of this market is being claimed by health food supplements of herbal origin, or (perhaps more troublesome) by off-label prescriptions for old standbys like the amphetamines.

In neuropharmacology, the difficult question of treatment versus enhancement arises immediately. It now appears plain that methylphenidate and newer drugs can improve executive function in patients with attention-deficit hyperactivity disorder (ADHD). The more difficult question is whether it should be prescribed for others who hope or believe that it may provide cognitive enhancement. The same issues are emerging as the molecular biology of learning suggests drug targets for improving knowledge acquisition or memory. Similarly, we have no difficulty in prescribing human growth hormone for a growing child who lacks stature because of a deficiency in it. As Parens (Chapter 6) points out, a case that might trouble us is whether it is acceptable for a fairly short child, who desperately loves basketball but is not medically deficient, to take human growth hormone. As for the use of steroids to enhance shot-put performance or mile times, that is so clearly an abuse that it is just not ethically interesting. Track and field is an activity conducted under widely understood rules of competition, and violating those rules plainly makes the playing field anything but level.

Where the brain is involved, the enhancement issue takes on a different and somehow more critical form. Much success in modern meritocratic societies depends on cognitive capacity in a competitive world (see Chapters 18, 19, 21). If, by taking the right drug, some people can improve their position, questions should arise about whether the playing field is level—especially if the treatment is expensive and not available to some competitors. The social justice issue here is one that we need to take seriously. That might be called a soft objection to enhancement. There is also a hard objection; it is the position sometimes taken by the President's Council on Biomedical Ethics that pro-cognitive therapy is interfering with something that could be called our 'nature.' I find it difficult to distinguish between this and other interventions into transmitter biochemistry, like the use of serotonin-reuptake inhibitors to treat depression. At a more fundamental level, I find a kind of naive nativism in the view that there is a natural state with which we are somehow interfering in these interventions. To find a natural state, i.e. one that is innocent of change through cultural intervention, one would have to rewind our evolutionary tape—perhaps to early hominids with cranial capacities about half that of modern humans. The subsequent history is marked by an explosive positive relationship between culture and brain evolution; in short, natural selection and culture have been interacting for all this time.

But the levelness of the playing field cannot be employed to make the ethical issues go away. The Chairman of the President's Council makes a thought-provoking argument on this point. Suppose the playing field was to be made level: every athlete in the race gets the steroids, and every test-taker gets the pro-cognitive drug. Will we feel the same way about the result? Will society wonder about the durability of the outcome? Will the winner feel like a winner, or be asking instead: 'Was that really me?'

The neuropharmacological enhancement/treatment issue has also surfaced in a real-world setting in connection with the children diagnosed as having ADHD. The study on Neuroethics and the Enhancement of Cognition and Learning sponsored by the National Science Foundation and the New York Academy of Sciences (www.nyas.org/neuroethics) (Farah, Illes *et al.* 2004) points out that several drugs targeting the dopamine and norepinephrine systems can improve executive function in laboratory tests on healthy young volunteers. However, the study's authors also emphasize that these have not been demonstrated to improve cognitive performance in real non-laboratory situations. Nevertheless, it is clear that many young people believe it will work; the estimates of illicit use of methylphenidate, for example, exceed the highest estimates of actual ADHD prevalence. Most of us will be ethically comfortable with the treatment use of methylphenidate in the case of bona fide ADHD in adults and children. The enhancement issue is more difficult to resolve, and is especially troublesome when the treatment is obtained illicitly and thus raises legal questions.

One final, and for me unexpected, aspect of the treatment/enhancement problem is not explicitly addressed in this volume. One can find thoughtful objectors even to treatment-inspired interventions in unexpected places. Consider, for example, the use of cochlear implants in deaf children. In a number of cases, deaf parents have said that they do not wish their deaf child to receive an enhancement of that kind. They have their reasons. The family has built an effective communication network based on shared capacities and limitations, and may have already invested heavily in building that network. On the other hand, one might argue that families do not stay together forever, and that the child needs to be equipped to deal effectively with hearing adults. Should society make a rule to deal with this situation? I pose the question without suggesting an answer, only to illustrate the complexity of finding distinctive ethical high ground in this area. Further discussion on this can be found in Parens (1998).

## Neuroimaging, privacy, and self-knowledge

The field of opportunity opened up by these technological advances is broad indeed, and it raises two different kinds of questions for us. The first have to do with how much we could learn about really higher functions with this technique. These are interesting questions, but for me, at least now, they do not raise difficult ethical issues. For example, we may learn enough about different patterns of neural activation in the brain, or possibly of their pharmacological sensitivities, to classify individuals as to behavioral phenotype. Would that raise ethical questions? Surely it would with respect to the applicability of such knowledge in social policy, for example if the knowledge could be employed in the insurance context or in the criminal justice system. But that kind of knowledge would not, in itself, change our view of what our individuality means, or of our humanity, and reshape the ethical landscape as a result.

Stealth fMRI technology is surely a bridge we can cross when, if ever, it comes. But I do not want a record of how my brain works trailing after me. That might not be a worry if, like the long-lived cookie I leave with Amazon about my reading preferences, it simply recounted some of my consumer choices. However, a spate of mainstream media treatments has been devoted to the use of brain imaging technologies for economic purposes. In the *New York Times Magazine* of 26 October 2003, an interesting piece by Clive Thompson was charmingly entitled 'There's a Sucker Born in Every Medial Prefrontal Cortex'. It and other articles describe various commercial ventures, some of them with academic links, to commercialize fMRI. It is now being applied actively, sometimes together with electroencephalography, in at least two areas. In the first, regional patterns of neural activation are recorded in response to television or print advertisements, or to demonstrations of particular products, in an effort to obtain evidence about consumer preferences. This is pretty straight-up marketing. In a second, more academic, kind of exercise, subjects are asked to make decisions about economic choices; the setting usually involves comparison between competing choices, one of which is good and has been standardized in terms of its evoked neural responses. The practitioners are calling this second project area neuroeconomics, a term now in such common use that it suggests widespread potential applications.

Now, I am not introducing the commercial side of neuroimaging because I think it raises serious ethical questions. Indeed, the whole notion struck me as shaky enough to make me wonder who is buying the service. It turns out that Daimler–Chrysler, Johnson and Johnson, and other firms that presumably know how to spend their money have been clients, so perhaps we can leave this universe alone with a *caveat emptor* proviso. I would be willing to let matters stay right there—except for the fear that the politicians are bound to get hold of it. How will we feel when the next candidate for Governor (of California, say) has been selected through the use of consumer-preference videos? It certainly influences my view of the ethical landscape that underlies knowing what our brains are doing. I will return to this point in connection with concerns about personal privacy; here I will just say that making sociopolitical arrangements on the basis of regional neural activity is post-modern phrenology, and we should not try it.

## A case to ponder

One more example in this domain may help us map it. In May 2003 the Lasker Forum tried to look at the gray area that lies between innovative medical practice, on the one hand, and more formal medical research conducted under formal ethical constraints (Common Rule, Helsinki Declaration) and the usual panoply of research regulation on the other (Kennedy 2003). We tried to do that by challenging interdisciplinary workshop panels with hypothetical scenarios. One was on the use of fMRI to evaluate a patient—let us call him Patton and assume that he is 17 years old—who had given some indication of sociopathic behavior. The case is set in the year 2008. In one of the evaluation scenarios, the simulated video showed Patton's mother and father engaged in a disagreement so intense that his mother strikes his father, an incident that Patton had previously reported in detail to his physician-neuroimager as one that had triggered a a typical anger reaction toward his mother. Watching the scenario, Patton reports anger with his mother, and the fMRI study shows intense activity in the amygdala but none in the orbitofrontal cortices, areas thought to be responsible for regulating anger responses. Together, these findings suggest that young Patton has functional brain patterns that predispose him to react strongly to anger stimuli with a diminished ability to control his behavior in response to anger. Therefore Patton is considered to be at high risk for violent behavior in the future. While this kind of prognosis had typically been imprecise, based only on traditional psychiatric evaluations and behavior tests, studies had shown that obtaining consistent fMRI data greatly enhanced the confidence with which such a prognosis can be made.

fMRI experts should not be bothered by some liberties we have taken here; the focus is on questions like the following, which sparked some lively discussion among the Lasker workshop participants.

Is the manipulation of images in the scene justified? Is it ethical? What about its combination with fMRI imaging technology? Is this an evaluation scenario that would, were it done in the research setting, have required IRB approval? What validation standards should exist for this kind of diagnostic use of neuroimaging?

What standards should be in place before fMRI is used to diagnose behavior disorders? Who should be involved in developing them?

Assume that, if they know in advance that such scenarios will be presented, patients will be able to modify their reactions to them. Therefore the physician wants to avoid giving patients a precise advance description of the assessment scenarios. In clinical practice, how should a psychiatrist obtain consent for this kind of assessment? Are warnings required?

What are the ethical implications of creating a video that reinvents the past and puts parents of already troubled adolescents in a negative light?

We went on and created some additional episodes. The evidence comes to indicate that Patton has a real potential for a pattern of abnormal behavior that will continue and worsen over time. What should he be told? When we accumulate more information about fMRI, it might give us confidence that it can be used in classifying people for behavioral risk. How can and should this be used? Suppose that Patton is now in his twenties and hurts someone in an outburst of anger, and is charged with assault and battery. What access would the courts have to the information from the clinic, including the fMRI data? Does the physician have any liability here?

## Knowledge we should do without

As I look around the corner to guess at where we are headed, I am concerned that it may be toward an individualized knowledge of brain work: a cognitive or 'thinking' phenotype, or perhaps a 'feeling' phenotype. Through some future fMRI technology, it just might be possible to derive for an individual, just to take a few examples, a predictive moral choice profile; an executive skill assessment, and an estimate of the capacity to repress or retrieve old memories. Perhaps worse, it might generate a capacity to peer into intentions, or value systems, or behavioral predilections of various kinds.

That is why the above scenario, hypothetical though it is, suggests some disturbing future possibilities. Privacy protection is already important in a few contexts; for example, we would not want information about the way our brains process information or make decisions to fall into the hands of our insurance company, or of a prospective employer. The larger future worry is the prospect that information from this or an even better technology might be used in a court procedure, perhaps as tests of truth telling or in examining the propensity of defendants to commit violent acts.

Of course, one can always say that society can arrange for such things to be protected. Because I am unconfident about such promises, neuroethics now becomes for me a privacy issue. I already do not want my employer or my insurance company to know my genome, and I have strongly supported legislation to prevent that from happening. As to my brainome, I do not want anyone to know it, for any purpose whatever including those offered in my own interest. It is far too close to who I am, and it is my right to keep that most intimate identity to myself.

One may argue that these are just imaginary risks. After all, there is no prospect that someone could spy on our thoughts or feelings by looking into our brains—as I have said, stealth fMRI technology is not here. But our future will hold many occasions in which people's brain images are stored and kept for other purposes. If these said something about my tendency to anger under different kinds of stress, or accounted for the ways in which I make moral choices, or how strangely I perform on certain intelligence tests—then I would be troubled if there were not robust rules preventing their distribution or use. This prospect, I hope, will also trouble the readers of this volume.

## Final note

This final note will focus on how what we might learn could change our sense of ourselves, and of where we fit in the world. Suppose that our knowledge of neural function leads us to a more reliably deterministic picture of how we make decisions, treat our loved ones, and evaluate the difference between right and wrong. Will we lose something? The more we know, does the will seem less free? This has been a subject of endless philosophical argument. Having paid my obligatory respects to a hard problem, I would leave it to others, except for this: I have so much respect for the complexity of our neural architecture and for the molding capacity of culture and experience that I find it difficult to take the determinist position. Thus I see no threat either to the 'freedom' of our wills, or to the particularity of the decisions each of us makes, individually, in different situations. And even if I did, I would see no reason to extend the issue into the domain of personal responsibility, which should remain as a social construct independent of our views of how the brain works.

There is a different question, though, and it has to do with our humanity. There are only a few great shared narratives of the human experiences. One is that we live on a special unique planet. Another is that we are a special unique species. Still another is our urge to explore. Thirty thousand explorers attend the annual meeting of the Society for Neuroscience each year, and as they seek understanding in the brains of humans and animals, we are sure to learn more about what is common to both and what is unique to each. How much convergence can we expect? I am seeing more and more glimmerings of similarity in the explorations of animal awareness or, if you prefer, consciousness. It is impossible to read Bernd Heinrich's *Mind of the Raven* (Heinrich 2000) without wondering whether the only thing we can do that they cannot is talk about things.

So what do we do if the similarities come to outweigh the differences? I find great inspiration in the unity of Nature, and anything that draws our species into a closer relationship with the rest of life strikes me as a gain in wisdom. Darwin wrote in his journal, one starlit night in Patagonia, 'We may be all one—we may be all blended together'. His insight came as a consequence of realizing continuity over time—fossils resembling contemporary species that he found. How profoundly exciting it would be if a similar understanding emerged from the neurosciences—and if, better yet, it provided some incentive to take better care of that special unique planet.

## Acknowledgement

Adapted from the Dana Lecture, Society for Neuroscience, New Orleans, 2003.

## References

Farah MJ, Illes J, Cook-Deegan R, *et al.* (2004). Neurocognitive enhancement: what can we do and what should we do? *Nature Reviews Neuroscience* 5, 421–5.

Heinrich B (2000). *Mind of the Raven: Investigations and Adventures with Wolf-birds.* New York: Ecco.

Kennedy D (2003). The Lasker Millenium Ethics Forum on Ethical Challenges in Biomedical Research and Practice, 15 May 2003.

Marcus S (ed.) (2002). *Neuroethics: Mapping the Field.* New York: Dana Foundation.

Parens E (ed.) (1998). *Enhancing Human Traits: Ethical and Social Implications.* Washington, DC: Georgetown University Press.

# Index

abortion 116, 117
access 107–8
accountability 9–10, 161–2
acetylcholine 13
action
  concept 34–7
  justificatory 70
  law 36
  reflex 62–3
active-controlled trials,
    limitations 127–30
actuarial information 113, 114
Adderall 255
ADHD 316
adolescent killers, death penalty 33–4, 49
agency, rational 69
alignment 270–1
alternative therapies 128
Alzheimer's disease
  autonomy 98–9
  capacity to value 88, 95, 98–9
  critical interests 90–1
  documentary film 304
  experiential interests 90
  hippocampus 94
  memory 94
  neuronal damage 94–5
amniocentesis 107
amygdala 144, 176
animals, implantable electrodes 196
anterior cingulate cortex 174
antisocial behavior 177
Aristotle
  morality 4
  responsibility 9
Armstrong, D. 64–5
artificial intelligence 65
atomic bomb 7
attitudes, neuroimaging 58–9
auditory brainstem implants 185–6
authenticity 81, 82
autism 305–6
autonomy 88–9, 96–9
  Alzheimer's disease 98–9

contemporaneous 99
decision making 89
enhancing 99
fundamentals 96–7
values 89, 97–8

*Beautiful Mind, A* 305
behavior
  electrical control 190
  mechanistic accounts 35, 36
  prediction 171–5
  reason-giving explanations 35
behaviorism 64
beliefs 35, 36, 146–7
beneficence 131
biases 230–1
bilinguals 268
biological causation 40, 41
brain
  automatic 145–6
  beginning of life 117
  beliefs 146–7
  causal mechanism 5
  computer interfaces 188–90, 194
  death 117
  development 141–4
  emotional system 19
  implants, ethical implications 193–7
  'interpreter' 146
  metaphysics 117
  mirror neurons 147
  moral reasoning 147
  plasticity 208–9, 285–6
  prejudice 144
  reading 57–9
  religion 293–5
  reward system 4, 30
  split-brain 64, 146
  ventromedial frontal damage 18–22, 25–8
Brain Communicator 189
Brain Fingerprinting Laboratories 177
Braingate 189
BRCA 110–11
breast cancer 110–11

cat, implantable electrodes 196
causes 5–6
central nervous system, development 141–4
*Charly* 307
child development, poverty 278
choices 6–8, 36
clinical equipoise 125–6, 130–2
clinical research 130–1
cochlear implants 185, 195, 256, 316–17
coercion 38, 109, 236, 258–9
cognitive stimulation 282–3
cognito 62
Commercial Alert 179
communication 230
compatibilism 45, 46–7
*Complaints of a Dutiful Daughter* 304
compulsion 38
computer
    interface with brain 188–90, 194
    mind as 65
confidentiality 291
conscious, illusion 41
consciousness
    beginning of life 142
    divide/diminished 42
    false 82
    neural correlate 66
    rationality 53–5
    responsibility 39–40
consent 106, 109; *see also*
    informed consent
content shifting 26
context 143–4
continuity 143
contra-causal free will 6–8, 45
control
    in control/not in control
        10–15, 53, 55–6
    parameter space 13–15
    self-control 39
conventional norms 27
Cooper, I. 216
cosmetic surgery 81–2
creativity framework 76, 77
Crick 66
criminal investigations 177
criminal justice 9–10
critical interests 89–91
culture 239
curing disease 106–7
cystic fibrosis 112

*Daubert* test 251
death penalty 33–4, 49
deception 57
decision making 4–5
    autonomy 89
    legal 47–9
    moral 3–16
decisions 4–5
*Deconstructing Harry* 303
deep brain stimulation 186–7, 217
    informed consent 137
    pain relief 218
    placebo-controlled trials 128–30
    side effects 194–5
Delgado, J. 185
deliberation 22
dementia, *see* Alzheimer's disease
depression, vagus nerve stimulation 187
Descartes, R. 62
desires 35, 36, 91–2
determinism 44, 111–15
    hard 45–6
    metaphysics 45–7
Dewey, J. 62–3
difference, not disease 113
diminished responsibility 9–10
disclosure
    genetic testing 234–5
    neuroimaging 233
discontinuity arguments 143
discrimination 105–6
distributive justice 259
diversity 81, 82
DNA
    analysis 106, 107–8
    databases 106
    fingerprinting 112–13
documentary films 303–6
Donoghue, J. 189
dopamine 13
Dresser, R. 88–9
drug trials 129
duress 38
duty to warn 108
Dworkin, R. 88–9
dyslexia 268

economics, functional neurosurgery 223–4
Edelman, G. 66
education
    alignment 270–1

enterprise 266–7
  good work 269–73
  'hat' problem 272–3
  moral 29–30
  neuroeducation 273–4
  neuroethics 239, 265–75
  neuroscience 267–9
  overarching goals 266–7
  policy 164
  profession 269–70
  twofold purpose 29
  value-laden profession 265, 266–7
efference copy 7
electroencephalography 150, 151
  brain fingerprinting 177
  computer control 189
electromagnetic mind control 191–2
eliminative materialism 41
ELSI program 105
embryo
  moral status 141–4
  research 116, 117
emotion 19, 27, 28–9
emotional reactivity 169–70
end-of-life care 238
enforcement
  enhancement 261
  mind reading 254–5
  predictions 247
enhancement 236–7
  banning 261
  coercion 258–9
  dangers 67–8
  distributive justice 259
  drift towards 107
  enforcement 261
  film portrayals 307–8
  flourishing 83–4
  frameworks 76–7
  functional neurosurgery 224
  genuine and fake 83
  legal issues 255–61
  neuropharmacology 315–17
  pediatrics 237, 259–60
  religion 291–2
  safety 256–8
  transcranial magnetic stimulation 107, 207–8
  unnatural or unholy 260–1
epilepsy 217
epinephrine 13
epoche 70

ethical frameworks 75–7, 132–5
ethical implications of neuroscience 18
Ethical Legal and Social Implications (ELSI)
    program 105
ethical relativism 239
ethics
  neuroscience of 18, 51, 75, 116
  of neuroscience 18, 51, 75
  of practice 18
eugenics 115–16
evil 71
experience 63
experiential interests 89–91
extinctions 78
extraversion 170

films
  documentaries 303–6
  frontier neurotechnologies 306–8
  madness 299–300
  mental illness 300–1
Fletcher, J. 125
flourishing 83–4
folk psychology 35, 36, 53, 54
forensics 106
forgiveness 293
frameworks 75–6
  creativity 76, 77
  gratitude 76, 77
freedom 81–2
free will 145
  contra-causal 6–8, 45
  metaphysics 45–7
frontal lobotomy 219
*Frye* test 250–1
functional magnetic resonance imaging (fMRI)
  activation maps 160–1
  BOLD contrast 156
  boundaries 155–6
  cerebral blood flow 156
  characteristics and trade-offs 152
  data display 161
  emotional word Stroop test 172–4
  experimental design 158–60
  general linear model regression 160
  hemodynamic response 156
  increasing rate and range of studies 150
  individual differences 169
  marketing strategies 164
  personality 170
  population inference 160

functional magnetic (*cont*).
  preprocessing data  160
  spatial resolution  156–7
  statistical data analysis  160–1
  studies with ethical, legal and social
    implications  153–5
  task design  158–9
  temporal resolution  156–7
  voxel size  157
functional neurosurgery
  economics  223–4
  enhancement  224
  epilepsy  217
  ethics  220–6
  future  219–20
  informed consent  220–2
  innovation  224–6
  last-chance therapy  222
  movement disorders  216–17
  neuromodulators  221
  pain relief  217–18
  psychiatric disorders  218–19
  research  224–6
  risk-benefit  222–3
  society  223–4
  therapeutic privilege  220–1
fundamental psychological error  40

Gage, Phineas  19, 55, 218–19
gate control theory  218
gene–environment interactions  176
Genesis  76
genetic engineering  78
genetics and genetic testing
  bearing children  235
  consent  106, 109
  determinism  111–15
  disclosure  234–5
  discrimination  105–6
  forensics  106
  information  105–6, 108–9
  insurance risk assessment  113
  interpretation  234
  learning disability  268–9
  metaphysics  115–18
  physicians and ethics  233–4
  polymorphisms  175–6, 177
  pre-employment  113, 178
  pre-implantation diagnosis  107, 235
  privacy  105–6, 234–5
  stigmatization  105–6

  therapeutic gap  110–11
genomic imaging  176
good and evil  71
good work  269–73
Google chip  191
gratitude framework  76, 77

habits  75
hard determinism  45–6
'hat' problem  271–2
heuristics  230–1
hippocampus
  Alzheimer's disease  94
  prosthetic  188
Hiroshima bombing  7
histamine  13
HLA status  107
HOME  284
homeland security  177
homicidal maniacs  301
5-HTT  175–6
human behavior, *see* behavior
human genome
  modularity  112
  soul  116
  variation  113
human intervention, Nature  77–9
humanistic view  52
humanity  319
human potential  285–6
Hume, D.  7, 8, 22
Huntington's disease  110
hyper-responsibility  40

images  149; *see also* neuroimaging
incompatibilism  45
incompetence  135–7
individual differences  169–71
infectious disease  238
information  105–6, 108–9
informed consent
  capacity to give  135–7
  deep brain stimulation  137
  functional neurosurgery  220–2
  genetics  109
  placebo-controlled trials  134–5, 136
  surgery  215
innovation  224–6
insurance risk assessment  113
intelligence, predictive  307
intention  35, 36, 143

internalism 22–8, 31
interpretation 231–2, 234
'interpreter' 146
intervention, Nature 77–9
intrinsically motivating 23
iron deficiency 281

James, W. 62–3, 124, 294–5
journalism 270
justificatory action 70

Kandel, E.R. 66
knowledge 318–19
Koch, C. 66

law
    human action 36
    nature 34
    personhood and responsibility 34–41
    practical reason 37
    right and wrong 30
    system of rules 37
    *see also* legal issues
lead toxicity 282
learning 267–8
learning disability 268–9
legal issues 245–63
    decision making 47–9
    enhancement 255–61
    mind reading 249–55
    neuroimaging 144, 150, 155
    prediction 246–8
    *see also* law
Levinas, E. 70–1
libertarianism 6, 45, 46
Libet, B. 42–3, 145
lie detectors 57–8, 250, 251–2
life
    beginning of 117, 142–3
    gift of 76
limbic system 12, 13, 19
long-term depression/potentiation 207

magnetic resonance imaging 150; *see also*
    functional magnetic resonance imaging
magnetoencephalography 150, 151
*MAOA* 177
marketing sector 164, 178–80
mastery of language 24–5, 26
materialist theory 64–5
McGinn, C. 65

McNaghten rule 10
mechanism 35, 36, 45, 80–1
media 297–311
medical care, ethics 130–1
medicalization 79
medicine, as an intervention 78–9
meditation 294
memory 68–9
    Alzheimer's disease 94
*mens rea* 9, 43
mental illness, media portrayals 298–303
mereological fallacy 58
metaphysical libertarianism 45, 46
metaphysics 45–7, 115–18
microchips, implantable 196
mind
    control 191–3
    humanistic/scientific view 52–3
    reading 249–55
mind–body problem 36, 62
*Minority Report* 306–7
mirror neurons 147
modafinil 255
Moniz, E. 219
moral absolutism 125–7
moral concepts 25, 27
moral decision making 3–16
moral education 29–30
morality
    Aristotelian concept 4
    nature 34
moral judgment 17–32
moral norms 27
moral reasoning 147, 293
morals, personhood and responsibility 34–41
motivation 24
motive internalism 22
movement disorders 216–17
movies, *see* films

Nagel, T. 65
nanotechnology 190–1
nanotechnology, biotechnology, information
    technology and cognitive science (NBIC) 191
Nash, J. F. 305
Nature, human interventions 77–9
Nazi eugenics 116
NBIC 191
near-infrared optimal imaging (NIR) 150
neural networks 8
neural prostheses 185–6

neuroeconomics 317
neuroeducation 273–4
neuroelectric interfaces 256
neuroenhancement, *see* enhancement
neuroethics
    challenges in the clinical setting 230–1
    coining of term 141
    coming paradigm 3
    culture 239
    definition 141
    education 239, 265–75
    neuroimaging 161–5
    religion 290–2
    structure 17–18
neuroimaging 57–9
    accountability 161–2
    attitudes 58–9
    behavior prediction 171–5
    commercial side 163, 317
    diagnosis 231
    disclosure 233
    equating structure and function 157–8
    forensic applications 106
    individual differences 169–71
    information 109
    interpretation of findings 231–2
    legal issues 144, 150, 155
    lie detection 57–8
    marketing 178–80
    neuroethics 161–5
    non-clinical, unexpected findings 163
    pediatrics 233
    personality 169–71
    preferences 58–9, 317
    privacy 233, 317–18
    prospective responsibility 164–5
    public involvement 163–4
    recruitment 178
    reproducibility 162
    responsiveness 162–3
    self-knowledge 317–18
    statistical data 180–1
    therapeutic gap 110
    treatment 232–3
neuromarketing 164, 178–80
neuromodulation 186, 221
neuropharmacology 107, 315–17
neuroscience
    challenge to personhood and responsibility
        41–7

education 267–9
ethical implications 18
ethics of 18, 51, 75
of ethics 18, 51, 75, 116
soul 292–3
neurosurgery, *see* functional neurosurgery
neurotheology 293–5
neuroticism 170
neurotransmitters 13
'no action thesis' 42
noesis 70
nonmaleficence 131
non-medical intervention 79
non-specific neurotransmitter projection
    systems 13
norepinephrine 13
normalcy 26, 27
nutrition 281–2

orbitoclast 219
orientation association area (OAA)
    294
'ought' judgments 27

P300 57
pain management 217–18, 236
parameter space 13–15
Parfit, D. 64
paternity issues 106
pediatrics
    enhancement 237, 259–60
    neuroimaging 233
    transcranial magnetic stimulation 206
perception 27–8
person, concept 34–7
personality 169–76
personhood
    morals and law 34–41
    neural test 117
    neuroscience challenge 41–7
phenomenology 70
Pinker, S. 66, 292
placebo-controlled trials 127
    adverse events 128
    clinical equipoise 126, 131–2
    deep brain stimulation 128–30
    ethical framework 132–5
    informed consent 134–5, 136
    methodological rationale 132–3
    risk assessment 133–4

risk minimization 134
  subject numbers 128
  surgical interventions 126
plasticity 208–9, 285–6
plausibility 28
pleiotropy 112
polygraphs 250, 251–2
polymorphisms 175–6, 177
positron emission tomography (PET)
  150, 151, 169
potentiality 143
poverty 277–87
  child development 278
  cognitive stimulation 282–3
  iron deficiency 281
  lead toxicity 282
  neurocognitive correlates 280–1
  neurocognitive profile 279–80
  nutrition 281–2
  protein energy malnutrition 281
  stress 283
  substance abuse 282
practical reason 37
pragmatism 123–7
prediction 6, 171–5, 246 –8
predictive intelligence 307
pre-employment testing 113, 178
preferences, neuroimaging 58–9, 317
prefrontal cortex 12, 13, 19
prefrontal lobotomy 219
pre-implantation diagnosis 107, 235
prejudice 144
prenatal diagnosis 107
prevention 106–7
prions 238
privacy
  genetic testing 105–6, 234–5
  mind reading 253–4
  neuroimaging 233, 317–18
  religion 291
probabilities 230
profession, education 269–70
profit-making sector 163
prospective responsibility 164–5
protein energy malnutrition 281
Provigil 255
Prozac 107
psychiatric disorders 218–19
psycho-ethical framework 75
psychotherapy 235–6
punishment 5

qualia 63
quantum physics 8

*Rain Man* 305
randomized controlled trials 127
rational agency 69
rationality
  consciousness 53–5
  responsibility 38, 40
rationing 223–4
readiness potential 145
realism constraint 44
reasons 7, 35
  practical 37
recruitment 178
reductionism 41, 53–4
reflex action 62–3
regulation 67
relational understanding 80–1
religion 289–96
  brain 293–5
  confidentiality 291
  enhancement 291–2
  neuroethics 290–2
  privacy 291
  science and 289, 290
  transcranial magnetic stimulation
    294
reproducibility 162
research 123–5
responsibility 33–50
  Aristotelian concept 9
  concept 37–8
  criteria 38–41
  diminished 9–10
  hyper-responsibility 40
  law 34–41
  morals 34–41
  neuroscience challenge 41–7
  prospective 164–5
responsiveness 162–3
retina, artificial 186, 256
reward 4, 30
risk
  functional neurosurgery 222–3
  placebo-controlled trials 133–4
Ritalin 80, 82–3, 114, 255
Robo-Rat 190, 192
*Roper* v. *Simmons* 33–4, 49
rules 37
Russell, B. 63–4

safety
   enhancement 256–8
   transcranial magnetic stimulation 206
savant-like qualities 208
savior children 107
schizophrenia 305
science
   mind 52
   religion 289, 290
   taboo 67
science fiction 306–7
Searle, J. 65–6
second-language learning 268
security issues 177
selective serotonin-reuptake inhibitors
      (SSRIs) 107
self-awareness, 63
self-control 39
self-creation 81
self-knowledge 317–18
self-worth 92
sensitivity 180–1
serotonin 13
sex offenders, anti-androgen therapy 109
sex selection 107
sham surgery 126
single-photon emission computed tomography
      (SPECT) 150, 151
skin-conductance response 20, 24
Skinner, B.F. 64
*SLC6A4* 175–6
social sciences 36
society 223–4
socio economic status 277
   child development 278
   neurocognitive correlates 280–1
   *see also* poverty
soul
   existence 5
   genes 115–16
   neuroscience 292–3
specificity 180–1
split-brain 64, 146
St John's wort 128
status quo bias 81
stem cells 116, 117, 143, 237
stereotactic surgery 216–17
stigmatization 105–6
Stimoceiver 190
stress 283
stroke 146

structure and function 157–8
subjectivity 68
substance abuse 282
substantive internalism 22–3
surgery
   ethics 213–16
   informed consent 215
   placebos 126
   stereotactic 216–17
   *see also* functional neurosurgery
syndrome 41

technology 79–81
television 302
terrorism 114
therapeutic gap 110–11
therapeutic misconception 163
therapeutic privilege 220–1
Tourette's syndrome 304
transcranial magnetic stimulation (TMS)
      187–8, 201–11
   basic neuroscience research 207
   brain effects 204
   clinical neurophysiology 204–5
   clinical research 205–6
   contraindications 206
   design 202
   enhancement 107, 207–8
   ethics 205
   neurobehavioral studies 204–5
   pediatrics 206
   principles 201
   religion 294
   safety 206
   seizures 206
   side effects 206
   stimulating coils 203
   therapeutics 205–6
transcutaneous electrical stimulation 187
'trolley problem' 21
Truman, President 7
*Twitch and Shout* 304

Ulysses contracts 221
unconscious, oddity 69
unholy 260–1
*United States* v. *Scheffer* 251–2
unnatural 260–1

vagus nerve stimulation 187
values

assessments of one's life as a whole
    93–4
autonomy 89, 97–8
capacity in Alzheimer's disease 88, 95,
    98–9
education 265, 266–7
self-worth 92
understanding 91–3
variant CJD 238
ventromedial frontal damage
    18–22, 25–8

VeriChip 196
violence 39
vision and vestibular
    substitution systems 186
visual prostheses
    186, 256

Warwick, K. 190
well-being 89–96